INTERVENTIONAL RADIOLOGY SECRETS

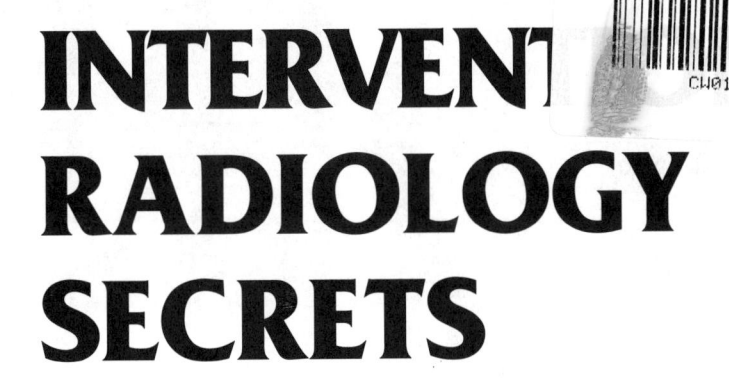

David L. Waldman, MD, PhD
Professor and Chair
Department of Radiology
University of Rochester Medical Center
Rochester, New York

Nikhil C. Patel, MD
Assistant Professor
University of Rochester Medical Center
Rochester, New York

Wael E.A. Saad, MBBCh
Instructor
Mallinckrodt Institute of Radiology
St. Louis, Missouri

HANLEY & BELFUS, INC.
An Imprint of Elsevier

HANLEY & BELFUS, INC.
An Imprint of Elsevier

The Curtis Center
Independence Square West
Philadelphia, Pennsylvania 19106

Note to the reader: Although the techniques, ideas, and information in this book have been carefully reviewed for correctness, the authors, editors, and publisher cannot accept any legal responsibility for any errors or omissions that may be made. Neither the publisher nor the editors make any guarantee, expressed or implied, with respect to the material contained herein.

Library of Congress Control Number: 2004103677

INTERVENTIONAL RADIOLOGY SECRETS   ISBN 1-56053-609-8

© 2004 by Hanley & Belfus, Inc. All rights reserved. No part of this book may be reproduced, reused, republished, or transmitted in any form, or stored in a database or retrieval system, without written permission of the publisher.

Printed in the United States of America

Last digit is the print number: 9 8 7 6 5 4 3 2 1

CONTENTS

I. GENERAL TOPICS

1. History and Famous People of Interventional Radiology 1
   Ian Wilson, MD

2. Interventional Radiology Nursing 4
   Chrissie Copoulos, RN, MS

3. Management of Contrast Reaction 7
   Lisa Kilejian, MD

4. Tools of the Trade for Interventional Radiologists 11
   Craig B. Glaiberman, MD

5. Gene Therapy 21
   Ian Wilson, MD

6. Coding in Interventional Radiology 24
   David L. Waldman, MD, PhD

II. VASCULAR INTERVENTIONS

7. Vascular Anatomy 27
   Ian Wilson, MD

8. Vascular Anomalies 35
   Wael E. A. Saad, MBBCh

9. Noninvasive Vascular Testing 44
   David L. Waldman

10. Aortoiliac Disease and Aorta Aneurysms 47
    David L. Waldman, MD, PhD

11. Peripheral Vascular Disease: Diagnosis and Intervention 69
    Bulent Arslan, MD

12. Carotid Artery Angiography and Intervention 82
    Wael E.A. Saadm MBBCh

13. Bronchial Artery Angiography and Intervention 92
    Arun Basu, MD

14. Renovascular Disease and Intervention 99
    Kalpesh C. Patel, MD

15. Mesenteric Angiography and Intervention 113
    Wael E.A. Saad, MBBCh, and William Kuo, MD

16. Uterine Artery Embolization for Fibroids 124
    Nikhil C. Patel, MD

17. Endovascular Management of Trauma 139
    David E. Lee, MD

18. Treatment of Tumors with Interventional Radiology Techniques 146
    Talia Sasson, MD, and Marlon Maragh, MD

19. Vascular Closure Devices 153
    Labib Syed, MD

20. Venous Access 158
    Waqar A. Shah, MS, MD

21. Arteriovenous Hemodialysis Access 171
    John Fitzgerald, MD

22. Deep Venous Thrombosis and Clinical Management 181
    Vicken N. Pamoukian, MD

23. Venous Syndromes and Management 186
    Nikhil C. Patel, MD

24. Pulmonary Angiography and Intervention 198
    Bulent Arslan, MD

25. Inferior Vena Cava Interruption 206
    Nikhil C. Patel, MD

26. Varicose Veins and Endovascular Management 216
    Wael E. A. Saad, MBBCh

27. Varicoceles and Testicular Vein Embolization 220
    Wael E. A. Saad, MBBCh

28. Portal Hypertension and TIPS 225
    Wael E.A. Saad, MBBCh

29. Vascular Intervention in Renal Transplantation 241
    Wael E.A. Saad, MBBCh

30. Vascular Intervention in Liver and Pancreas Transplantation 245
    Wael E. A. Saad, MBBCh

III. NONVASCULAR INTERVENTION

31. Tracheoesophageal and Gastrointestinal Intervention 253
    Wael E. A. Saad, MBBCh

32. Hepatobiliary Intervention 268
    Wael E. A. Saad, MBBCh

33. Nonvascular Intervention in Solid Organ Transplantation 280
    Wael E. A. Saad, MBBCh

34. Genitourinary Intervention 285
    Ryan K. Lee, MD

35. Percutaneous Management of Abnormal Fluid Collection 293
    Wael E. A. Saad, MBBCh

36. Catheter and Tube Management 304
    Wael E. A. Saad, MBBCh

37. Musculoskeletal Intervention 311
    Wael E. A. Saad, MBBCh

38. Image-guided Biopsy 319
    Wael E. A. Saad, MBBCh

INDEX 329

CONTRIBUTORS

Bulent Arslan, MD
Assistant Professor, Radiology, University of Arizona, Head, Vascular and Interventional Radiology, Tucson Veterans Hospital, Tucson, Arizona

Arun Basu, MD
Department of Radiology, University of Rochester Medical Center, Rochester, New York

Chrissie Copoulos, RN, MS
Department of Radiology, University of Rochester, Strong Memorial Hospital, Rochester, New York

John M. Fitzgerald, MD
Resident, Department of Radiology
Strong Memorial Hospital, Rochester, New York

Craig B. Glaiberman, MD
Instructor, Mallinckrodt Institute of Radiology, Vascular and Interventional Radiology, Washington University, Barnes-Jewish Hospital, St. Louis Children's Hospital, St. Louis, Missouri

Lisa Kilejian, MD
Radiology, University of Rochester Medical Center, Rochester, New York

William T. Kuo, MD
Chief Resident, Radiology, University of Rochester Medical Center, Rochester, New York

David E. Lee, MD
Assistant Professor of Radiology, Diagnostic Radiology, University of Rochester Medical Center, Rochester, New York

Ryan K. Lee, MD
Radiology, University of Rochester Medical Center, Rochester, New York

Marlon R. Maragh, MD
Diagnostic Radiology Resident, Diagnostic Radiology, University of Rochester, Strong Memorial Hospital, Rochester, New York

Vicken Nichan Pamoukian, MD
Clinical Instructor, Vascular Surgery, Surgery, Lenox Hill Hospital, New York, New York

Kalpesh Patel, MD
Resident, Radiology, University of Rochester Medical Center, Rochester, New York

Nikhil C. Patel, MD
Assistant Professor of Radiology, Diagnostic Radiology, University of Rochester Medical Center, Rochester, New York

Wael E. A. Saad, MBBCh
Instructor, Mallinckrodt Institute of Radiology, Washington University, St. Louis, Missouri

Talia Sasson, MD
Assistant Professor, Radiology, University of Rochester Medical Center, Rochester, New York; Dotter Interventional Institute, Portland, Oregon

Waqar A. Shah, MD
Resident, Vascular and Interventional Radiology, Radiology, University of Rochester Medical Center, Strong Memorial Hospital, Rochester, New York

Labib Syed, MD
Resident, Department of Radiology, University of Rochester, Rochester, New York

David L. Waldman, MD, PhD
Professor and Chair, Radiology, University of Rochester Medical Center, Rochester, New York

Ian Wilson, MD
Chief Resident, Radiology, University of Rochester Medical Center, Rochester, New York

PREFACE

This book is inspired by our medical students, residents, fellows, technologists, and nurses. Their questions and thirst for knowledge motivate and inspire us all to keep learning. The organization of this book includes detailed organ-based and procedural questions as well as practical how-to issues that are often not found in standard journals or textbooks. These facts are nonetheless encountered in daily practice of vascular and interventional radiology. The intention of our topics is to improve the reader's understanding of vascular and interventional radiology and the ever-increasing role that it plays in patient care. We welcome our reader's comments and questions as we explore the future secrets that vascular and interventional radiology holds.

This book is dedicated to all the patients who are seen and treated by the interventional radiologists. In medicine we sometimes forget that our patients are the true teachers of medicine. It is quite clear that the role of the interventional radiologist is moving from a procedure-based specialist to a clinician.

We would like to take this opportunity to thank Shirley Cappiello for her secretarial assistance in the preparation of this manuscript. We would also like to thank Margaret Kowaluk for her assistance in preparing the images for this book. In addition, our sincere thanks go to Stan Ward at Hanley & Belfus for his assistance in coordinating the production of this book.

David L. Waldman, MD, PhD
Nikhil C. Patel, MD
Wael E.A. Saad, MBBCh

I. General Topics

1. HISTORY AND FAMOUS PEOPLE OF INTERVENTIONAL RADIOLOGY

Ian Wilson, MD

1. Who is the father of psychosurgery?

Egas Moniz (1874–1955), who was born in Avanca, Protugal and earned a medical degree from the University of Coimbra. He trained in neurology in Paris under Babinski, Marie, and Sicard. Moniz sought a less hazardous means of intracranial tumor localization as an alternative to pneumoencephalography (a technique developed by the American neurosurgeon, Walter Dandy). He first introduced angiography into clinical practice in 1927, using sodium iodide to localize and size a patient's brain tumor. Moniz published extensively about normal and pathologic cerebral angiography. In 1949 he shared the Nobel Prize in medicine with Walter Rudolf Hess for "the discovery of the therapeutic value of leucotomy in certain psychoses," also known as the frontal lobotomy.

2. Who developed the percutaneous entry technique used in interventional radiology?

Sven Ivar Seldinger (1921–1999), who was born in Mora, Sweden and earned a medical degree from the Karolinska Institute. The technique, published in 1953 in *Acta Radiologica*, can be summarized as "needle in, wire in, needle out, catheter in, wire out."

3. Who is Lopo De Carvalho?

Lopo De Cavalho, a key figure early angiography, collaborated in angiography with Egaz Moniz. He worked at the Portuguese School of Angiography.

4. Who is the father of interventional radiology?

Charles Dotter, who was born in Boston. He earned a medical degree and subsequently trained in radiology at Cornell University. He served as a professor and chairman of the Department of Radiology at the University of Oregon Health Sciences Center. Dotter first described transluminal angioplasty in 1964 (via serial dilation of stenotic lesions with catheters of gradually increasing size). He worked closely with William Cook to make some of the first tools of interventional radiology commercially available. Dotter was nominated for Noble Prize in Medicine in 1978.

5. Who is Eberhart Zeitler?

Eberhart Zeitler is responsible for disseminating in Europe the technique of percutaneous transluminal angioplasty, which would later result in renewed enthusiasm for such therapy as a viable means of treatment in North America. He introduced Dotter's technique to Andreas Gruentzig, who later developed interventional cardiology.

6. Who developed the balloon dilation catheter for peripheral angioplasty?

Andreas Gruentzig, a Swiss cardiologist. Gruentzig worked closely with John Abele, founder of what was then Medi-Tech, to manufacture dual-lumen balloon catheters for angioplasty. He also introduced the registry concept to track procedures and performed the first coronary balloon angioplasty in May 1977 in San Francisco.

7. Summarize the contributions to interventional radiology of Josef Rosch.

Born in Pilsen, Czechoslovakia, Josef Rosch received a medical degree from Charles University in Prague. He immigrated to the United States and became a research associate at the Health Sciences Center of the University of Oregon, Portland. He was a professor of radiology and the head of cardiovascular radiology from 1970 to 1990. Rosch was active in the development of novel vascular and interventional radiologic techniques since the 1950s. He pioneered development of splenoportography and visceral angiography, especially for the diagnosis and treatment of gastrointestinal bleeding. Rosch also introduced vasoconstrictor infusion and selective embolization as treatments. He developed and introduced techniques for transjugular liver biopsy, transjugular intrahepatic portosystemic shunt, and transcervical fallopian tube catheterization and was an early investigator of expandable wire frame endovascular prostheses.

8. Who is Cesare Gianturco?

Born in Naples, Italy, Cesare Gianturco earned a medical degree from the University of Naples in 1927. He trained in radiology at the University of Rome and was a radiology fellow at the Mayo Clinic. He also did postgraduate study in radiology and physiology at University of Minnesota. Gianturco is the creator of occlusive coils for embolotherapy, inferior vena cava filters (Bird's Nest Filter), and expandable stents.

9. Who introduced the technique of transhepatic emoblization for the treatment of variceal bleeding?

Anders Lunderquist, who was born in Sweden in 1925 and earned a medical degree from the University of Lund in 1955. He wrote "Angiography in Carcinoma of the Pancreas" as Ph.D. thesis and published extensively about procedural complications of angiography, portography, and balloon catheter dilatation in the vascular system. Lunderquist introduced the technique of transhepatic embolization for the treatment of variceal bleeding in the mid 1970s.

10. Who is Kurt Amplatz?

A pioneering figure in cardiac angiography, Kurt Amplatz was a prolific developer of novel interventional devices such as guidewires, dilators, foreign body retrieval systems, and thrombectomy devices.

11. Who is John Doppman?

John Doppman was one of the first to use embolization for the treatment of tumors and vascular malformations.

12. Who discovered the technique of computed tomography?

Sir Godfrey Newbold Hounsfield, who was born on August 28, 1919. He is a Nobel laureate and Commander of the Order of the British Empire, knighted in 1981. He led the EMI, Ltd. team that invented the first all-transistor computer in 1957. Hounsfield discovered the technique of computed tomography, used extensively for the purposes of guidance during interventional procedures, for which he received the Nobel Prize.

13. Who founded Cook, Inc.?

William Cook, a former Army medic. He collaborated closely with Charles Dotter during the company's humble beginnings. With his wife, he fashioned early products—guidewires, catheters, and needles—in their apartment. Cook was the first to manufacture devices for pioneering angiographers, and his company is the largest manufacturer of interventional radiology products. Along with Josef Rosch, he was instrumental in the creation of the Dotter Institute at the Health Sciences Center of the University of Organ.

14. Who is John Abele?

Founder of Boston Scientific (formerly known as Medi-Tech), Abele was an early collaborator with Andreas Gruentzig in the development of the balloon dilation catheter for percutaneous transluminal angioplasty.

15. Who is Julio Palmaz?

Julio Palmaz earned a medical degree from the National University of La Plata in Argentina in 1971 and trained in radiology at the University of California, Davis. He invented the widely used Palmaz balloon-expandable stent—the basis for many endovascular therapeutic strategies.

16. Who pioneered angiography with carbon dioxide?

Irvin F. Hawkins. Carbon dioxide is widely used as an alternative or supplemental contrast agent.

17. Who was the first president of the Society of Cardiovascular and Interventional Radiology (SCVIR)?

Stanley Baum, MD, who served as president from 1974 to 1976.

18. How many founding members of the SCVIR were there?

Forty-eight.

19. In what year was the SCVIR founded?

SCVIR was founded in 1973 and formally organized in 1974. It was initially called the Society of Cardiovascular Radiology. The name was changed in 1983 to the Society of Cardiovascular and Interventional Radiology. In 2002 the society had a second name change; it is now called the Society of Interventional Radiology (SIR).

2. INTERVENTIONAL RADIOLOGY NURSING

Chrissie Copoulos, RN, MS

1. Who works in interventional procedure rooms?
A registered nurse (RN) and a radiology technologist (RT) assist the interventional radiologist (IR) with the procedure.

2. Describe the role of the RN in interventional radiology.
In the procedure room itself, the RN administers moderate sedation (or conscious sedation) to the patient. This procedure involves attaching monitoring equipment to the patient (heart monitor, pulse oximeter, and blood pressure cuff), monitoring the patient's vital signs throughout the procedure, and giving sedation.

3. What is moderate sedation?
Moderate sedation consists of the administration of pain medication and a sedative with continuous vital sign monitoring. Fentanyl and midazolam (Versed) are frequently used because of their short half-life and the ability to reverse their effects, if needed. Another commonly used pain medication is meperidine (Demerol). All of these medications are given intravenously in individual doses throughout the procedure. Midazolam has the added benefit of causing some amnesia; patients frequently do not remember details during the procedure and may not remember the procedure at all.

4. What medications are used to reverse the sedation and why would the sedation need to be reversed?
Flumazenil (Romazicon) and naloxone (Narcan) are used to reverse midazolam and fentanyl, respectively. If the patient becomes too deeply sedated and respirations are not spontaneous, reversal is needed. This scenario is no longer moderate sedation and is beyond the scope of the RN's practice. Changes in vital signs and patient responsiveness are used to determine the level of sedation and the need for reversal, if indicated.

5. How much sedation is given?
The amount varies for each patient and each procedure. Age and medical condition affect patient response to sedation, and each patient is treated as an individual. Some procedures tend to be more painful than others and require more sedation.

6. Which procedures are more painful?
Any procedure requiring balloon inflation or insertion of a new catheter is generally more painful (angioplasties or stent placements, biliary tubes, nephrostomy tubes). Bone biopsies can also be painful and more traumatic because of the sound of the hammer against bone. However, each patient responds to pain individually and must be continuously assessed during the procedure.

7. What else does the RN do in interventional radiology?
Before the procedure patients must be properly prepared. RNs obtain and review the patient's medical history, including allergies and medications, and the necessary lab work. The patient also receives teaching about the procedure.

After the procedure the patient requires monitoring until the sedation wears off, usually an hour after the last dose given. Some patients need further monitoring. For example, patients undergoing liver biopsies need monitoring for bleeding, and patients undergoing biliary tube and nephrostomy tube placement need monitoring for sepsis. Some patients require home care for care of tunneled central lines, peripherally inserted central catheter (PICC) lines, and drainage tubes. The radiology RN arranges for home care as needed (if not arranged by the ordering service).

8. What lab tests are needed? Why?

Any patient undergoing an invasive procedure in interventional radiology requires recent coagulation studies with results that are within normal limits. These lab values include prothrombin time (PT), partial thromboplastin time (PTT), international normalized ratio (INR), and platelet count. Any existing coagulopathy needs to be corrected before the procedure to avoid bleeding complications during and after the procedure. Patients receiving a contrast medium must have a recent assessment of blood urea nitrogen (BUN) and creatinine levels as well. These laboratory values are indicators of renal function and preexisting renal impairment. Because contrast mediums can cause nephrotoxicity, it is important to know precontrast renal function.

9. How are patients prepared for procedures?

All patients must have the appropriate lab work (as described previously), must avoid oral ingestion (NPO status) for at least 4 hours before the procedure, and should take their regular medications (with the exception of anticoagulants, aspirin products, and nonsteroidal anti-inflammatory drugs [NSAIDs]). Blood pressure control is especially important in angiogram procedures; thus, prescribed antihypertensives should be taken before the procedure. Outpatients must have a driver to take them home, because they are not allowed to drive after receiving moderate sedation. Consideration must be given to the patient's ability to lay flat, ability to follow commands, and level of orientation. Angiography patients must be on flat bed rest without moving the affected extremity for several hours. Some patients must lie prone on the procedure table; this requirement must also be taken into consideration.

10. What happens if the patient has not been NPO for the appropriate time?

The procedure is postponed until at least 4 hours after the meal, or the patient is offered the option of proceeding without sedation.

11. What happens if a patient with poor renal function must have contrast?

Some treatments include pre-, intra- and/or postprocedure hydration with intravenous fluids and administration of acetylcysteine before and after the procedure.

12. What if the patient is allergic to contrast or has an allergic reaction to the contrast during the procedure?

If the allergy is known before the procedure and is of mild-to-moderate severity (nausea/vomiting, hives), the patient is premedicated with prednisone and diphenhydramine. Patients with a history of a severe reaction to contrast (respiratory arrest, throat swelling, or extreme wheezing) should be carefully considered and may be given an alternate contrast (such as the contrast given in MRI), or carbon dioxide may be injected into the vessel.

If the patient begins to have a reaction during the procedure, reaction medications should be available in the procedure room and are given immediately. These medications include solumedrol, diphenhydramine, epinephrine, antiemetics, and albuterol. Resuscitation equipment is also in the room as a precaution (ambu bags, oxygen, nebulizers, with an emergency cart nearby).

13. What types of allergic reactions do patients have?

Patients can exhibit the following reactions: nausea, vomiting, hives, itching, wheezing, swollen tongue/airway, decrease in blood pressure, and/or respiratory arrest. Reactions may begin gradually or appear suddenly and must be treated immediately.

14. Does the RN assist with the procedure?

No. The sole responsibilities of the RN are patient monitoring and administration of sedation. Some procedures require close monitoring of the heart rhythm for ectopy, and the RN is the only person in the room to monitor vital signs. Some patients also require blood product transfusions, initiation of thrombolytics, blood pressure control medication, measuring of fluid drainage, documentation of vascular pressures, fluid boluses, blood glucose monitoring, postprocedure wound care, and/or neurologic assessment. The RN is responsible for these aspects as well. The physicians are updated about changes in vital signs or patient condition as appropriate. The RT is present in the room to run the equipment and assist with the procedure.

15. What else may be done by the RN before specific procedures?

For angiography procedures, the pulses distal to the puncture site are located, marked, and documented. They are also rechecked after the procedure is completed. Some patients require a Foley catheter, which is inserted by the RN. Any required antibiotics are given. Neuroradiology procedures require preprocedure neurologic assessment as well as intra- and postprocedure assessment. This assessment includes but is not limited to pupil check, level of orientation, hand grasps, ability to follow commands, and lower extremity strength. Neurologic assessment should be done with any neurologic case, including carotid studies. The RN also sets the patient at ease, describing what will happen and what the RN will be doing during the procedure.

16. Why does the angiography patient have to lie flat for so long?

Most angiography patients receive a groin puncture. Any flexion of the affected leg can potentially cause bleeding and/or hematoma at the site. Length of bed rest or immobility varies by institution but is intended to promote stability for the forming clot at the puncture site.

17. What if the groin is not punctured?

The axilla is the next location for arterial puncture. Patients with this access site must not use the affected arm and must also stay on bed rest.

18. Which procedures require the patient to lie prone on the procedure table? Which require that the patient lie on his or her side?

Prone: nephrostomy tube insertions or changes, thrombolysis of deep venous thrombosis, vertebroplasty, vertebral bone biopsy, and kyphoplasty.

On side: nephrostomy tube insertions or changes. Varying degrees of position may also be required during lung biopsies, radiofrequency ablations, and biliary tube insertions or changes.

19. What happens to the patient after the procedure?

Inpatients are monitored in a recovery area until they have returned to their preprocedure status (vital signs and level of alertness). The inpatient RN receives a report from the radiology RN, and postprocedure orders, if appropriate, accompany the patient to the inpatient unit.

Outpatients go home with a designated driver. Some stay to recover from the procedure for several hours (uterine artery embolizations, angiogram, liver biopsy, vertebralplasty, vertebral bone biopsy), whereas others receive additional antibiotics before leaving (e.g., patients receiving replacement of existing biliary tubes). Others may go home as soon as the sedation wears off (tunneled central lines, Port-a-Caths, paracentesis). Outpatients are given written discharge instructions that include diet, activity, medication, wound care, and emergency instructions.

BIBLIOGRAPHY

1. American Radiological Nurses Association: Guidelines of Radiology Practice and Standards of Radiology Nursing Practice. Oakbrook, IL, American Radiological Nurses Association, 2000.
2. Caridi R: Carbon dioxide digital subtraction angiography: Potential complications and nursing intervention. Images 17(1):4–7, 1998.
3. Knight CD: Radiology nurses keep pace with interventional technology. Images 20(4):10–11, 2001.
4. Morgan LK, Nunnelee J (eds): Core Curriculum for Radiological Nursing. Oakbrook, IL, American Radiological Nurses Association, 1999.
5. Oran NT, Oran I, Memis A: Management of patients with malignant obstructive jaundice: Nursing perspective from the interventional radiology room. Cancer Nurs 23(2):128–133, 2000.
6. Whitlock D: Scheduling guidelines for vascular and interventional procedures: Tools for the radiology nurse. Images 19(2):8–9, 2000.
7. Young S (ed): Patient Care in Interventional Radiology, 2nd ed. Gaithersburg, MD, Aspen Publishers, 2002.

Website

American Radiological Nurses Association: www.arna.net.

3. MANAGEMENT OF CONTRAST REACTION

Lisa Kilejian, MD

1. **What is a contrast reaction?**
   Contrast reaction includes various physical manifestations categorized as mild, moderate, or severe. The pathogenesis is multifactorial, involving histamine release and complement activation; however, the precise mechanism is unknown.

2. **Is treatment of a contrast reaction always necessary?**
   Treatment varies with the severity of the reaction. A mild contrast reaction does not require pharmacologic intervention, whereas a severe reaction requires prompt medical intervention. All contrast reactions require prompt assessment, beginning with the standard airway, breathing, and circulation (ABC) guidelines.

3. **Summarize the incidence of contrast reactions.**
   - Ionic high-osmolality contrast: 5–12%
   - Nonionic contrast material: 1–3%

4. **List the specific types of reactions.**
   - Anaphylactoid (idiosyncratic)
   - Chemotoxic (nonidiosyncratic)
   - Local

5. **What are anaphylactoid reactions?**
   Anaphylactoid reactions are unexpected, and the etiology is uncertain. They are also known as idiosyncratic reactions. Because they mimic allergic, anaphylactic reactions, the likelihood increases in persons with a history of asthma, food/drug allergies, or previous contrast reactions. Use of low-osmolality media decreases the number of reactions.

6. **What are chemotoxic reactions?**
   Chemotoxic side effects relate to the ionic nature and osmolality of the contrast media.

7. **What chemotoxic side effects are related to ionic contrast material?**
   Neurotoxicity, electrocardiogram changes, arrhythmia, cardiac depression, renal tubular injury, and vascular injury are chemotoxic side effects. These side effects are related to the ionic nature, specifically the cation content of the contrast material. There are fewer chemotoxic reactions with nonionic contrast media.

8. **Discuss osmotoxic side effects.**
   Osmotoxic side effects are related to the dose or concentration of the contrast material. The side effects include arrhythmia, hypotension, changes in plasma volume, and changes in vascular permeability, vasodilation, and vasomotor instability. Low-osmolality contrast material reduces the number of these effects.

9. **How can contrast reactions be avoided?**
   - Ensure that the appropriate study is requested. Ultrasound, noncontrast CT, or noncontrast MR may be a more appropriate study.
   - Properly evaluate all patients for potential high risk.
   - Premedication of high-risk patients who need a contrast CT study should be considered.

10. List the potential symptoms of mild contrast reactions.

Mild contrast reactions include nausea, vomiting, cough, warmth, headache, dizziness, shaking, altered taste, itching, pallor, flushing, chills, sweats, rash, hives, nasal stuffiness, swelling of eyes and face, and anxiety.

11. How should mild symptoms be treated?

If these signs and symptoms do not progress, only observation is necessary.

12. Define moderate contrast reactions.

A moderate degree of clinically evident focal or systemic signs or symptoms includes tachycardia/bradycardia, hypertension, pronounced cutaneous reaction, hypotension, dyspnea, bronchospasm, wheezing, and laryngeal edema.

13. Should moderate symptoms be treated?

Yes. Immediate treatment is necessary. Close observation is essential to evaluate for progression to a life-threatening event.

14. Define severe contrast reactions.

Severe reactions are life-threatening. Examples include laryngeal edema, convulsions, profound hypotension, arrhythmias, unresponsiveness, and cardiopulmonary arrest.

15. How are severe symptoms treated?

Prompt recognition and treatment are essential. Hospitalization is always indicated.

16. How common are contrast reactions in children?

Contrast reaction is less frequent in children than in adults.

17. What minor reactions may be seen in children?

Hives, rhinorrhea, sneezing, nausea and vomiting, and facial edema.

18. How are minor reactions in children treated?

Observation is essential since small children cannot verbalize their symptoms. Diphenhydramine or chlorpheniramine is appropriate for treatment. If the reaction is progressing, subcutaneous epinephrine (1:1000) is suggested.

19. What more severe reactions may be seen in children?

Bronchospasm, laryngeal edema, anaphylactic shock, pulmonary edema, and cardiac arrest.

20. How are more severe reactions treated in children?

Prompt evaluation, intravenous epinephrine (1:10,000), oxygen, and intravenous fluids are the mainstays of treatment. A beta-agonist inhaler should be administered for bronchospasm. A child who is asthmatic can also use his or her own inhaler. Although steroids are not helpful for an acute reaction, they are beneficial for long-term stabilization.

21. What must every radiology department have readily available when children are given contrast?

Pediatric emergency equipment is essential to proper care of a pediatric contrast reaction. Specifically, pediatric-sized oxygen delivery devices, from partial nonrebreathers to intubation equipment, must be readily available.

22. Summarize the pediatric dose schedule.

- Antihistamine: diphenhydramine (Benadryl): 1–2 mg/kg IV, up to 50 mg
- Corticosteroid: methylprednisolone (Solu-Medrol): 2 mg/kg IV loading dose
- Diuretic: furosemide (Lasix): 1 mg/kg per dose IV, maximum of 40 mg

- Epinephrine (1:10,000): IV, 0.1 ml/kg; repeat every 5–15 min, as needed
- Epinephrine (1:1000): subcutaneous, 0.01 mg/kg, repeated every 15–30 min; maximum dose, 0.3 ml/dose
- Albuterol inhaler (Proventil, Ventolin): 2 puffs every 20–30 min, as needed (90–180 μg)
- Vagolytic: atropine: 0.02 mg/kg IV of the 0.1 mg/ml solution, with minimal dose of 0.1 mg; maximal dose for infant/child = 0.5 mg; maximal dose for adolescent = 1.0 mg

23. How is urticaria treated?

Discontinue the injection if it has not been completed. Although no treatment is needed in most cases, an H_1 receptor blocker, such as diphenhydramine (25–50 mg orally [PO], intramuscularly [IM], or IV) or hydroxyzine (5–50 mg IM), may be used. An H_2 receptor blocker may be added, such as cimetidine (300 mg PO or IV, diluted in 10ml D5W solution, given slowly) or ranitidine (50 mg PO or IV, diluted in 10 ml D5W solution, given slowly).

24. What agents may be used if the above agents are not adequate?

- Alpha agonist (arteriolar and venous constriction)
- Epinephrine SC (1:1000) or 0.1–0.3 ml (= 0.1–0.3 mg) if no cardiac complications are present

25. Describe the treatment for facial or laryngeal edema.

1. Administer alpha agonist (arteriolar and venous constriction)
   - Epinephrine SC (1:1000), 0.1–0.3 ml (= 0.1–0.3 mg); repeat as needed up to a maximum of 1.0 mg

   or
   - If hypotension is evident, epinephrine (1:10,000) slowly IV 1.0 ml (= 0.1mg), given slowly IV; repeat as needed to maximum of 1.0 mg
2. Oxygen, 6–10 L/min (via mask)
3. If the patient does not respond to therapy or acute laryngeal edema is obvious, seek appropriate assistance (e.g., cardiopulmonary response team).
4. Consider intubation.

26. How is bronchospasm treated?

1. Give oxygen, 6–10 L/min (via mask).
2. Monitor electrocardiogram, oxygen saturation (pulse oximeter), and blood pressure.
3. Use beta-agonist inhalers (bronchiolar dilators, such as metaproteronol [Alupent], terbutaline [Brethaire], or albuterol [Proventil]).
4. Give epinephrine SC (1:1000), 0.1–0.3,ml (=0.1–0.3mg)

   or

   If hypotension is evident, epinephrine (1:10,000), 1.0 ml (= 0.1 mg), slowly IV. Repeat as needed (maximum of 1.0 mg).
5. Alternatively, use aminophylline: 6.0 mg/kg IV in D5W over 10–20 min (loading dose), then 0.4–1.0 mg/kg/hr, as needed. Watch for hypotension. Terbutaline (0.25–0.5 mg IM or SC) also may be used.
6. Call for assistance (e.g., cardiopulmonary arrest response team) for severe bronchospasm or if oxygen saturation < 88% persists.

27. What if the patient experiences hypotension with tachycardia?

1. Legs elevated 60° or more or Trendelenburg position.
2. Monitor electrocardiogram, pulse oximeter, and blood pressure.
3. Give oxygen, 6–10 L/min (via mask).
4. Rapid administration of large volumes of isotonic Ringer's lactate (or normal saline) if the patient is poorly responsive.
5 If poorly responsive, give epinephrine (1:10,000), 1.0 ml (0.1 mg) slowly IV. Repeat as needed up to a maximum of 1.0 mg.
6. If still poorly responsive, transfer to intensive care unit for further treatment.

28. Describe the treatment of a vagal reaction (hypotension with bradycardia).
1. Monitor vital signs.
2. Legs must be elevated 60° or more (preferred) or Trendelenburg position.
3. Secure airway; give oxygen, 6–10 L/min (via mask).
4. Secure IV access; rapid fluid replacement with Ringer's lactate or normal saline.
5. Administer atropine, 0.6–1.0 mg IV slowly. Repeat atropine to a total dose of 0.04 mg/kg (2–3 mg) in adults.

29. How do you manage severe hypertension?
1. Monitor electrocardiogram, pulse oximeter.
2. Nitroglycerine, 0.4-mg tablet sublingually (may repeat 3 times), or topical 2% ointment (apply 1-inch strip).
3. Give sodium nitroprosside. Solution must be further diluted with 5% dextrose before infusion. It is essential to maintain proper monitoring for potential precipitous decreases in blood pressure; review complete dosage and administration instructions before use. An infusion pump may be necessary to titrate.
4. Transfer to ICU or emergency department.
5. For pheochromocytoma, give phentolamine, 5.0 mg (1.0 mg in children) IV.

30. What if the patient has a seizure?
1. Give oxygen, 6–10 L/min (via mask).
2. Consider diazepam, 5.0 mg, or midazolam, 2.5 mg.
3. If longer effect is needed, obtain consultation; consider phenytoin infusion, 15–18 mg/kg at 50 mg/min.
4. Monitor vital signs carefully.
5. Consider cardiopulmonary arrest response team for intubation, if needed.

31. How is pulmonary edema managed?
1. Elevate torso; use rotating tourniquets (venous compression).
2. Give oxygen, 6–10 L/min.
3. Give diuretic: furosemide, 40 mg IV, slow push.
4. Consider morphine.
5. Transfer to ICU or emergency department.
6. Corticosteroids are optional.

32. How is extravasation of contrast treated?
Elevation of the affected extremity above the level of the heart decreases capillary hydrostatic pressure and thereby promotes resorption of extravasated material.

Both warm and cold compresses are effective. Warm compresses promote vasodilation and resorption, whereas cold compresses decrease cellular uptake of the toxic contrast material, allowing local vascular and lymphatic systems to disperse the agent.

33. When is a surgical consultation needed?
Immediate surgical consultation is needed with extravasation of 50 ml or more of high-osmolality or 100 ml of low-osmolality contrast material. In the wrist, ankle, or dorsum of hand, the amounts requiring surgical consultation are 30 ml of high-osmolality and 60 ml of low-osmolality contrast material. Other indications include swelling and or pain after 2–4 hours, altered tissue perfusion as noted by decreased capillary refill at time of event, skin ulceration or blistering or change in sensation of the affected limb.

BIBLIOGRAPHY

1. Committee on Drugs and Contrast Media: Manual of Contrast Media, 4th ed. [CITY?], American College of Radiology, 2001.
2. Dunnick NR, Sandler CM, Newhouse JH, Amis ES: *Textbook of Uroradiology, 3rd ed.* [PUBLISHER?], Philadelphia, 2001.

4. TOOLS OF THE TRADE FOR INTERVENTIONAL RADIOLOGISTS

Craig B. Glaiberman, MD

1. **Does needle size increase or decrease with increasing gauge size?**
   Decrease.

2. **How many French (F) to one millimeter?**
   3 F = 1 mm.

3. **What size wire will fit through a 21-gauge micropuncture needle?**
   0.018 in.

4. **What size wire will fit through an 18-gauge Potts needle?**
   0.035 or 0.038 in.

5. **What is the mandril of a guidewire?**
   The mandril is the inner tapered wire that is wrapped by the stainless steel or hydrophilic coil.

6. **What is the difference between Rosen and Bentson wires in terms of tip characteristics?**
   The Rosen wire has a J-tip or curved configuration, whereas the Bentson has a straight tip.

7. **What is the advantage of the curved tip of the Rosen wire over the floppy tip of the Bentson wire?**
   Although the Bentson has a very floppy tip, the curved end of the Rosen helps prevent dissection of the wire tip under atherosclerotic plaques.

8. **What is the advantage of a stiff Amplatz wire compared with a Bentson wire?**
   A stiff Amplatz wire (Fig. 1) provides more "body" to advance drainage catheters through soft tissues that otherwise might buckle when placed over a Bentson wire.

9. **What is the purpose of hydrophilic coating on glide/Terumo wires?**
   To make them more slick and easier to pass through catheters and blood vessels.

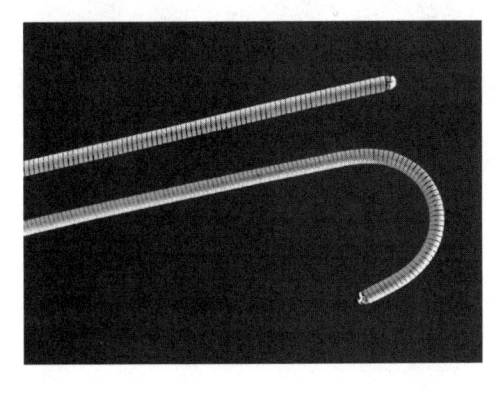

FIGURE 1. Amplatz stiff straight and curve tip wire. (Courtesy of Cook, Inc.)

10. What is a torque device? How do you use it?
When using a hydrophilic wire, it is not easy to steer it alone with a gloved hand. A torque device (Fig. 2) slips over the end of the wire and is tightened to improve steerability of an angled glide wire.

11. Why do you have to be careful not to force glide/Terumo wires through vessles?
Because they can easily dissect the vessel or soft tissues through which you are working.

12. Why should you not advance a hydrophilic wire through an 18-gauge needle?
It is not recommended because you may shear off the hydrophilic coating, which can embolize.

13. What is the first thing you should do to a hydrophilic wire before using it?
Flush or wet it.

14. What is the difference between a side-hole and an end-hole catheter?
A side-hole catheter (Fig. 3A) has multiple side holes and is used for contrast injections when a large-volume, tight bolus is needed to opacify vessels such as the aorta or inferior vena cava (IVC). End-hole catheters (Fig. 3B) are used for directed, smaller vessel selection and injection.

15. When withdrawing a wire from an end-hole catheter, what complication should you keep in mind? How might you prevent it?
A vacuum can be created inside the catheter when you withdraw a wire from an end-hole catheter. This vacuum may cause small air embolisms that can be disastrous when you are working in the aortic arch. This complication can be prevented by withdrawing the wire slowly while filling the hub of the catheter with heparinized saline.

16. What is the typical size of an angiographic catheter?
5F or 1.8 mm. Both 4- and 6-F catheters can be used as well.

17. Explain the purpose of double-flushing. How is it done?
Double-flushing is most often used during work in the aortic arch or across any blood vessel that feeds the brain. Two syringes of heparinized saline are used. The first is used simply to aspirate any small clots that may have formed inside the catheter. After a wet-to-wet hook-up, the second syringe is used to clear the blood from the catheter with heparinized saline. Bubbles should be meticulously cleared from the syringes before hooking up.

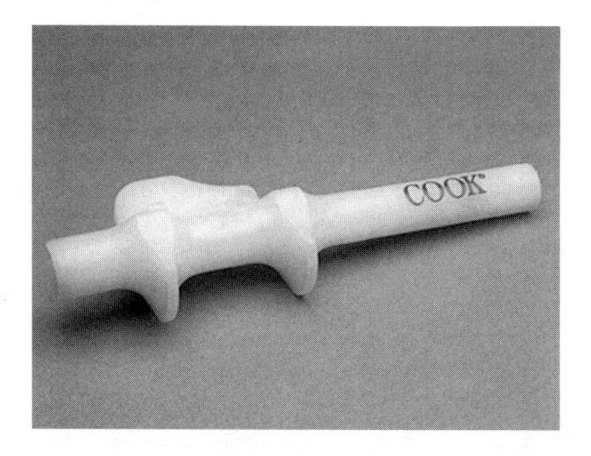

FIGURE 2. Torque device. (Courtesy of Cook, Inc.)

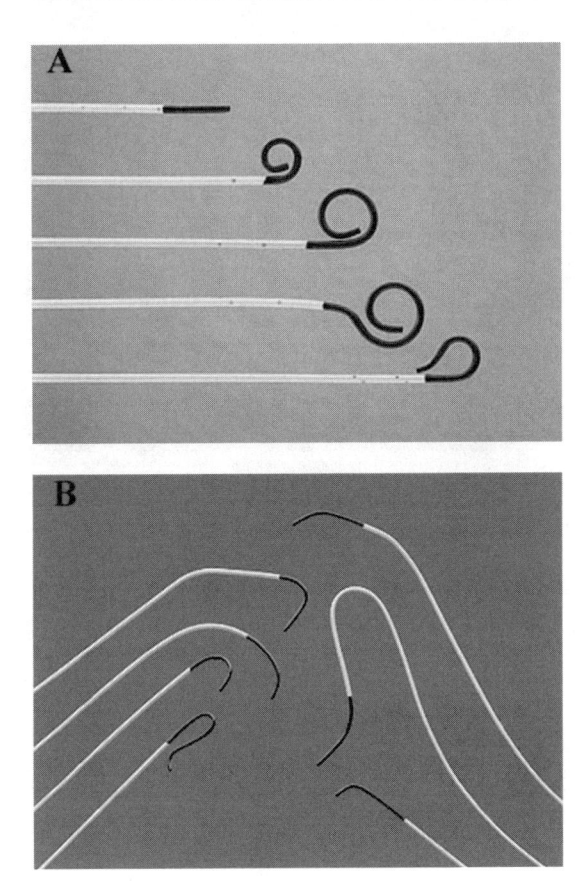

FIGURE 3. A, Side-hole catheters. **B,** End-hole catheters. (Courtesy of Cook, Inc.)

18. Explain the difference between the primary and secondary curve of an angiographic catheter.

In catheters with multiple curves, the first or primary bend in the catheter establishes the direction in which the catheter will point and provides a "backstop" from which to work. Compare the Simmons 1, 2, and 3 catheters to get a feel for the size of the primary curve. The size of the vessel determines the size of the primary curve. The secondary curve then becomes vessel selective. The angle of the origin of the vessel to be selected determines the angle of the secondary curve. Now compare the Simmons style catheter with a Cobra or H1 catheter.

19. What is the major determinant of which catheter to use?

The target vessel to be catheterized. Often many different catheters can be used for a single vessel and becomes operator dependent. For example, the superior mesenteric artery (SMA) can be selected with a Sos, RC-1, or Simmons-style catheter.

20. What is the purpose of a sheath?

The sheath (Fig. 4) protects the catheterized vessel from injury during long procedures when many catheter exchanges are anticipated. It can also facilitate catheter manipulation if scarring is present at the access site. It is also required during embolization procedures.

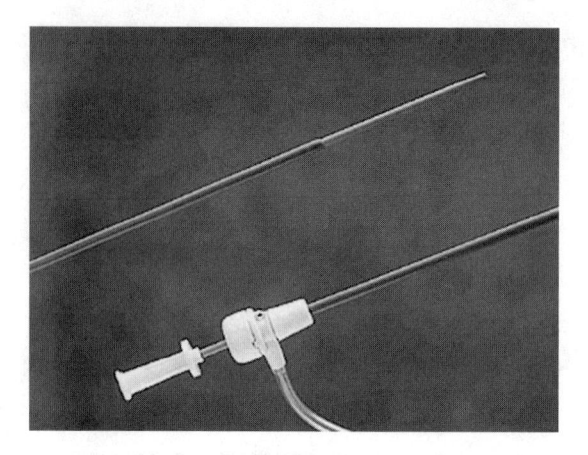

FIGURE 4. Access sheath. (Courtesy of Cook, Inc.)

21. Why is it important to always hook the sheath up to a heparinized flush bag?

Thrombus would form in the sheath and may embolize during catheter exchange or manipulation.

22. Are sheaths measured by the inner or outer diameter? Why is this knowledge important?

Sheaths are measured by the inner diameter. Catheters, stents, and balloons are measured by the outer diameters. This distinction helps to determine what size equipment will fit through the sheath.

23. What is a guiding catheter?

A guiding catheter is a specialized sheath that is typically longer than a regular sheath and curved to supply directional capability. It is often used to protect stents, balloons, and devices. An example is a Balkan sheath (Fig. 5), which can be used for iliac and renal intervention.

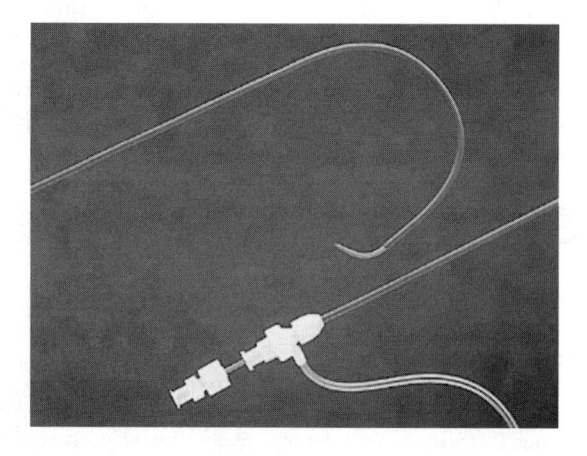

FIGURE 5. Balkan sheath (Courtesy of Cook, Inc.)

24. What is the importance of a safety wire? How is it used?

A safety wire maintains access across a lesion that has been the target of intervention. If dissection or rupture of a vessel occurs, a balloon can be quickly placed across the lesion to tamponade rupture or tack down flow-limiting dissection flaps.

25. What is the difference between a stent graft and a bare stent?

Stent grafts are bare stents covered with material such as Gore-Tex (Fig. 6A) that are used to exclude aneurysms, bile ducts, or the intimal lining of venous structures. **Bare stents** have open interstices (Figs. 6B-6D).

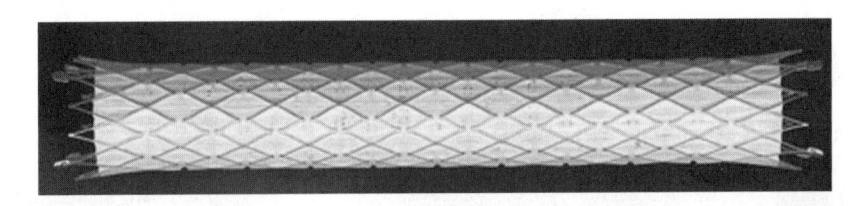

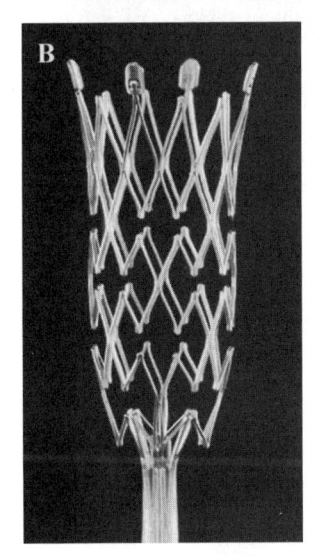

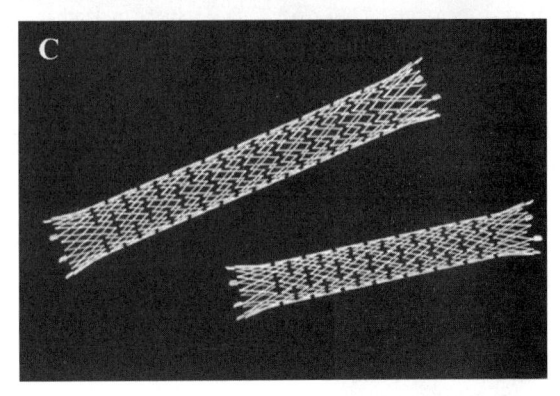

FIGURE 6. A, Covered Fluency stent graft. **B, C,** and **D,** Luminex bare stents. (Courtesy of Bard, Inc.)

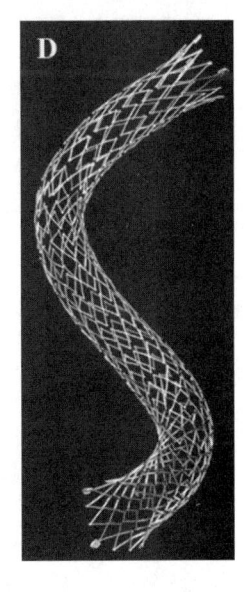

26. What is the theoretical benefit of placing a stent graft in an abdominal aortic aneurysm? In a vein?

Stent grafts are used to exclude blood flow into the aneurysm sac, allowing it to thrombose around the graft (Fig. 7). Intimal hyperplasia is a common cause for stenosis of stented vessels from ingrowth through the interstices of bare stents. It is thought that the graft material will exclude intimal hyperplasia and provide longer patency rates.

27. With regard to stent deployment, what is meant by self-expanding? Balloon-expandable?

A self-expanding stent, such as a Wallstent, opens on its own when deployed and requires subsequent placement of a balloon to dilate it. Balloon-expandable stents are already mounted on balloons and are deployed by inflating the balloon.

28. What does foreshortening imply? Why is it important in choosing stents to deploy?

When some stents are deployed or balloon-dilated, they shorten. The Wallstent (Boston Scientific, Natick, MA) has the largest degree of foreshortening of any stent currently on the market.

29. When is the Trerotola device used? What does PTD stand for?

The Trerotola device (developed by the doctor of the same name) is a percutaneous thrombectomy device (PTD) that is used to lyse clot in dialysis grafts (Arrow International, Reading, PA). It is a motorized "egg-beater" that can be placed into polytetrafluoroethylene (PTFE) grafts through a short sheath to break up thrombus.

30. What is the largest IVC in which one can safely place a Greenfield filter?

28 mm.

31. Where does the lysed clot from PTFE grafts often go if not contained by a stenosis at the venous anastamosis?

Lysed clots often go to the lungs as small pulmonary emboli.

32. What is Nitinol? Describe its special characteristic.

Nitinol, which stands for nickel-titanium alloy, was developed by NASA. It has thermal memory such that, when it is heated, it returns to its original shape. This characteristic allows

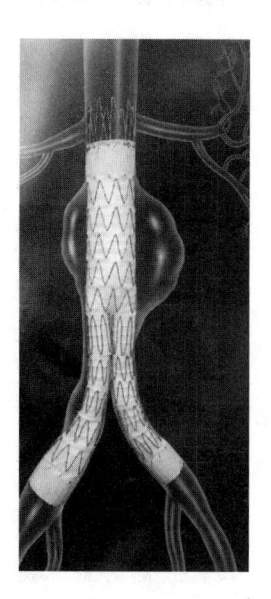

FIGURE 7. Zenith AAA stent. (Courtesy of Cook, Inc.)

packaging into a small delivery system. Normal body temperature returns Nitinol to its original shape.

33. Explain the difference between a temporary and a permanent embolic agent.

Temporary embolic agents resorb or allow recanalization of vessels, whereas **permanent embolic agents** cause irreversible occlusion. Temporary agents such as gelfoam are useful in trauma cases when the goal is to reduce the pressure head to bleeding vessels rather than induce ischemia.

34. Explain the difference between a distal and a proximal embolic agent.

The difference is relevant to both size and feeding vessel. **Distal agents** are very small and reach the capillary-arteriolar level (300–500 microns). **Proximal agents,** such as coils, are often large (2–15 mm) and come in a variety of lengths. One must be cognizant of collateral vessels when using proximal agents because flow to the lesion can persist through numerous other channels.

35. What is PVA?

Polyvinyl alcohol (Fig. 8).

36. What characteristic of PVA makes it a good permanent agent?

PVA incites an inflammatory reaction, rendering it highly thrombogenic.

37. Of what are coils typically made? What is added to make them more thrombogenic?

Coils are made of stainless steel or platinum constructed with polyester threads to make them more thrombogenic (Fig. 9).

38. What is the advantage of using gelfoam as an embolic agent?

Gelfoam is a resorbable temporary agent that can be cut to varying sizes. Vessel recannalization occurs approximately 2 weeks after embolization.

39. What is meant by nontarget embolization? Why is it an important concept?

Nontarget embolization is a complication that results in the entrance of embolic materials into vessels not intended for occlusion. Coils can be retrieved, whereas other agents cannot. Ischemia and infarction of adjacent tissues are undesired effects. The concept is especially important with

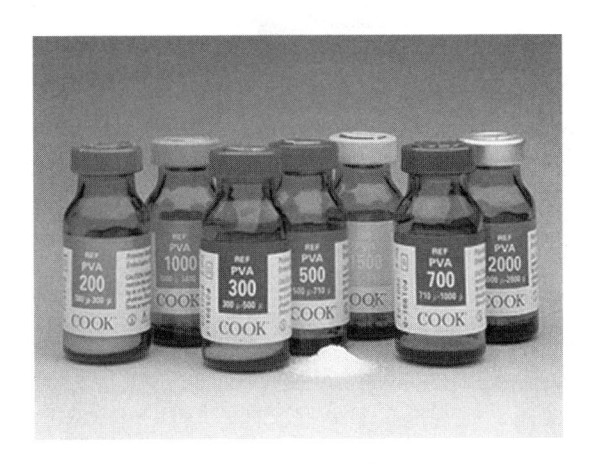

FIGURE 8. PVA particles in different sizes. (Courtesy of Cook, Inc.)

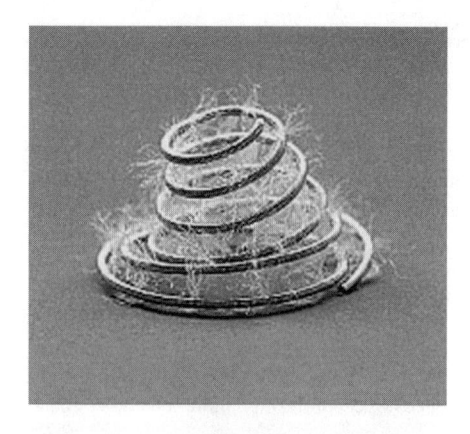

FIGURE 9. Tornado coils. (Courtesy of Cook, Inc.)

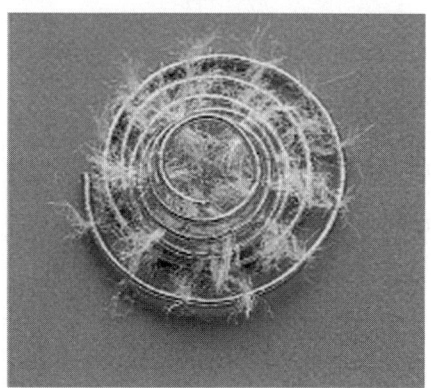

chemoembolization of the liver. Nontarget embolization to the pancreas, stomach, or gallbladder can cause pancreatitis, duodenal ulceration, gastric ulceration, or cholecystitis.

40. What is meant by trocar technique with regard to abscess drainage?

Trocar technique is a one-step placement of a drainage catheter over a stiff inner needle. Once into a fluid collection, the catheter is fed off of the needle, which is withdrawn. No guidewire is used in this technique.

41. What is the purpose of the inner stylet in trocar needles?

The trocar provides the sharp point with which to puncture the organ or vessel of choice. It is then withdrawn to allow passage of a guidewire while maintaining access. The trocar also prevents occlusion of the access needle by a core of the tissues through which it is passed.

42. Explain the differences among a percutaneous nephrostomy tube (PCN), a nephroureteral stent (NUS), and a double-J stent (DJS)?

The **PCN** is an external drain that enters the posterior flank and collecting system. It is usually coiled in the renal pelvis and drains urine externally to a bag.

The **NUS** is an internal-external drain that enters from the posterior flank, but it is longer than the PCN and extends into the bladder to allow both external drainage to a bag and internal drainage to the baldder (Fig. 10).

The **DJS** is strictly internal and extends from the renal pelvis into the bladder. It can be placed from either an existing PCN/NUS or from the bladder.

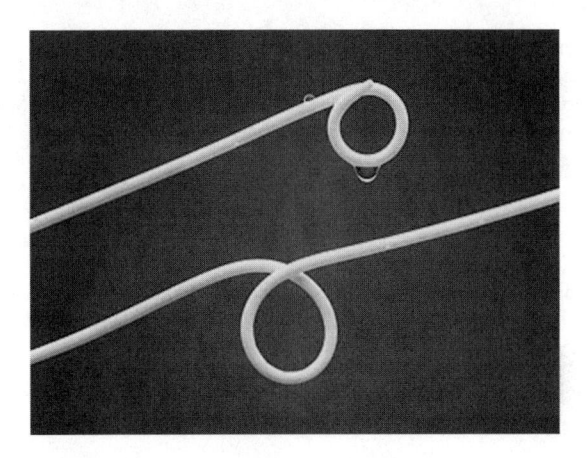

FIGURE 10. Nephroureteral stent. (Courtesy of Cook, Inc.)

43. Other than coming all the way off magnification, what two strategies can the interventionalist use to see more of the patient?

By raising the patient away from the x-ray tube, or by lowering the image intensifier. Often both are done in combination to reduce scatter and operator exposure.

44. List six characteristics of guidewires.
- Length
- Diameter
- Tip configuration
- Torqueability
- Stiffness
- Outer coating

45. When doing hand-injection digital subtraction angiography (DSA), when should you inject contrast?

Only after the "mask" has been obtained. This is usually when the screen goes "blank".

46. What is meant by "forming" the angiographic catheter?

When catheters are inserted over a wire, they enter the vessel in a straight line. The size of the vessel that they enter determines how much of the shape they regain from inherent material memory. Often the catheters need to be pushed and turned to form them in the aorta. Some of the larger curved catheters require formation in the arch or off other vessels, such as the contralateral iliac artery.

47. What is meant by a "waist" in the balloon? What does it imply?

The waist is the impression formed upon the balloon by the stenotic atherosclerotic plaque or intimal hyperplasia. It is either completely reduced or diminished to a point where no residual pressure gradient remains or a good angiographic result is obtained.

48. How does absolute alcohol work as a sclerosing agent?

Alcohol denatures proteins, causing inflammation and fibrosis.

49. Which size syringe generates a higher-pressure hand injection: 3 cc or 20 cc?

A 3-cc syringe generates more pressure.

50. What is a microcatheter? How is it used?

Amicrocatheter is a small (3-F) catheter used to cannulate very small vessels to deliver precise embolic materials or perform angiography of specific arteries and veins. Microcatheterse are often introduced coaxially through 4-F or 5-F angiography catheters.

BIBLIOGRAPHY

1. Baum S: Abrams' Angiography: Vascular and Interventional Radiology, 4th ed. Philadelphia, Lippincott Williams & Wilkins, 1996.
2. Castaneda-Zuniga W: Interventional Radiology. Philadelphia, Lippincott Williams & Wilkins, 1996.
3. Kandarpa K: Handbook of Interventional Radiology, 3rd ed. Philadelphia, Lippincott Williams & Wilkins, 2003.
4. Kaufman J: Vascular and Interventional Radiology: The Requisites. St. Louis, Mosby, 2004.
5. Valji K: Vascular and Interventional Radiology. Philadelphia, W.B. Saunders, 1999

5. GENE THERAPY

Ian Wilson, MD

1. What is gene therapy?
Gene therapy is the introduction of recombinant genes into selective somatic cells to treat acquired or inherited disorders.

2. Describe the radiologist's role in gene therapy.
Radiologists are uniquely situated to use interventional techniques and diagnostic imaging modalities to deliver genes and subsequently assess the functioning of delivered genes in vivo.

3. How can the vascular endothelium be exploited for the purposes of gene therapy?
Vascular endothelial cells can be transduced or transfected to express gene products that have local or regional effects. For example, endothelial cells induced to overexpress tissue plasminogen activator (t-PA) or hirudin may treat thrombosis. Endothelium induced to express vascular endothelial growth factor (VEGF) can increase regional blood vessel density in ischemic conditions.

4. Which diseases are potentially amenable to vascular gene therapy?
- Cardiac and limb ischemia
- Vasculoproliferative disorders
- Hypercholesterolemia
- Atherosclerosis
- Thrombosis
- Hypertension

5. What gene products are being investigated for the treatment of restenosis?
Thymidine kinase, cytosine deaminase, retinoblastoma gene product, p21 cyclin-dependent kinase inhibitor 1, c-Myc, c-Myb, cyclo-oxygenase. In addition, genes coding for thrombomodulin, hirudin, t-PA, and a urokinase-type plasminogen activator are being investigated for the vascular gene therapy of thrombosis.

6. What gene products are being investigated for their role in angiogenesis?
VEGF, hepatocyte growth factor (HGF), leptin, and thrombopoietin.

7. What gene product promises to play a wide role in the treatment of many cardiovascular diseases?
Nitric oxide synthetase.

8. Define molecular imaging.
Molecular imaging is defined as the in vivo detection, characterization, and/or quantification of biologic processes at the cellular and molecular level.

9. How can ultrasound be exploited for gene therapy?
Ultrasound can be used to guide the delivery of genes via endovascular or percutaneous extravascular approaches. Ultrasound contrast agents have been used to deliver genetic material as a nonviral method. The cavitation phenomenon of ultrasound contrast agents has been shown to induce varying degrees of local endothelial disruption to enhance the uptake and expression of the exogenous genes.

10. How can magnetic resonance imaging (MRI) be exploited for gene delivery and surveillance?

High spatial resolution cross-sectional images of vessel walls have been obtained using receiver coils incorporated into catheters. Functional MR, MR spectroscopy, and novel paramagnetic contrast agents can be used to assess the effects of gene therapy in vivo.

11. What specific drug delivery devices are available for endovascular use?

Passive diffusion balloons (double-occlusion and spiral balloons), pressure-driven balloons (microporous, hydrogel-coated, coaxial, and perfusion balloons), and mechanical devices (needle injection catheter and stent systems) have been manufactured by several companies.

12. How does gene therapy work?

The delivered therapeutic genes augment the host's genome or inhibit endogenous gene expression.

13. Explain the central dogma of gene expression.

The central dogma explains the process of gene expression. DNA is replicated enzymatically. DNA codes for the production of messenger RNA (transcription). Messenger RNA (mRNA) is processed and transported to the cytoplasm, where it is translated by ribosomes into a gene product (protein).

14. What are the two broad categories of gene delivery?

In vivo and ex vivo.

15. Describe the process of in vivo gene therapy.

In vivo gene therapy involves the administration of recombinant genes to a patient via viral or nonviral vectors.

16. Describe the process of ex vivo gene therapy.

Ex vivo gene therapy involves the introduction of recombinant genes to a patient's harvested somatic cells, followed by the administration of the altered cells back to the patient.

17. Define reporter gene.

A reporter gene encodes for a product (protein) that is easily identifiable. The product of reporter genes may be either intracellular or located on the cell surface. An example of an intracellular marker gene is tyrosinase. Among other actions, tyrosinase catalyzes the oxidation of dopa to dopaquinone, which undergoes cyclization and polymerization to yield melanin. The high affinity of melanin for iron accounts for the high signal intensity of melanin-containing structures on T1. They can be detected in vivo using MR. The somatostatin receptor gene is an example of a reporter gene whose produce resides on the cell surface. The somatostatin receptor gene product can be detected in vivo using radiolabeled octreotide, a nuclear medicine imaging agent in clinical use.

18. What are viral vectors?

Noncellular biologic vehicles for the delivery of a gene that can only reproduce and express the gene within a host cell.

19. List the advantage of viral vectors vs. nonviral gene delivery schemes.

Viral vectors usually have greater transfection efficiency.

20. What is the most commonly used viral vector?

Retroviruses account for the majority of viral vectors (53%) employed in clinical trials of gene therapy. The second most frequently used viral vector is the adenovirus (19%).

21. Explain the difference between transduction and transfection.

The difference lies in the vehicle of delivery. **Transduction** is accomplished when viral vectors are used to delivery genetic material. **Transfection** is the process by which genes are delivered using nonviral means such as liposomes.

22. What are liposomes?

Liposomes are cationic unilamellar phospholipids that can form complexes with DNA by electrostatic interactions between positively charged lipid residues and negatively charged phosphates of nucleotides.

23. What are microbubbles? How do they work?

Microbubbles are microscopic spheres that usually contain a fluorocarbon bound by lipid, protein, or a polymeric lattice. At a certain ultrasonic frequency the microbubbles cavitate. Cavitation releases their contents.

24. What are stem cells?

Progenitor cells that give rise to differentiated cell types.

BIBLIOGRAPHY

1. Li T, et al: Gene transfer with echo-enhanced contrast agents: Comparison between Albunex, Optison, and Levovist in mice—initial results. Radiology 229:423–428, 2003.
2. Weissleder R, Mahmood U: Molecular imaging. Radiology 219:316–333, 2001.
3. Yang X: Imaging of vascular gene therapy. Radiology 228:36–49, 2003.

6. CODING IN INTERVENTIONAL RADIOLOGY

David L. Waldman, MD, PhD

1. What is HCFA?
Health Care Financing Administration, which in 2001 was renamed the Center for Medicare and Medicaid Services (CMS).

2. What is RBRVS?
Resource-based relative value scale.

3. Define CPT.
CPT refers to the current procedural terminology coding method.

4. For what does S&I stand?
Supervision and interpretation code.

5. For what does E&M stand?
Evaluation and management codes.

6. What is meant by ICD9?
International classification of disease, ninth revision.

7. What is RVU?
Relative value unit.

8. What is the most important feature to keep you out of trouble during coding?
Documentation.

9. Describe the basis of angiography coding.
Angiography coding is based on vascular anatomy and requires knowledge of the coding anatomy. A vascular family is defined as a group of blood vessels arising from a single branch off the aorta. Each artery arising from the aorta or each vein draining directly into the inferior vena cava begins its own vascular family (parent vessel).

10. What is meant by nonselective arterial catheterization?
A catheter placed directly into an artery or moved from an arterial access site into the aorta is considered nonselective. The most frequently used code for a nonselected arterial catheterization is 36200, which is defined as introduction of a catheter into the aorta (Fig. 1).

11. What is meant by selective arterial catheterization?
A catheter moved from the aorta or punctured vessels into one of the branches off the aorta is considered selective. The code that should be used depends on whether the artery catheterization is above or below the diaphragm. Selective arterial catheterization can be defined as first order (i.e., catheterization of a parent vessel or a vascular family) or second order (i.e., catheterization of a branch of the parent vessel). You can also have third order and above catheterizations.

12. If you perform angiography in a nonselective method and then move the catheter into the parent vessel, can you code for both the nonselective and selective angiogram?
You can only code for the highest order of blood vessel. Remember that the report needs to document what is done. If it is not documented, it was not done.

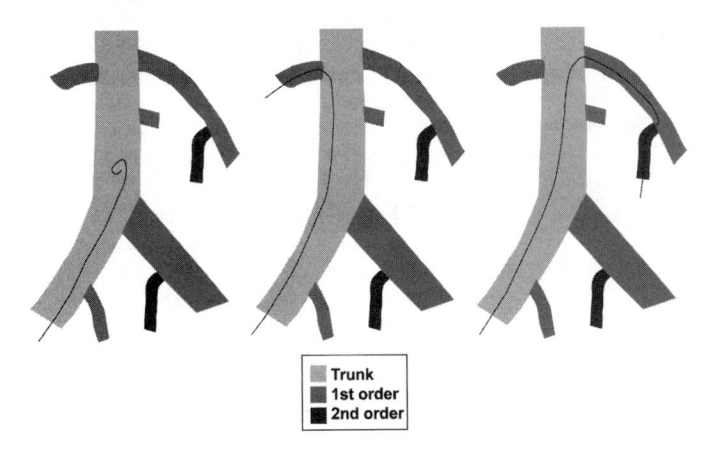

FIGURE 1. Three examples of vascular coding. In the first example, the catheter is placed only in the aorta. The CPT code for a nonselective angiogram is 36200. The second example is catheterization of the renal artery, a branch directly from the aorta. It is considered first order, and the CPT code is 36245. In the final example, the catheter is placed into a branch off the superior mesenteric artery. This is considered second order; the CPT code is 36246. You can code for only the highest order vessel that you cannulated. Remember: if you did not do it, you cannot bill for it—and if you did not document it, you did not do it.

13. What is a modifier?

A modifier is a subcode placed on the CPT code that helps further define what was done. Modifiers help the insurance companies further understand the work performed. For example a modifier 50 would be placed on an examination in which bilateral procedures were performed. If you did bilateral renal angiograms, the CPT coding would be 36245–50. This coding means that bilateral first-order selective renal angiograms were performed. The S&I code that goes with this CPT code is 75724, defined as bilateral selective renal arteriogram, including flush aortography..

14. If a code does not exist for the service, may I use the best fit?

If a code does not exist for the services provided, use caution in attempting a best fit. Instead use the unlisted procedural code.

15. Can E&M coding be billed by interventional radiologists?

E&M services may or may not be included. A routine periprocedural E&M is always bundled into the procedure; however, there are always payer-specific rules. Specfic modifiers are critical, based on the timing of the E&M service. It is important to understand the specific global periods for each defined procedure.

16. Where is the best place to learn more about accurate coding?

The Society of Interventional Radiology's manual on coding. Because coding is highly complex, it is important that you understand the rules. Remember, once you understand the rules, CMS will change them.

17. What are the levels of E&M service?

Problem focused (brief), expanded problem focused, detailed, and comprehensive.

18. What is the most important factor for E&M coding?

Documentation. All E&M services must be documented and dated in the complete and legible medical record. You must include the reason for the encounter and relevant history, examination findings, and correlative prior tests. An assessment and a plan for care are also required. If it is not documented, it has not happened. If documentation is not legible, it did not happen.

19. What are the codes used for E&M services?
- 99211: Problem focused (requires presence of a physician), approximately 5 minutes.
- 99212: Expanded medical focus, approximately 10 minutes.
- 99213: Detailed visit, minimum of 15 minutes.

Codes 99212 and 99213 require two of the three components, including history, physical examination, and medical decision.

20. What E&M codes are used for inpatient services?
99221, 99222, and 99223. The level of service follows the above code. These codes are to be used by the admitting physician and not by a consultant. E&M codes apply to all services on the date of admission by the admitting physician.. The codes depend on the level of care for the entire encounter.

21. Which codes are used for subsequent hospital care?
99231, 99232, and 99233. These codes can be used by consulting physicians. They are used by the physician who has initiated treatment or participates in the patient's management. No interventional procedures are required. This code is also used when a global period of several days is involved.

22. Which codes are used for inpatient consultation services?
99251, 99252, and 99253. Use these codes when an opinion or advice about the evaluation or management of a patient has requested by the managing physician. The opinion and/or services must be documented in the medical record.

23. Define HIPAA.
HIPAA stands for the Health Insurance Portability and Accountability Act, which was passed in 1996. The law deals with transaction standards, including privacy and security standards. The goal is to promote the efficiency and effectiveness of the health care system.

24. When do organizations need to be in compliance?
October 16, 2003 was to deadline for all covered parties to comply with HIPAA's electronic and code set standards.

25. Who is responsible for code enforcement?
CMS is responsible for enforcing the electronic transactions and code sets provision of the law.

26. What is the "minimum necessary" standard for HIPAA compliance?
The privacy rules require a physician to make reasonable efforts to limit the amount of protected health information used or disclosed to the minimum amount necessary to accomplish the purpose of the use or disclosure.

27. Where can learn about HIPAA?
Multiple good governmental and nongovernmental websites are available for information. The below list is by no means inclusive.

Governmental Website
http://cms.hhs.gov/default.asp

Nongovernmental Websites
http://www.wedi.org
http://www.nchica.org
http://www.hipaadvisory.com

II. Vascular Interventions

7. VASCULAR ANATOMY
Ian Wilson, MD

1. What anatomic variant can simulate acute aortic injury?
Ductus diverticulum. The most distal segment of the embryonic right arch manifests as a fusiform dilatation of the ventromedial aspect of the proximal descending thoracic aorta (Fig. 1).

2. What anatomic variant can simulate acute great vessel injury?
Diverticulum of Kommerell—a bulbous remnant of the dorsal aortic root.

3. What is aortic coarctation?
Aortic coarctation is a congenital localized narrowing of the aorta, usually located adjacent to the ductus arteriosus and distal to the origin of the left subclavian artery. Aortic coarctation is traditionally classified into preductal and postductal types.

4. How does aortic coarctation develop?
The ductal, malunion, and differential growth theories are proposed mechanisms. The **ductal theory** states that the existence of circumferential ductal tissue and its subsequent fibrotic obliteration leads to constriction.

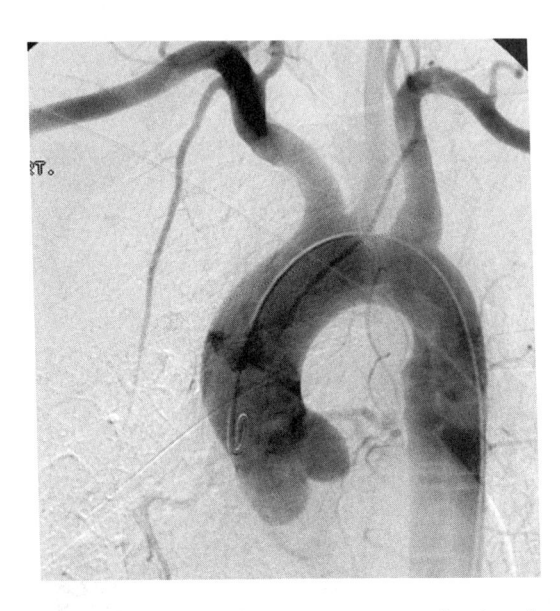

FIGURE 1. Left anterior oblique angiogram demonstrates two normal variants: bovine arch, in which the brachiocephalic and left carotid ateries have a common trunk, and prominent ductus bump, which must no' be mistaken for an aortic transection.

The **malunion theory** postulates that the obstructive lesion localizes to an embryologic communication between the fourth aortic arch and the cephalic aspect of the dorsal aorta. The consequent alteration in hemodynamics results in hypoplasia. The malunion theory is the suspected etiology of aortic coarctation at sites distal to the ligamentum arteriosum.

The **differential growth theory** implicates developmental changes in great vessel position (i.e., the migration of the subclavian artery from the sixth to the fourth arch), which presumably result from differential growth.

5. **What collateral pathways are found in the setting of aortic coarctation?**
   - Internal thoracic artery-descending thoracic aorta via anterior and posterior intercostal arteries
   - Superior epigastric-inferior epigastric arteries
   - Verterbral-anterior spinal arteries
   - Thyrocervical and costocervical trunks-internal thoracic via first two intercostals

   Other unnamed collateral pathways also exist.

6. **What are the common, clinically important variants in the aortic arch?**
   Right subclavian aberrancy (Fig. 2), right aortic arch, and ductus diverticulum.

7. **What is the thyroidea internal mammary artery (IMA)?**
   A variant artery occurring in 6% of people, the thyroidea IMA supplies the thyroid isthmus and medial portions of the thyroid lobes. In most cases, it arises from the brachiocephalic artery. In 1% of cases, the thyroidea IMA arises between the brachiocephalic and left subclavian arteries. It arises from the right common carotid in 1% of cases.

8. **Which aortic arch variants are associated with other defects?**
   Right aortic arch and mirror-image aortic arch.

9. **What are the common anatomic variations of the celiac axis?**
   Classic anatomic branching occurs in 65–75% of the population (Fig. 3). Trifurcation occurs in 25% of people, and 5–10% of people exhibit classic branching plus a dorsal pancreatic or middle colic artery.

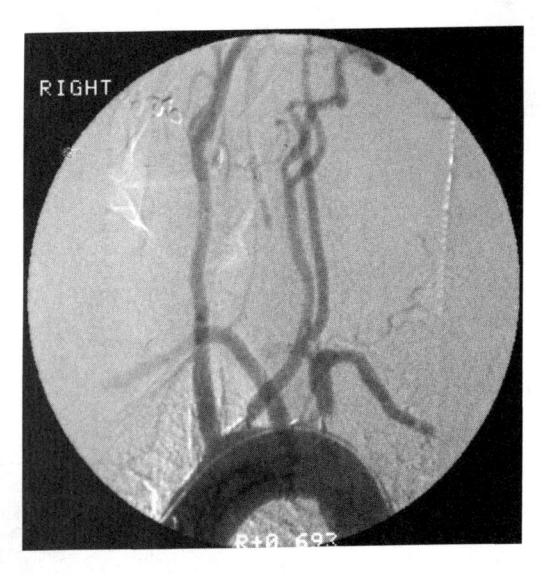

FIGURE 2. Left occipitoanterior angiogram of the aortic arch demonstrates a left-sided aortic arch with an aberrant right subclavian artery.

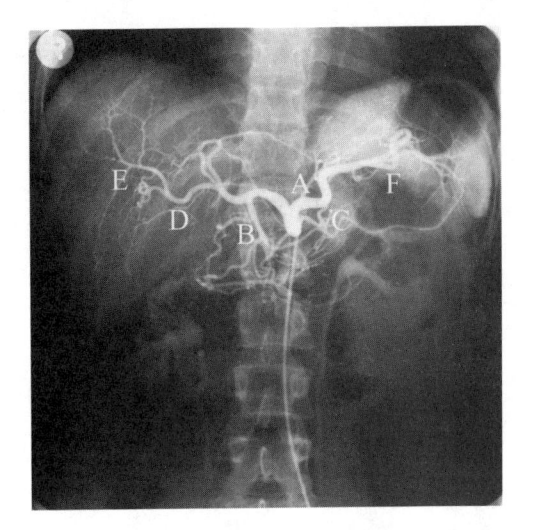

FIGURE 3. Selective view of the celiac trunk (A) demonstrates the gastroduodenal artery (B), gastroepiploic artery (C), proximal (D) and distal (E) hepatic arteries, and splenic artery (F). This is a normal branch pattern.

10. **Describe the usual branching pattern of the bronchial arteries.**
    - Three bronchial arteries (45%): two left and one right bronchial artery (40%); two right and one left (5%).
    - Four bronchial arteries (24%): two left and two right bronchial arteries (20%); three left and one right (4%).

11. **In aortic occlusion, what collateral pathways allow distal perfusion?**
    - Abdominal aorta–posterior intercostal and lumbar arteries-deep circumflex iliac artery–external iliac artery (Fig. 4)
    - Abdominal aorta–lumbar artery–iliolumbar–internal iliac–external iliac artery
    - Abdominal aorta–superior mesenteric artery (SMA)-arc of Riolan–IMA–superior and inferior hemorrhoidals–internal pudendal artery–internal iliac artery–external iliac artery (Fig. 5)

12. **In iliac occlusion, what collateral pathways allow distal perfusion?**
    Lumbar-hypogastric-cross-pelvic collateral arteries.

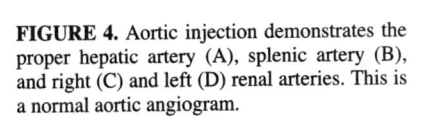

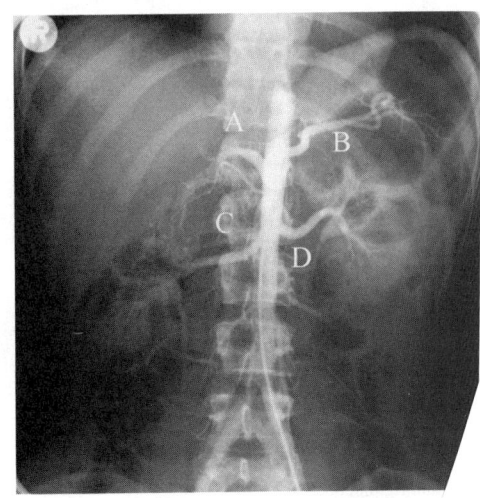

FIGURE 4. Aortic injection demonstrates the proper hepatic artery (A), splenic artery (B), and right (C) and left (D) renal arteries. This is a normal aortic angiogram.

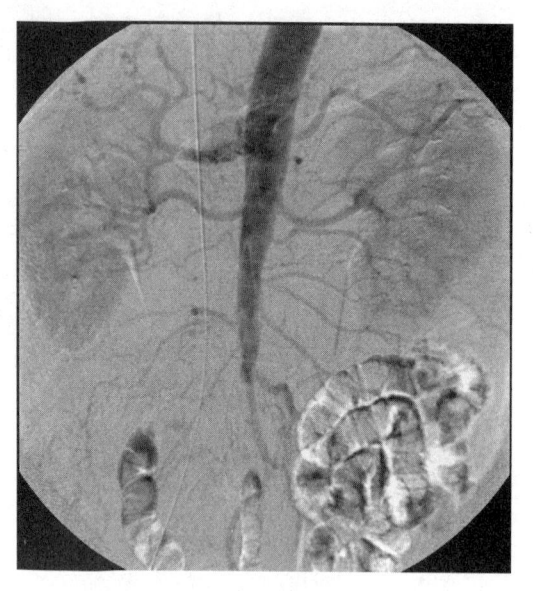

FIGURE 5. Infrarenal aortic occlusion, also known as Leriche syndrome, is typically defined as the clinical triad of impotence, buttock claudication, and thigh claudication. It occurs in young males. The angiographic appearance is a smooth tapering of the infrarenal aorta with distal occlusion. Collateral pathways are present to maintain the blood supply of the pelvis and lower extremities.

13. What is the Winslow pathway?

A collateral pathway that manifests in the presence of aortoiliac occlusion. The pathway is as follows: subclavian-external iliac via the internal mammary-superior and inferior epigastric anastomosis.

14. What are the major visceral collateral arteries?
- Arc of Riolan
- Arc of Buhler
- Marginal artery of Drummond
- Arc of Barkow

See Figures 6 and 7.

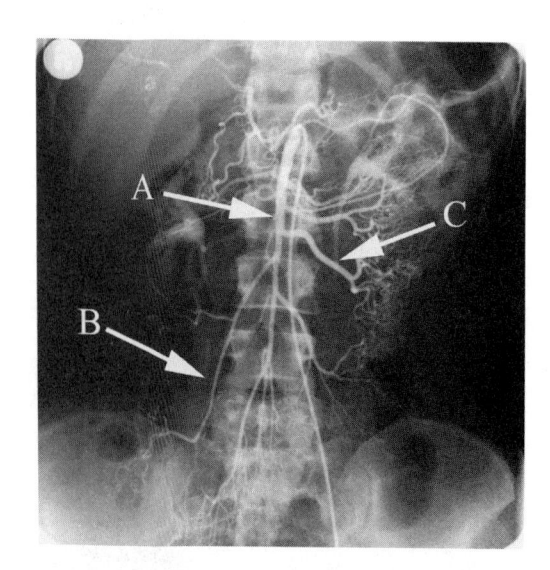

FIGURE 6. Selective injection of the superior mesenteric artery illustrates the main trunk (A) as well as the iliocolic (B) and jejunal (C) branches. This is a normal branch pattern.

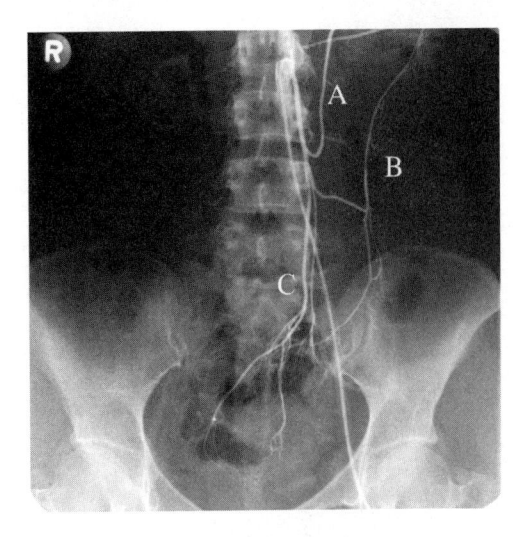

FIGURE 7. Selective injection injection of the inferior mesenteric artery illustrates the left colic branch (A), marginal branch (B), and main trunk (C).

15. What is the arc of Riolan?
A direct connection between the SMA and IMA via the middle and left colic arteries at the splenic flexure.

16. What is the marginal artery of Drummond?
Series of longitudinal anastomoses adjacent and parallel to the colon and originating from the arcades of the ileocolic, right, middle, and left colic arteries.

17. What is the arc of Buhler?
Persistence of the embryonal ventral anastomosis—a communication between the celiac and superior mesenteric arteries.

18. What is the arc of Barkow?
An epiploic anastomosis, composed of left and right arcs, that provides branches to the transverse colon from the left epiploic artery (left branch) and the right epiploic arteries (right branch). The left and right epiploic arteries arise from the left and right gastroepiploic arteries, respectively.

19. Describe the usual arterial supply to uterine fibroids.
Uterine fibroids are predominantly supplied by branches of the internal iliac artery—more specifically, branches of the anterior division of the internal iliac artery. The uterine artery is typically the first branch of the anterior division.

20. Describe the important pelvic anatomic variants with regard to uterine artery embolization for fibroids.
Forty percent of patients exhibit trifurcation of the internal iliac artery into anterior, posterior, and uterine branches. In approximately 5% of patients, the uterine artery arises proximal to the bifurcation. There is a reported 10–15% occurrence of uterine-ovarian artery anastomosis. In 1% of patients, the uterine artery may be absent or discontinuous. In the 0.3% of patients with bilaterally absent uterine arteries, myometrial perfusion is provided by branches of the ovarian artery.

21. What bony landmarks can be used in performing angiographic evaluation of the aorta and its branches?
- Inferior phrenic: T12
- Celiac axis: T12–L1

- SMA: L1–L2
- Renal arteries: L1–L2
- IMA: L3–L4

22. What is the adductor hiatus?
A common site of superficial femoral artery stenosis.

23. Describe popliteal artery entrapment.
Popliteal artery entrapment is a a congenital abnormality that may manifest clinically as acute-onset lower extremity claudication. The condition may progress to intermittent complication and may be complicated by popliteal artery thrombosis, aneurysm formation (with or without thromboembolic phenomena), and lower extremity ischemia.

24. What anatomic structures are involved in popliteal entrapment?
Popliteal artery entrapment syndrome is classified into four main types:
- Type I: medial arterial course; normal insertion of medial head of gastrocnemius muscle
- Type II: medial arterial course; lateral insertion of medial head of gastrocnemius
- Type III: compression and medial deviation of popliteal artery secondary to plantaris muscle or accessory fasicles from the medial head of the gastrocnemius
- Type IV: normal artery course; extrinsic compression by the popliteus muscle.

25. Explain hypothenar hammer syndrome.
Hypothenar hammer syndrome is characterized by numbness, paresthesias, stiffness, coldness, and blanching of digits secondary to ulnar artery occlusion or aneurysm formation resulting from repetitive trauma (Fig. 8).

26. What is thoracic outlet syndrome (TOS)?
TOS is a neurovascular compression syndrome of the upper extremity resulting from compression of the brachial plexus, subclavian artery, or subclavian vein (Fig. 9) between the clavicle and first rib. Anatomically, the thoracic outlet is defined as the region traversed by the brachial plexus, subclavian artery, and subclavian vein. The costoclavicular space, interscalene triangle,

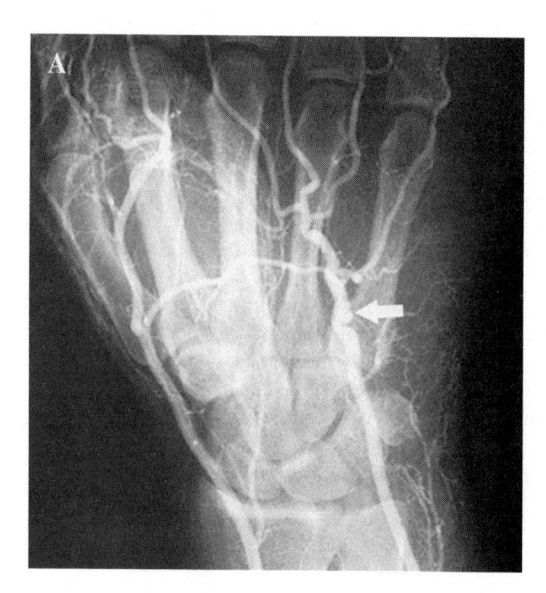

FIGURE 8. A 40-year-old man who works at a copy center presents with a positive Allen test. He gives a history of repetitive trauma on the ulnar aspect of the hand secondary to using the hypothenar aspect of the hand to staple papers. Angiogram of the hand demonstrates aneurysm formation of ulnar artery consistent with hypothenar hammer syndrome. The position of the ulnar artery in the hypothenar eminence crossing the hamate bone makes it vulnerable to repetitive occupational or recreational trauma. The arterial lesion may appear angiographically as spasm, occlusion, aneurysm, or a combination thereof.

Vascular Anatomy

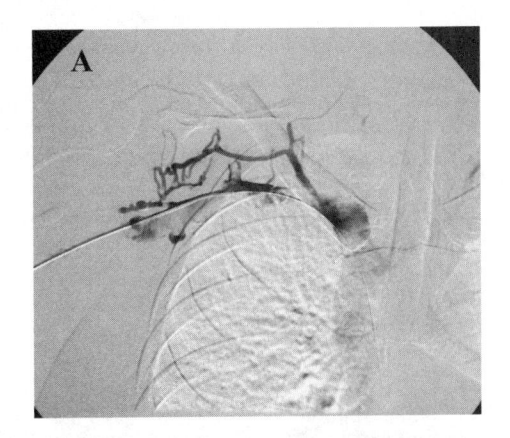

FIGURE 9. A, Venogram of right upper extremity shows occlusion of right subclavian vein with thrombosis. **B,** After thrombolysis, underlying focal occlusion is consistent with thoracic outlet syndrome.

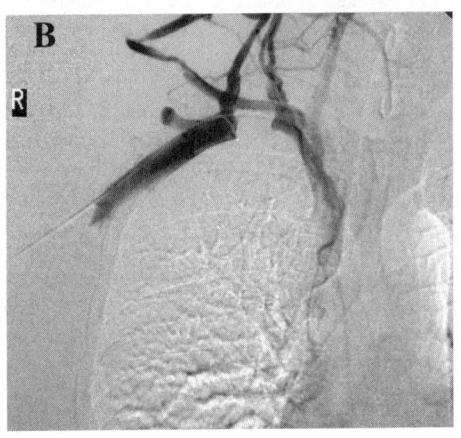

and angle between the pectoral muscle insertion and the coracoid process of the scapula are potential compression sites.

27. Discuss the signs and symptoms of TOS.

Clinically, patients usually present with pain localizing to the C8 or T1 dermatome. Angiographically, extrinsic compression of the subclavian artery (often with poststenotic dilatation), aneurysm formation (often with thromboembolic complication), or steal may be seen.

28. Which veins are primarily used for the placement of peripherally inserted central catheters (PICCs)?

Basilic, brachial, and cephalic veins.

29. What venous anomaly must be excluded before of an inferior vana cava (IVC) filter?

IVC duplication, which results from persistence of the right and left supracardinal veins. This anomaly occurs in approximately 2% of people. The left IVC drains into the left renal vein and would provide a ready conduit for the transit of a lower extremity deep venous thrombus despite placement of an IVC filter into the infrarenal right IVC.

30. Explain total anomalous pulmonary venous return (TAPVR).

TAPVR a defect resulting from failure of the pulmonary veins to fuse with the right atrium. Radiographically, this defect manifests as a "snowman" configuration of the cardiomediastinal silhouette.

31. Explain partial anomalous pulmonary venous return (PAPVR).

Also known as scimitar syndrome, PAPVR involves abnormal communication between one or several pulmonary veins and a systemic vein such as the superior or inferior vena cava. PAPVR is occasionally associated with ventricular septal defect, tetrology of Fallot, pulmonary valve atresia, coarctation of the aorta, common atrium, and single ventricle.

32. What are the components of the lower extremity deep venous system?
- Anterior tibial vein
- Posterior tibial vein
- Peroneal vein
- Popliteal vein
- Superficial femoral vein
- Common femoral
- External iliac veins

The anterior tibial vein drains the dorsum of the foot and anterior compartment of the lower extremity; it crosses the interosseous membrane to join the posterior tibial vein at the level of the fibular head. The posterior tibial vein drains the deep muscles of the posterior compartment. The peroneal vein, which arises from ankle tributaries, drains the lateral and posterior compartments. Along with the muscular veins of the gastrocnemius and soleus, these veins merge to form the popliteal vein, which continues cephalad as the superficial femoral vein at the level of the adductor canal.

33. Describe the three major divisions of the superficial venous system.

The three major division of the superficial venous system are the greater saphenous, lesser saphenous, and lateral venous systems. Reflux within these regional venous systems and/or their respective tributaries manifests clinically as varicose veins. The greater saphenous vein is the longest vein, coursing from the anterior aspect of the medial malleolus until its junction with the femoral vein approximately 3 cm below the inguinal ligament. The lesser saphenous vein courses from posterior to the lateral malleolus to approximately 3 cm above the knee, where it empties into the popliteal vein.

34. Explain the clinical importance of perforating veins.

Perforating veins (venae comitantes) link the superficial venous system to the deep venous system. They usually contain valves and course obliquely through the musculature, which assists in unidirectional blood flow toward the deep venous system.

35. What are the clinically important groups of perforating veins?

Hunterian, Dodd's, Boyd's, and Cockett perforators drain into the greater saphenous system.

36. What sonographic feature helps to identify the greater saphenous vein?

The greater saphenous vein courses toward the saphenofemoral junction in its own fascial sheath. This anatomic feature is exploited during ultrasound-guided endovenous ablation as the interventionalist administers perivenous local anesthesia.

BIBLIOGRAPHY

1. Baum S (ed): Abrams' Angiography, 4th ed. Boston, Little, Brown. 1997.
2. Kadir S: Atlas of Normal and Variant Angiographic Anatomy. Philadelphia, W.B. Saunders, 1991.
3. McGraw JK: Ablation of venous varicosities: Patient selection and anatomic considerations. In Proceedings of the 28th Annual Scientific Meeting of SIR, 2003, pp 140–143.
4. Neiman HL, Yao JST: Angiography of Vascular Disease. New York, Churchill Livingstone, 1985.
5. Tamm EP: The Little Green Book: Questions for Radiology Conference and Examination Preparation. Philadelphia, Lippincott Williams &Wilkins, 2000.
6. Worthington-Kirsch [initials?]: [title of presentation]. In Proceedings of the 28th Annual Scientific Meeting of SIR, 2003, p 63.

8. VASCULAR ANOMALIES

Wael E. A. Saad, MBBCh

1. **Describe the classification of congenital vascular lesions.**
   Congenital vascular lesions are broadly classified (based on clinical and biologic vascular criteria) into **hemangiomas** and **vascular malformations**. Vascular malformations are classified as follows:
   1. Venous
   2. Venular
   3. Capillary
   4. Lymphatic
   - Microcystic lesions
   - Macrocystic lesions
   5. Arteriovenous
   6. Mixed
   7. Venous-lymphatic
   8. Venous-venular

2. **Describe the natural history of hemangiomas.**
   Hemangiomas first appear soon after birth (although as many as 30% may already be apparent at birth). They typically proliferate during the first year of life and then involute during the childhood years. Although considerable variation is seen with respect to rate of proliferation and involution, both features are constant.

3. **Where can hemangiomas occur?**
   Hemangiomas can occur in most organs (almost anywhere). However, the vast majority are found in or just deep to the skin.

4. **How are cutaneous or subcutaneous hemangiomas classified?**

New Classification	Old Classification
Superficial hemangioma	Capillary or strawberry hemangioma
Deep hemangioma	Cavernous hemangioma
Compound hemangioma	Capillary cavernous hemangioma

5. **What are vascular malformations? Discuss their natural history.**
   Unlike hemangiomas, vascular malformations are present at birth (although they may not be clinically apparent) but present at a later stage. In addition, vascular malformations do not proliferate (histopathologically), nor do they involute. Instead, slow but continuous expansion and evolution is the expected course. Trauma, sepsis, hormonal modulation, and changes in blood and/or lymph flow and/or pressure may temporarily speed this process.

6. **Compare the growth of vascular malformations and hemangiomas.**
   Hemangiomas enlarge by a process of hyperplasia (increasing cell numbers). However, vascular malformations enlarge by vascular ectasia and cellular hypertrophy (cells increase in size but not in number).

7. **What are arteriovenous malformations? Describe their histopathogenesis.**
   Arteriovenous malformations (AVMs) are a subtype of vascular malformations. Their underlying abnormality is at the level of the capillary bed (hypothesized to be lack of innervation of the precapillary sphincters) across which the arteriovenous shunting takes place. All other find-

ings, hypertrophy of the afferent arterial system and dilation of the draining system, are secondary effects resulting from the altered flow dynamics across this primary abnormality.

8. How do you differentiate between hemangiomas and vascular malformations angiographically?

Both hemangiomas and vascular malformations can exhibit high-flow arteriovenous shunting. This feature (although important) does not distinguish between the two groups. However, hemangiomas appear angiographically as organized, gland-like vascular neoplasms with vessel staining/blush. This pattern is usually not seen in vascular malformations, which consist of a collection of abnormal vessels without a stain/blush (Fig. 1).

9. Why is it important to know the syndromes associated with congenital vascular lesions and lymphatic malformations?

Knowledge of associated lesions aids in obtaining appropriate imaging studies to examine for additional vascular malformations or other lesions.

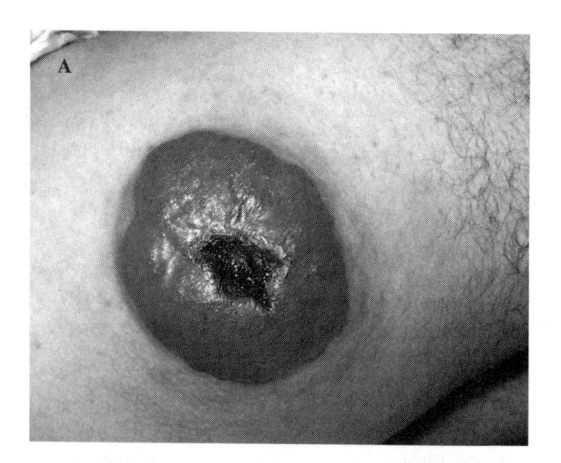

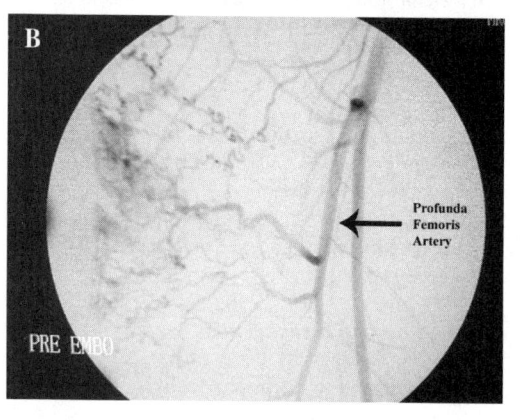

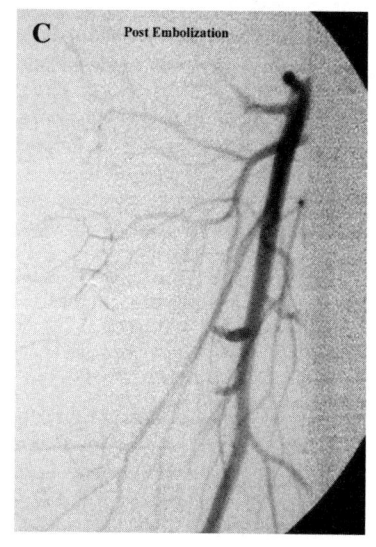

FIGURE 1. A, Long-standing cutaneous vascular malformation on the right lateral upper thigh of a 16-year-old boy. The patient tolerated the lesion until recently when it ulcerated and began to bleed occasionally. He also states that he is unable to wear jeans due to friction and bleeding. He was referred for presurgical embolization of the vascular malformation to minimize bleeding. **B,** Selective angiogram of the right profunda femoris demonstrates abnormal tortuous branches supplying the cutaneous vascular malformation. **C,** The lesion was successfully embolized using PVA particles. The patient underwent surgery on the following day without significant blood loss.

10. List the syndromes associated with congenital vascular lesions.

Maffucci syndrome: venous malformations and/or hemangiomas and multiple enchondromatosis.

PHACE syndrome: post-fossa anomalies, facial hemangiomas, arterial abnormalities, cardiovascular defects, eye abnormalities.

Klippel-Trenaunay syndrome: combined capillary (AVM)-lymphatic-venous malformations of the trunk or extremities in association with limb overgrowth.

Sturge-Weber syndrome: capillary malformations with intracranial abnormalities.

Proteus syndrome: cutaneous and visceral vascular malformation, hemihypertrophy, hand and foot overgrowth, exostosis and lipomatosis.

11. List the syndromes associated with lymphatic malformations.
- Turner's syndrome
- Down's syndrome
- Trisomy 13 and 18
- Klippel-Trenaunay syndrome

12. Describe Kasabach-Merritt syndrome and its potential consequences.

Kasabach-Merritt syndrome consists of consumptive coagulopathy with subsequent thrombocytopenia that is associated with a large vascular lesion/tumor. These lesions are usually of the Kaposiform, hemangioendothelioma variant, and not simple hemangiomas. The mortality rate associated with this syndrome is estimated to be 20–30% as a result of severe sepsis, coagulopathy, or invasion of vital organs.

13. List the advantages and disadvantages of evaluating vascular malformations with MR.
Advantages
- Noninvasive
- High sensitivity (90–100%)
- Best modality to determine the full extent of extensive lesions
- Can determine high-flow components, if any, of complex vascular malformations (flow voids)
- Determines relationship between vascular malformation and adjacent anatomic structures
- Standardized planes and sequences that are not operator-dependent (compared with Doppler ultrasound)
- Follow-up MR (compared with preoperative MR) easily detects residual lesions and their progression over sequential MR examinations

Disadvantages
- Expensive
- Poor specificity (24–33%)

14. How can the specificity of MR be augmented?
- Dynamic contrast-enhanced MR can improve the specificity by up to 95%
- Complementary Doppler ultrasound evaluation with or without angiography/venography

15. List the advantages and disadvantages of Doppler ultrasound in evaluating vascular malformations.
Advantages
- Inexpensive
- Noninvasive
- Can be done in clinic setting
- Adds to other imaging modalities (CT, MRI) a functional component by determining flow volume and resistive indices. By these criteria, functional improvement can be determined by subsequent postoperative Doppler evaluation

Disadvantages
- Operator-dependent
- May under estimate the full extent of the lesion
- Poor sensitivity, especially in low-flow vascular malformations (sensitivity can be improved by power-Doppler)

16. Describe the Doppler findings exhibited by vascular malformations before and after successful treatment.

	Before Treatment	After Treatment
Slow-flow AVM or venous malformation	• Slow-flow veins • Compressible • 20% no flow seen • Monophasic wave form	• No flow • Diminished compressibility
High-flow AVM	• High flow • Low resistive indices (RI)	• Reduces flow • Higher (normalized) RIs

17. Describe the MR findings exhibited by vascular malformations before and after successful treatment.

	Before Treatment	After Treatment
Slow-flow AVM or venous malformation	• Low T1, high T2	• Heterogenous T1 and T2 (reduced signal on T2) • Decreased lesion size
High-flow AVM	• Flow voids • High signal on T2 • Increased T2 edema	• Reduced flow void • Reduced T2 signal in lesion • Decreased T2 edema • Decreased lesion size

18. Describe the anatomic distribution of venous malformations.
- Head and neck: 40%
- Extremities: 40%
- Trunk: 20%

19. Describe the clinical picture of venous malformations.
- Usually asymptomatic
- Disfigurement
- Pain and discomfort (may be exacerbated in the early morning and/or on exertion)

Venous malformations tend to grow in proportion to the patient's growth and often enlarge during puberty and pregnancy.

20. List the advantages of direct percutaneous phlebography compared with catheter-directed phlebography in the evaluation and management of venous malformations.
- Determines venous architectural pattern
- Determines features and extent of venous drainage to the systemic circulation and thus determines safety of sclerosant administration and/or tourniquet placement
- Helps estimate the amount and rate of sclerosant administration

Endoluminal transcatheter phlebography/venography is usually not as good in fulfilling the above goals because it fails (at least in part) to opacify most of these lesions.

21. Describe the types of venoarchitecture of venous malformations as revealed by direct, percutaneous phlebography.

The phlebographic patterns of venous malformations may predict the treatment response of venous malformations to percutaneous sclerotherapy.

- Cavitary (varix) pattern with late venous drainage and no evidence of abnormal draining veins: good response to percutaneous sclerotherapy.
- Spongy pattern (small honey-comb cavities) with late venous drainage: difficult to treat (refractory) by percutaneous sclerotherapy.
- Rapid venous opacification of dysmorphic veins: transient good response with high recurrence after percutaneous sclerotherapy.

22. List the type of sclerosants used to treat venous malformations.
- Absolute alcohol
- Alcoholic solution of zein (Ethiblock, Ethicon, Norderstedt, Germany) mixed with contrast medium (popular in Europe)
- Lipiodol admixed with alcohol

Regular water-soluble contrast media precipitates with alcohol; the two cannot be admixed.

23. Describe the steps involved in treating venous malformations by direct percutaneous venous sclerosis.
1. Induce general anesthesia per anesthesiologist.
2. Use direct percutaneous phlebography to determine vascular architecture and draining veins and to estimate volume and rate of sclerosant administration.
3. Apply tourniquet or manual compression over draining veins to prevent escape of sclerosant to the systemic circulation.
4. Administer sclerosant via phlebography needle (20–23 gauge).
5. Wait for at least 10–15 minutes and release tourniquet, monitoring patient's vital signs.

24. How does ethanol induce AVM thrombosis?
- Denaturation of blood proteins
- Denaturating vascular endothelial damage
- Denuding the vascular wall of endothelium

25. Why is ethanol theorized to have more permanent results in the treatment of vascular malformations?
The hypothesis behind the more permanent results achieved by ethanol embolization is the damage that ethanol inflicts on the endothelium. The recurrence of vascular malformations is thought to be due to endothelial proliferation and recannulization of the AVM nidus. In addition, the endothelium is thought to release angiogenesis factors that promote neovascular recruitment.

26. Discuss the results of direct percutaneous ethanol sclerosis in the treatment of venous malformations.
- Technical success rate: 88–92%
- Rate of favorable clinical response after technical success: 96%

27. How many sclerosis sessions are required per treatment?
In one study, 71% of patients required one session, and 29% required two sessions. In another study, the mean number of sessions was 3.3 per patient.

28. What is the complication rate for direct percutaneous ethanol sclerosis?
The complication rate is 0–27%. Potential complications include the following:
- Ischemic bullae
- Tissue fibrosis
- Deep venous thrombosis and pulmonary embolus
- Nerve palsy

29. List the causes of failure of direct percutaneous sclerosis of venous malformations.
- Inaccessible lesions
- Rapidly draining veins that cannot be compressed
- Spongy lesions with multiple, small honeycomb compartments

30. What is the maximum ethanol dose that can be administered safely?
The maximum safe dose of ethanol is 0.5–1.0 ml/kg body weight. With such doses systemic ethanol contamination during sclerotherapy is found in 83% of patients.

31. What are the consequences if this dose is exceeded?
Doses over 1.0 ml/kg patient body weight may cause:
- Hypoglycemia and metabolic acidosis
- Seizures and/or coma
- Rhabdomyolysis with subsequent nephrotoxicity
- Cardiopulmonary collapse, including pulmonary hypertension, oxygen desaturation, atrial fibrillation (and other dysrhythmias), and systemic hypotension

32. How is ethanol toxicity managed?
1. General anesthesia and cardiopulmonary monitoring (including Swan-Ganz catheter) per the anesthesiology department result in early detection.
2. One of the early signs of cardiopulmonary collapse is a rise in pulmonary pressure. In response to this finding, stop ethanol injection and inject (per anesthesiologist) via the Swan Ganz catheter nitroglycerin or prostaglandin E_2 or adenosine.

33. Describe the clinical picture of high-throughput AVMs.
- High cardiac output failure (up to 18%)
- Pain localized to AVM (including rectal and/or testicular pain in pelvic AVMs)
- Pulsatile, disfiguring mass with or without thrill
- Progressive nerve deterioration/palsy
- Hemorrhage (up to 26% in pelvic AVMs)
- Ischemia due to steal phenomenon
- Mass effect (up to 35% in pelvic AVMs)
- Extremity swelling
- Extremity varicosities and stasis ulcerations
- Abortions in cases of pelvic/uterine AVMs (Fig. 2)

34. How do you clinically determine whether a high-flow AVM is affecting the heart?
The patient is tachycardic at baseline and has a high/wide pulse pressure. In addition, the patient exhibits reflex brachycardia on compression or occlusion of the AVM (Nicoladoni-Branham test).

35. What AVMs naturally cause hemorrhage?
- Cerebral and spinal AVMs
- AVMs of the alimentary tract
- Superficial AVMs with ulcerations

36. List the source vessels (feeders) that supply pelvic AVMs.
- Internal iliac artery (83%)
- Internal mammary artery (23%)
- Profunda femoris (17%)
- Common femoral artery (6%)

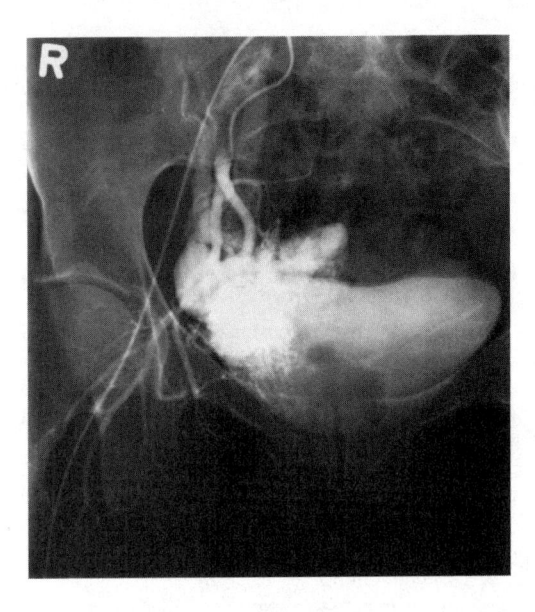

FIGURE 2. Pelvic angiogram with injection of the right hypogastric artery demonstrates ateriovenous malformation in a 29-year-old woman with a history of spontaneous abortions.

37. Discuss the results of endoluminal therapy for the treatment of high-flow vascular malformations.

Unlike low-flow vascular malformations and/or venous malformations, which have a therapeutic success rate of 88–92%, high-flow AVMs are more difficult to treat. From 43% to 83% (at best) are treated successfully. The therapeutic response depends on the complexity, extent, and location of the AVM. Up to 14% of pelvic AVMs treated with endoluminal therapy require subsequent surgery, and up to 56% of lower extremity AVMs treated with endoluminal therapy require eventual amputation. Repeat embolization procedures beyond the first embolization become successively more difficult.

38. What is the major predictor of inevitable lower extremity amputation in cases of AVMs?

The major predictor of amputation is AVM involving all three vessels below the knee.

39. What is the value of endoluminal therapy in such patients?

- Palliation. Endoluminal therapy can temporize limbs for 1–6 years (delay amputation).
- Preoperative endoluminal therapy for AVMs at the level of a planned amputation reduces AVM recurrence at the stump and does not adversely affect stump healing.

40. Describe the differences in prognosis between upper and lower extremity high-flow AVMs.

Upper Extremity High-flow AVMs	Lower Extremity High-flow AVMs
Presents at later age	Presents at earlier age
Less disabling symptoms	More disabling symptoms
More durable response to endoluminal treatment	Poor response to surgical and/or endoluminal treatment
Disfiguring excisions and amputations less likely	Amputations more likely (up to 56%)

41. List the causes of uterine AVMs.
By definition all AVMs are congenital. Those listed as acquired most likely represent AVMs diagnosed as a result of precipitating and/or accentuating factors:
- Gestational trophoblastic disease (74% of acquired AVMs)
- Previous uterine surgery
- Endometrial carcinoma
- Maternal diethylstilbestrol (DES) exposure

42. Explain the gender difference in success rates of endoluminal embolization of pelvic AVMs.
AVM recurrences are more common in women. Women require over three embolization sessions on average, whereas men on average require less than two sessions. Women usually have complex AVMs with multiple (and often bilateral) vascular supply, whereas AVMs in men have a simple (single), unilateral blood supply. In addition, pregnancy accentuates pelvic AVM recurrence.

43. Discuss the complications associated with endoluminal therapy of high-flow AVMs.
Complications are expected in more than 10% of patients and have been described in up to 30% of patients (10% are major complications). Examples include the following:
- Skin blisters and ulcerations
- Skin and tissue necrosis (sloughing)
- Necrosis of visceral organs in pelvis (rectum particularly sensitive)
- Motor and/or sensory nerve injury
- Auto amputation of digits
- Pulmonary embolization of embolic material (including coils)
- Ethanol toxicity, including cardiopulmonary collapse

44. List the embolic/sclerosing agents used to treat AVMs.
- Polyvinyl alcohol (PVA) particles
- Metal coils
- Gelfoam
- Tissue adhesives/glue (isobutyl-2-cyanoacrylate [IBCA]/NBCA)
- Boiling contrast
- Alcohol
- Autologous blood clot
- Detachable balloons
- Sotradecol
- Ethibloc
- The kitchen sink

45. Definfe truncation (skeletalization) of AVMs. Why is it not effective?
Truncation or skeletalization of AVMs refers to permanent endoluminal embolization of arterial feeders of the AVM (or surgical ligation). This procedure is totally futile because the AVM nidus is intact. Neovascular recruitment reconstitutes flow to the AVM nidus, and small (initially meniscal) arterial feeders hypertrophy and reestablish high flow within the AVM.

46. What is the ideal strategy for treating AVMs?
First you trap it. Then you kill it:
- Identify the AVM nidus by angiography.
- Shut down the circulation (super-selectively) to and from the nidus by using multiple occlusion catheters on the arterial side and occlusion balloons and/or tourniquets on the venous side. Coaxial and triaxial techniques may be required
- Ablate the nidus with a sclerosant, preferably alcohol. Try to maximize the duration of alcohol dwelling in the nidus.
- Release the circulation.

47. Define the role of the initial angiogram prior to endoluminal treatment.
1. To determine the angioarchitecture of the AVM:
   - Identify nidus if possible
   - Identify different compartments of the AVM
   - Identify inflow and outflow anatomy and caliber to plan for their occlusion
2. To determine flow characteristics with or without inflow and outflow occlusion.
   - Determine safety of ethanol administration
   - Determine volume and rate of ethanol injection

48. When is direct percutaneous treatment of AVMs required?
When the AVM is inaccessible endoluminally:
- Prior surgical ligation and/or resection
- Prior intraarterial coil placement
- Prior use of tissue adhesives
- Convoluted anatomy with failed endoluminal access

BIBLIOGRAPHY

1. Baker L, Waner M, Thomas R, Suen JY: The management of arteriovenous malformations. Arch Otolaryngol [VOL? PAGES?], 1998.
2. Burrows PE, Mulliken JB, Fellows KE, Strand RD: Childhood hemangiomas and vascular malformations: angiographic differentiation. AJR 141:483–488, 1983.
3. Claudon M, Upton J, Burrows PE: Diffuse venous malformations of the upper limb: Morphologic characterization by MRI and venography. Pediatr Radiol 31:507–514, 2001.
4. Dickey KW, Pollak JS, Meier GH III, et al: Management of large high-flow arteriovenous malformations of the shoulder and upper extremity with transcatheter embolotherapy. J Vasc Intervent Radiol 6:765–773, 1995.
5. Donnelly LF, Adams DM, Bisset GS III: Vascular malformations and hemangiomas: A practical approach in a multidisciplinary clinic. AJR 174:597–608, 2000.
6. Dubois F, Soulez G, Oliva VL, et al: Soft-tissue venous malformations in adult patients: Imaging and therapeutic issues. Radiographics 21:1519–1531, 2001.
7. Hammer FD, Boon LM, Mathurin P, Vanwijck RR: Ethanol sclerotherapy of venous malformations: evaluation of systemic ethanol contamination. J Vasc Intervent Radiol 12:595–600, 2001.
8. Jacobowitz GR, Rosen RJ, Rockman CB, et al: Transcatheter embolization of complex pelvic vascular malformations: Results and long-term follow-up. J Vasc Surg 33:51–55, 2001.
9. Lee BB, Kim DI, Huh S, et al: New experiences with absolute ethanol sclerotherapy in the management of a complex form of congenital venous malformation. J Vasc Surg 33:764–772, 2001.
10. Mason KP, Michna E, Zurakowski D, et al: Serum ethanol levels in children and adults after ethanol embolization or sclerotherapy for vascular anomalies. Radiology 217:127–132, 2000.
11. Mulliken JB, Glowacki J: Hemangiomas and vascular malformation in infants and children: A classification based on endothelial characteristics. Plast Reconstruct Surg 69:412–420, 1982.
12. Suh JS, Shin KH, Na JB, et al: Venous malformations: Sclerotherapy with a mixture of ethanol and lipiodol. Cardiovasc Intervent Radiol 20:268–273, 1997.
13. Van Rijswijk CSP, Von der Linden E, Van der Woude HJ, et al: Value of dynamic contrast-enhanced MR imaging in diagnosing and classifying peripheral vascular malformations. AJR 178:1181–1187, 2002.
14. Vin-Christian K, McCalmont TH, Frieden IJ: Kaposiform hemangioendothelioma: An aggressive, locally invasive vascular tumor than can mimic hemangioma of infancy. Arch Dermatol 133:1573–1578, 1997.
15. Vogelzang RL, Nemcek AA Jr, Skrtic Z, et al: Uterine arteriovenous malformations: primary treatment with therapeutic embolization. J Vasc Intervent Radiol 2:517–522, 1991.
16. White RI Jr, Pollak J, Persing J, et al: Long-term outcome of embolotherapy and surgery for high-flow extremity arteriovenous malformation. J Vasc Intervent Radiol 11:1285–1295, 2000.
17. Yakes WF, Rossi P, Odink H: How I do it: Arteriovenous malformation management. Cardiovasc Intervent Radiol 19:65–71, 1996.

9. NONINVASIVE VASCULAR TESTING

David L. Waldman, MD, PhD

1. Who was the first person to measure blood pressure directly?
The first direct measurement of blood pressure was performed by Steven Hales in 1714. In 1896, Scipione Riva-Rocci developed the first sphygnomanometer.

2. List the basic methods of noninvasive vascular testing.
- Pulse examination
- Doppler ultrasonography
- Plethysymography (PVR)
- Segmental blood pressures
- Transcutaneous oximetry

3. What basic principle underlies Doppler ultrasonography?
Doppler ultrasonography measures alterations in the frequency of the reflected signal that is used to measure blood velocity.

4. What happens as blood goes through a stenosis within a blood vessel?
As blood traverses down a stenosis within a blood vessel, velocity increases. Downstream turbulence may also be identified. Spectral waveform analysis may be used to determine the degree of disease.

5. Define the display modes of ultrasound.
- A-mode: amplitude mode
- B-mode: brightness mode
- M-mode: motion mode

6. What are the two most commonly used ultrasound tranducers?
Alinear array transducer is usually used for superficial structures. It produces a wider near field. The second type of transducer is a sector scanner, which has a wider far field. The sector scanner is more useful to image deeper structures.

7. Explain extremity pressure measurements.
Extremity pressure measurements are the noninvasive test most frequently used to detect the presence of hemodynamically significant stenosis. In the lower extremity, pressure gradients are evaluated. A gradient in excess of 20 mmHg between cuffs placed along the extremity indicates significant disease. In the upper extremity, a 10-mmHg drop indicates significant disease.

8. Define ankle brachial index.
An ankle brachial index is the systolic blood pressure of the arm divided by the systolic blood pressure of the leg. A normal ABI is approximately 1. An ABI of 0.9–0.7 indicates claudication, whereas an ABI of 0.07–0.04 usually indicates rest pain. An ABI less than 0.4 may represent tissue loss.

9. What is another name for pulse volume recordings?
Pulse volume recordings (Fig. 1) are also called arterial plesmythography. This is perhaps the most sensitive and reproducible test to evaluate patients for arterial insufficiency. Pulse volume recordings are obtained at multiple levels, including the high thigh, low thigh, calf, ankle, and transmetatarsal levels.

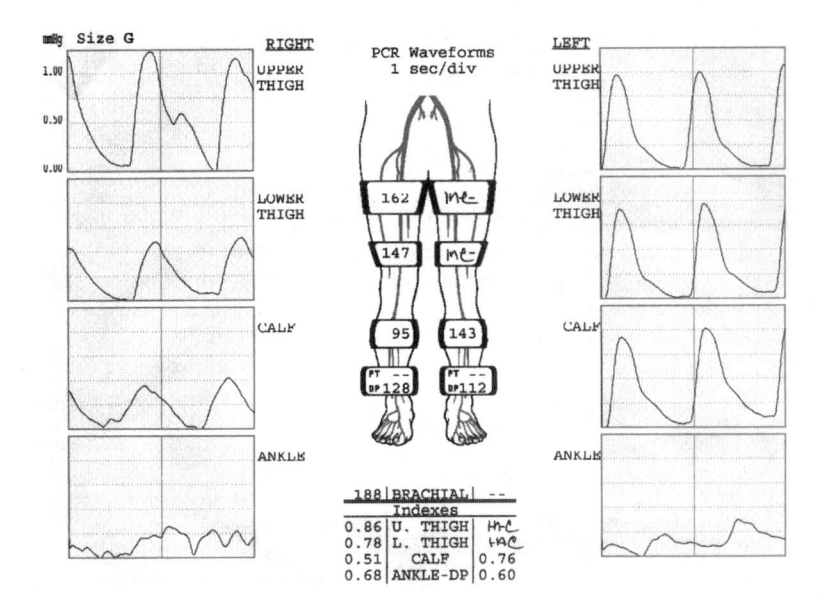

FIGURE 1. The left extremity has normal PVR waveforms and normal pressure measurements to the calf. There are abnormal waveforms within the ankle. The right extremity demonstrates flattened waves and a significant drop in pressure in the mid thigh. This finding is consistent with stenosis of the superior femoral artery, as found on angiogram.

10. Describe the theory that underlies pulse volume recordings.

As blood flows under the blood pressure cuff, changes in the cuff are recorded as waveforms. These waveforms are interpreted both qualitatively and quantitatively, but they are not the same as arterial Doppler waveforms. The cuffs are at constant pressure, and changes in volume create the waveforms.

11. Describe a normal Doppler waveform.

A normal Doppler waveform is triphasic in the lower extremities because of the high resistive system. As you move down the extremity, the velocity normally decreases.

12. What happens to Doppler waveform within a stenosis?

Within a hemodynamically significant stenosis (> 50% in diameter), waveforms become biphasic distal to the stenosis because of the loss of diastolic flow reversal. Spectral broadening is seen, along with a significant increase in the peak systolic velocity. As the stenosis increases, the waveform becomes flattened and monophasic.

13. Explain the role of the Intersocietal Commission for the Accreditation of Vascular Laboratories (ICAVL).

The ICAVL was established to provide a mechanism to recognize the quality and appropriateness of vascular laboratory testing and reporting. Over the past 5 years insurance carriers have linked reimbursement with accreditation.

14. What is the first step in the evaluation of a patient?

At a patient encounter, an appropriate history is the most important initial step. This history should guide the noninvasive examination. This history should be made available to physicians reading the examination so that they can correlate any clinical symptoms with the examination.

15. How is Doppler frequency shift (F_d) calculated?

$$F_d = \frac{2F \, V \cos\theta}{C}$$

where F = frequency of transmitted ultrasound, V = velocity of blood, θ = angle of the incident ultrasound beam, and C = speed of light

16. What evaluation or examination should be performed if a patient with continued claudication presents with normal ABIs and normal physical examination?

An exercise test should be performed. The usual choice is a treadmill test for claudication, which is similar to a cardiac stress test. As the patient exercises, blood requirements into the legs increase. A drop in the ABI indicates that the blood vessels cannot dilate and that there is a significant stenosis within the blood vessels.

BIBLIOGRAPHY

1. Ernst CB, Stanley JC (eds): Current Therapy in Vascular Therapy, 4th ed. St. Louis, Mosby, 2001.
2. Hallaett J, Mills J (eds): Comprehensive Vascular and Endovascular Surgery. St. Louis, Mosby, 2003.
3. Mercuri M, McPherson DD, Bassiouny H, Glagov S (eds): Developments in Cardiovascular Medicine. New York, Kluwer Academic Publishers, 1998.
4. Rutherford RB (ed): Vascular Surgery, 5th ed. Philadephia, W.B. Saunders, 2000.

10. AORTOILIAC DISEASE AND AORTIC ANEURYSM

David L. Waldman, MD, PhD

1. **What percentage of abdominal aortic aneurysms (AAAs) occur below the renal arteries?**
   Ninety-five percent of AAAs occur below the renal arteries.

2. **What percentage of AAAs occur in men vs. women?**
   Eighty-five percent occur in men. Women's aneurysms tend to rupture at smaller sizes.

3. **What is the risk of rupture of an aneurysm larger than 6 cm?**
   An aneurysm of 6 cm or above has a 70% chance of rupture within 5 years. AAA rupture is the thirteenth leading cause of death in the United States.

4. **When should AAAs be repaired?**
   This issue has become controversial because of the new, less invasive methods of repairing AAAs. Any aneurysm larger than 5 cm and all symptomatic aneurysms should be repaired. Aneurysms that grow at a rate of greater than 0.5 cm per year should also be repaired. One caveat is that larger AAAs tend to grow faster.

5. **What is the operative mortality rate of AAA repair?**
   Exact figures are difficult to ascertain. Within the literature, elective repair has a mortality rate as low as 1.7% and as high as 10%. Rates for repair of symptomatic aneurysms range between 10 and 20%. Mortality rates for ruptured aneurysms range between 22 and 48%. It is quite clear that the more aneurysm repairs the surgeon and hospital perform, the lower the mortality rates.

6. **What is the operative morbidity rate for open repair of AAAs?**
   The rate of myocardial infarction is approximately 5%. There is a 0.5–1% dialysis rate, along with a 6% rate of renal failure.

7. **Who first described an endoluminal repair of AAAs?**
   Juan Parodi first described endoluminal repair of AAAs in 1991. The basis for his approach was that enduluminal repair is less invasive with less blood loss and therefore should result in less morbidity and mortality as well as faster recovery times.

8. **Describe the goals of placing an endoluminal graft to repair AAAs.**
   The purpose the stent graft in patients with AAAs is to prevent death. In order to prevent death, you need to prevent rupture. In order to prevent rupture, you need to prevent growth. In order to prevent growth, you need to prevent pressure.

9. **List the three options for endoluminal graft placement.**
   1. Straight tube graft: no longer used because of graft movement as the aneurysm shrinks.
   2. The most widely used device is the aortic bi-iliac graft.
   3. Rapidly gaining popularity is the aortic uni-iliac device. This particular device requires a contralateral occluder along with a femoral-femoral bypass graft to maintain bilateral flow.

10. **How are the devices structured?**
    There are two types of design options: a one-piece design, which is unsupported with hooks at the ends, and a modular or multipiece design, which is built within the patient and fully stent-supported.

11. Which devices are currently approved by the Food and Drug Administration (FDA)?

Three devices are currently FDA-approved: (1) AneuRx (Medtronics, Minneapolis, MN), (2) Excluder (Gore, Newark, DE), and (3) Zenith (Cook, Bloomington, IN). Ancure (Guidant, Indianapolis, IN) was recently withdrawn from the market.

12. What is the most important factor in building a successful endovascular program for AAA repair?

The most important element for developing a successful program is patient selection. The patient's anatomy (Fig. 1) is extremely important to developing an endovascular program, along with the quality of the patient's blood vessels. A thrombus within the neck or severe tortuosity is a major deterrent to successful implantation. Occasionally the excitement of new technology pushes the programs to the limits. The author urges all practitioners to resist this temptation.

13. What is the maximum diameter of the aortic neck for AAA repair?

AneuRx and Gore have a maximum diameter of 28 mm. Zenith, which has a neck diameter of 32 with suprarenal fixation, allows treatment of patients with aortic necks of 28–30 mm.

14. Describe the preoperative work-up for endovascular repair of AAA.

Over the past several years, the initial work-up has changed significantly. We currently require only a thin-cut, contrast-enhanced CT scan (1.5–3 mm around the level of the renal arteries). The CT scan should undergo a three-dimensional reconstruction. We have found that the quality of three-dimensional reconstruction supplants the preprocedural angiogram.

15. Describe the current surveillance protocol after implantation.

We follow patients with a contrast-enhanced CAT scan with immediate and delayed imaging, using slices of 1.5–3 mm in thickness around the level of the renal arteries. The patients are imaged at 30 days, 6 months, and 1 year. They then are followed annually.

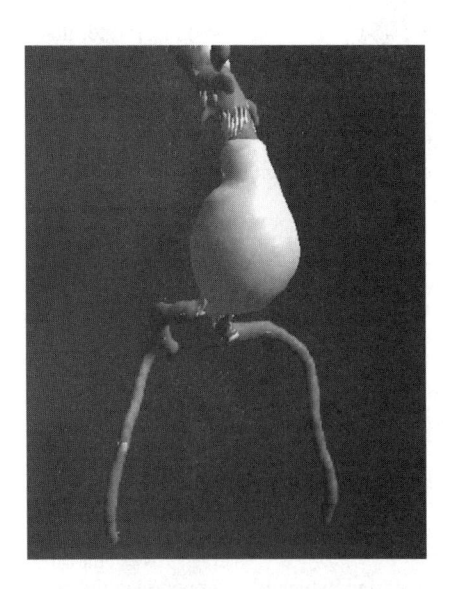

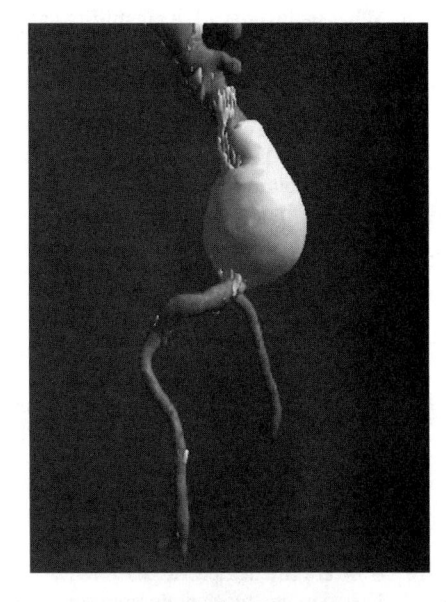

FIGURE 1. A and **B,** Two views from a three-dimensional aortic reconstruction. The reconstruction was done in preparation for endograft placement. Such reconstruction techniques will eventually replace diagnostic catheter angiography. They allow the physician to evaluate the degree of iliac tortuosity and the quality of the aortic neck during planning of therapy.

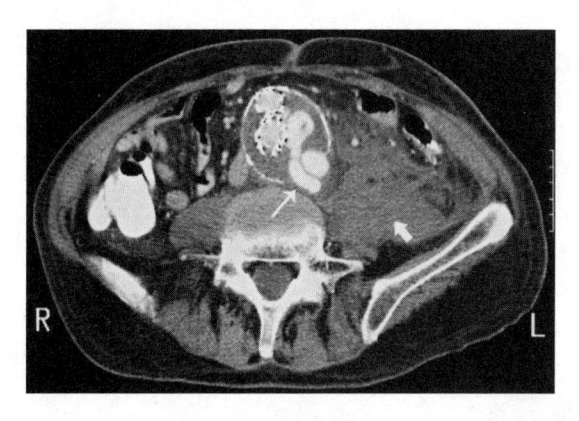

FIGURE 2. Axial CT scan indicates a type II endoleak *(thin arrow)* leading to rupture with retroperitoneal hemorrhage *(thick arrow)*.

16. What are the goals of surveillance?

Surveillance is used to detect endovascular leaks. AAA morphology is followed, along with aneurysm volume. It is important to evaluate device structure and positional changes for kinks and occlusions. Long-term follow-up can define fabric tears or junctional dehiscence.

17. What is the long-term durability of endovascular peri-AAA repair?

Currently the durability and long-term sequelae of aortic stent grafts are not known. Endograft AAA repair mandates follow-up at regular intervals for the lifetime of the patient.

18. Is endovascular repair safe?

The FDA trials of both Anurex and Ancure in comparision with surgical AAA repair demonstrate that endovascular repair can be safe and overall produces less morbidity than open repair. The mortality rates during the Ancure trial were similar to the mortality rates of open surgery.

19. How is the success of endovascular repair defined?

- Implantation success is defined as successful deployment of the device at the desired location.
- Technical success is defined as a successful deployment at 30 days with no persistent endovascular leak or need for surgical conversion.
- Clinical success is defined as no sack growth greater than 5 mm or endovascular leak at 6 months.
- Secondary clinical/continuing success is defined as maintenance of clinical and technical success with no sac growth or additional endovascular procedure to seal endovascular leaks or to treat any later complication.

20. Describe the various types of endovascular leaks.

- **Type I** is a leak at the attachment site (Fig. 3).
- **Type II** is a branch-to-branch leak. The most common branch-to-branch leak is from the hypogastric to a lumbar artery (Fig. 4).
- **Type III** leak is defined as a hole in the graft material or a junctional dehiscence (Fig. 5).
- **Type IV** is defined as graft porosity.
- Over the past several years a **type V** leak has been defined as endotension. It is characterized by no leak but continual growth of the aneurysm sac.

21. What are the most common endovascular leaks?

Type II leaks are the most common and usually account for 70–90% of all leaks.

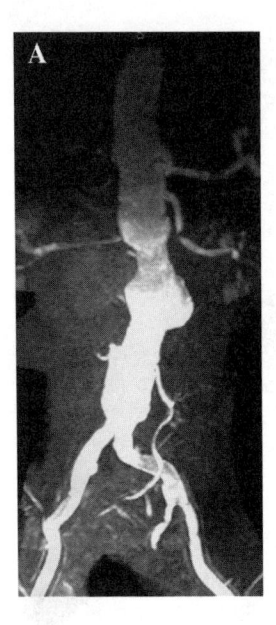

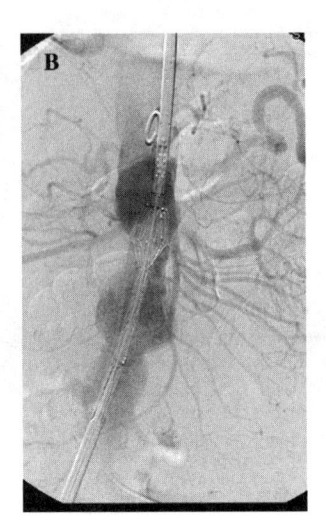

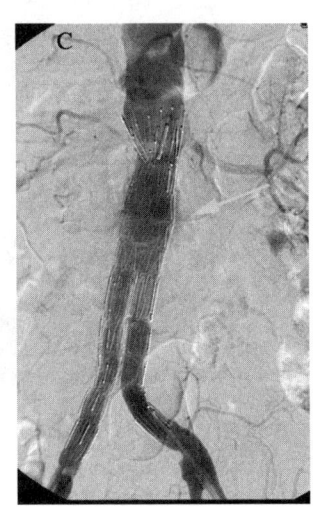

FIGURE 3. A, MRA of a patient with an infrarenal abdominal aortic aneurysm. **B,** Angiogram to identify the renal arteries before deployment of a Zenith graft (Cook, Inc., Bloomington, IN). **C,** Completion angiogram demonstrated evidence of type I endoleak *(arrow)*. The leak was repaired with a molding balloon and suprarenal fixation of the graft.

22. Which endovascular leaks need to be repaired?
- No patient should leave the operating room with a known **type I** leak.
- **Type II** leaks are highly controversial. In our practice type II leaks are followed and repaired only when interval sac growth is observed. Such patients need to be followed closely.
- **Type III** leaks require intervention (Fig. 6).
- **Type IV** leaks are usually self-limiting.
- **Type V** leaks require conversion or open repair.

The goal of endovascular repair is to prevent rupture. If the aneurysm continues to grow, the patient is not protected against aortic rupture.

23. What are the best methods for evaluating endovascular leaks?
We believe that a triphasic CT scan is the best method for evaluating endovascular leaks. A three-dimensional reconstruction may be necessary. MR angiography may also be used, along with transabdominal ultrasound. Transabdominal ultrasound, however, is highly operator-dependent. Catheter angiography may be useful in defining the exact type of endovascular leak. More recently direct sac punctures have been used to measure pressure within the sac and to perform therapy.

24. How common is peripheral vascular disease?
Peripheral vascular disease affects less than 5% of the patient population below the age of 60 years, whereas more than 20% of the population over the age of 75 is affected. Ten percent of the population greater than age 70 suffers from lifestyle-limiting problems causing intermittent claudication secondary to episodic obstruction.

25. List the most important risk factors for peripheral vascular disease.
- Tobacco abuse
- Hypercholesterolemia
- Hypertension

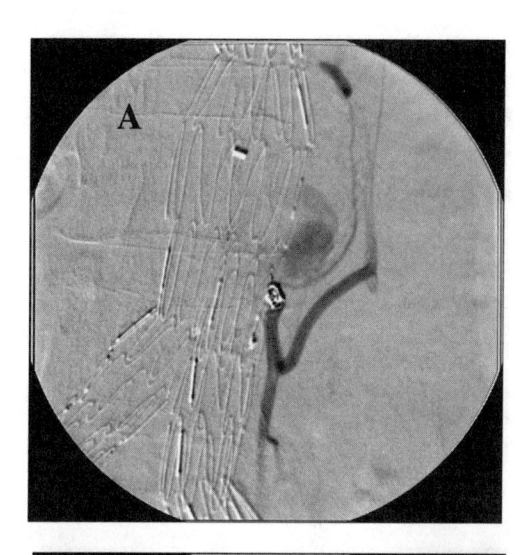

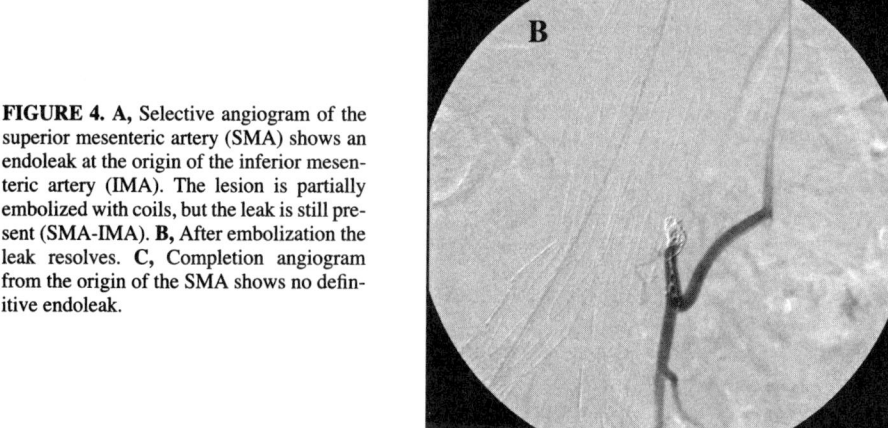

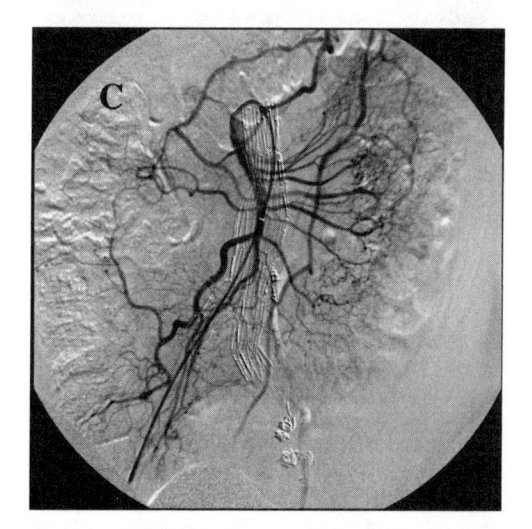

Aortoiliac Disease and Aortic Aneurysm 51

FIGURE 4. A, Selective angiogram of the superior mesenteric artery (SMA) shows an endoleak at the origin of the inferior mesenteric artery (IMA). The lesion is partially embolized with coils, but the leak is still present (SMA-IMA). **B,** After embolization the leak resolves. **C,** Completion angiogram from the origin of the SMA shows no definitive endoleak.

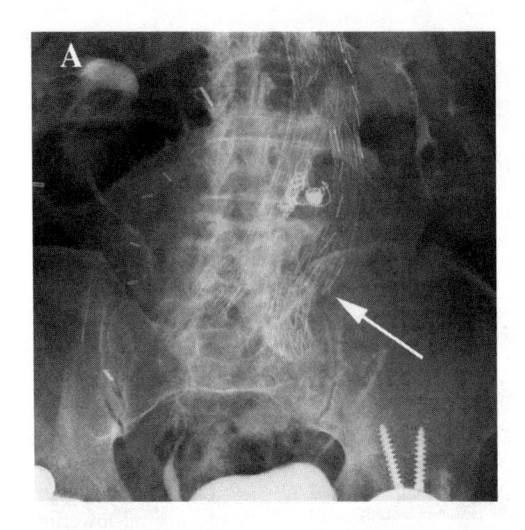

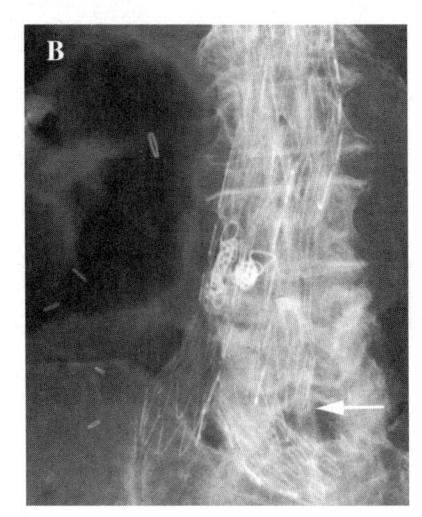

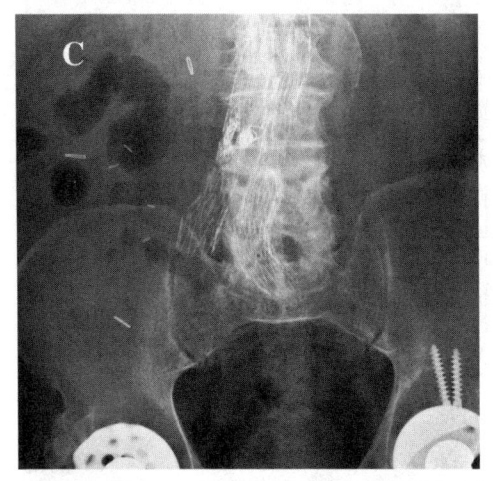

FIGURE 5. Three years after endograft repair of an abdominal aortic aneurysm, the patient developed a separation of the left liac limb (**A** and **B**). This type III endoleak requires repair. **C,** An iliac extension was used to seal the leak.

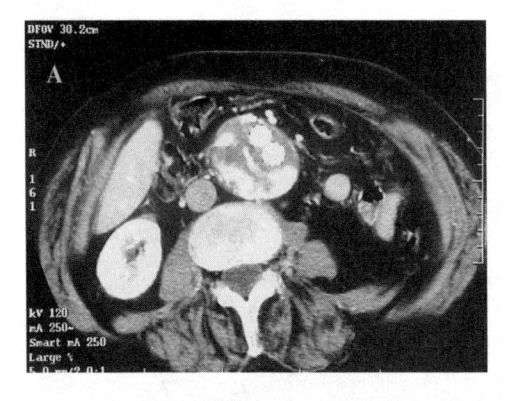

FIGURE 6. A, CT scan clearly demonstrates a significant endoleak. Angiography showed a leak from the posterior body of the graft. **B,** Graft explant illustrates a fabric tear (type III endoleak).

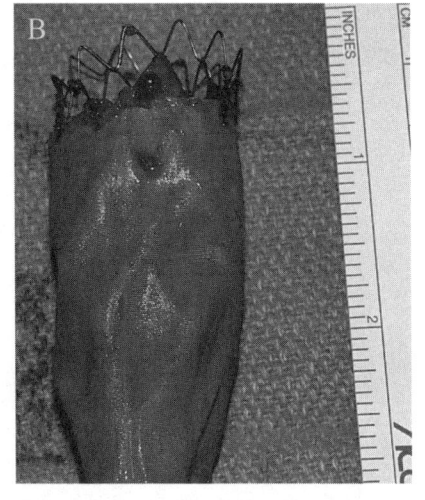

- Diabetes
- Obesity
- Sedentary lifestyle

26. How are mortality rates affected by peripheral vascular disease?
Life expectancy is reduced by approximately 10 years in patients with peripheral vascular disease. Seventy five percent of deaths are caused by cardiovascular events.

27. Describe the work-up of patients with peripheral vascular disease.
The work-up includes the patient history, physical examination, laboratory values, noninvasive studies, and possibly angiography.

28. Define ABI.
ABI is the ankle-brachial index, or ankle systolic pressure over brachial systolic pressure. The normal value is 1.0. Moderate disease is 0.7–1. Severe disease is less than 0.5.

29. What are the treatment options for peripheral vascular disease?
Treatment options include medical management with exercise programs, lipid-lowering medications or antiplatlet drugs. Minimally invasive techniques include angioplasty and possible vascular stenting. More invasive techniques include surgical bypass.

30. What is the technical success rate of stents for aortic iliac occlusion?
Technical success for most series is greater than 90%.

31. What is the 5-year patency rate for iliac stents?
The 5-year patency rate ranges from 54% to over 93% (Fig. 7), with most series averaging 72%. None of the series evaluated include all comers. Intention-to-treat rates are unknown.

32. Which lesions respond most favorably to balloon angioplasty?
Concentric focal lesions located in the common iliac artery respond most favorably to balloon angioplasty. Long stenosis or tandem lesions and chronic occlusions respond less favorably to balloon angioplasty.

33. What are the indications for metallic stent placement?
The indications for placement of vascular stents include long segmental disease, chronic occlusions (Fig. 8), and focal lesions that demonstrate suboptimal response to balloon angioplasty. Over the past several years, many practitioners have lowered their threshold for stent placement.

34. Which vascular stents are approved for use in the iliac system?
Currently, the large Palmaz (P308) (Johnson and Johnson Interventional Systems, Warren, NJ) systems and multiple sizes of the yellowbox Wallstent (Boston Scientific, Watertown, MA) iliac prosthesis are the only stents fully approved by the FDA for use in the iliac arteries.

35. Are there any FDA-approved stent grafts for the use in aortic iliac occlusive disease?
At this time there are no FDA-approved stent grafts.

36. When should a lesion be considered significant?
Hemodynamic evaluation is the best method for lesion evaluation. A systolic gradient greater than 10 should be considered significant. A mean gradient greater than 5 should is considered significant. If the patient complains of symptoms and the lesion does not appear hemodynamically significant, a challenge should be performed by administration of a vasodilator. Nitroglycerin or tolazoline (Priscoline) can be given through the catheter to dilate the vascular bed. Pressure gradient should be measured immediately after administration of the vasodilator.

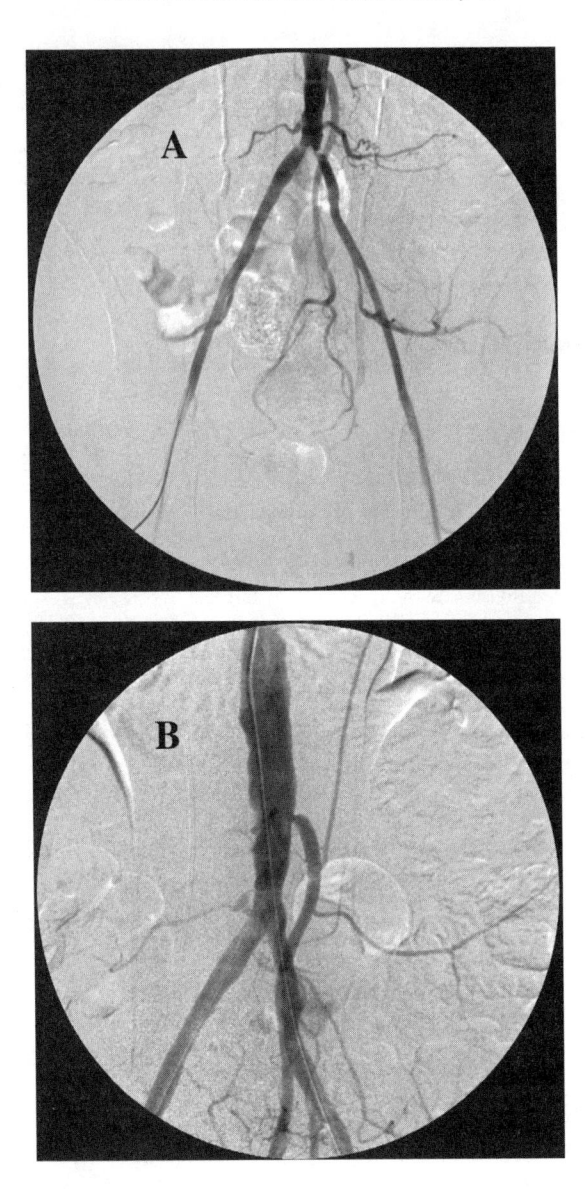

FIGURE 7. A, Bilateral narrowing is seen at the iliac bifurcation. **B,** Iliac stents were used with no residual pressure gradient.

37. How do you know a lesion has been successfully treated?

The end point for the procedure is based on hemodynamics. Ideally, waveforms should be measured above and below the treated segment. There should be no mean or systolic gradient after treatment.

38. How should patients be followed after treatment?

As an interventional radiologist, you must follow the patients whom you treat. You should consider them as your patients. A follow-up visit for an uncomplicated intervention should in-

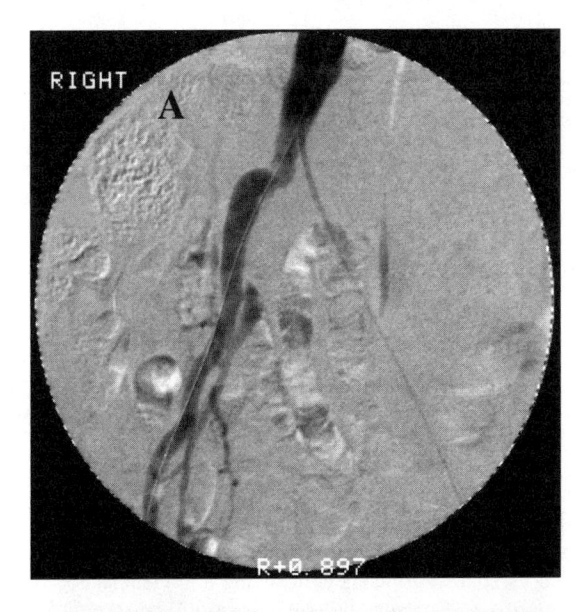

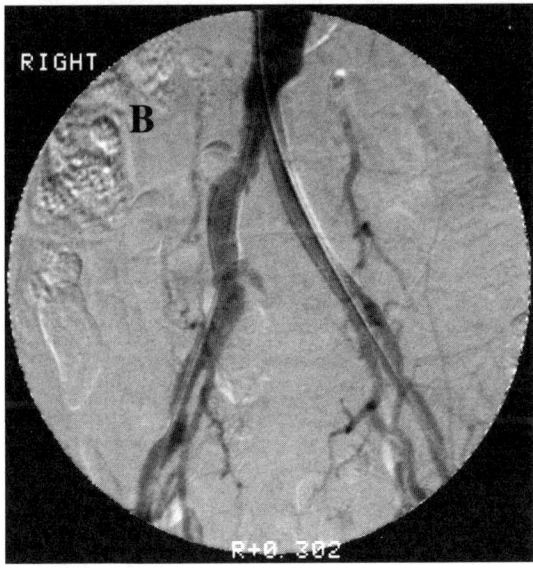

FIGURE 8. A, Angiogram shows right-sided common iliac occlusion. **B,** Wire was manipulated through the occlusion, and a stent was placed primarily. Heparin was given during the procedure.

clude discharge instructions. Discharge instructions should include a follow-up visit to your clinic in approximately 7–14 days. If the patient is doing well and shows improvement in ABIs and claudication, it is appropriate to follow the patient every 6 months for 2 years. This is the period during which restenosis is most likely to occur. There is no global period for percutaneous aortic iliac interventions. Billing of evaluation and management services is legitimate and highly recommended.

39. Categorize vasculitis.
There are multiple types of vasculitis. Commonly they are separated by vascular distribution.

Type of vasculitis	Typical Host	Vessels	Target Tissues
Takayasu (Fig. 9)	20-yr-old female	Aorta and main branches	Heart, brain, skeletal muscle
Polyarteritis nodosa	40-yr-old person	Small muscular branches	Small aneurysms, bifurcations within the kidney and gut
Giant-cell arteritis (Fig. 10)	60-yr-old person	Large elastic vessels. specifically temporal and subclavian arteries	Eye
Vasculitis associated with connective tissue disorder (e.g., SLE and RA)	35-yr-old female	Similar to polyarteritis nodosa or more commonly affecting the capillaries	Skin. predominantly in the extremities
Burger's disease (Fig. 11)	35-yr-old male smoker	Arterials	Skin and digits

SLE = systemic lupus erythematosus, RA = rheumatoid arthritis.

40. Describe the clinical manifestations of Takayasu arteritis.
The patient may present with systemic manifestations, including inflammation and fever, and symptoms of localized vascular insufficiency, including arm claudication or new-onset hypertension. Takayasu's arteritis is also called pulseless disease. When the disease affects both subclavian arteries, the radial or ulnar pulse in the arms is absent.

41. Describe the diagnostic evaluation of Takayasu arteritis.
Patients may present in the acute phase with an elevated sedimentation rate. They may also have an anemia with the possibility of an increased gammaglobulin production. No specific serologic markers are seen.

Definitive diagnosis is made by imaging. Previously catheter-directed angiography was performed, but now MR or CA gives a more global overview of the vascular status.

42. Are men or women affected more often by polyarteritis nodosa?
Men are affected twice as often as women.

43. Describe the angiographic appearance of polyarteritis nodosa.
Polyarteritis nodosa appears most commonly as aneurysms at vascular bifurcations. Usually they are punctuate aneurysms and occur within the kidneys and small bowel. Renal involvement is more common in patients who are positive for hepatitis B virus.

44. What are the treatment options for polyarteritis nodosa?
Polyarteritis nodosa is usually treated medically. Conventional therapy includes steroids.

45. Define fibromuscular dysplasia.
Fibromuscular dysplasia is a nonathrosclerotic disease that primarily affects the kidneys, carotid arteries (Fig. 12), and external iliac arteries. It is an uncommon disorder, accounting for slightly more than 1% of all patients who undergo angiography. This disorder is primarily found in women.

46. Define the types of fibromuscular dysplasia.
There are multiple classifications of fibromuscular dysplasia. The simplest approach separates fibromuscular dysplasia into three categories:

Type I includes intimal dysplasia. It is difficult to distinguish from medial dysplasia on angiography.

Type II is the most common type of fibromuscular dysplasia. Fibromuscular rings alternate

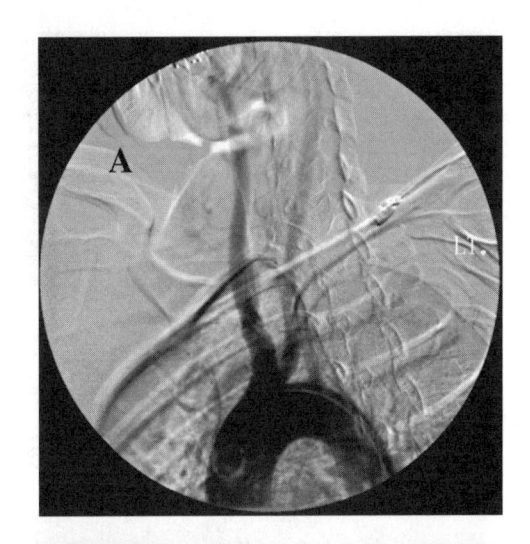

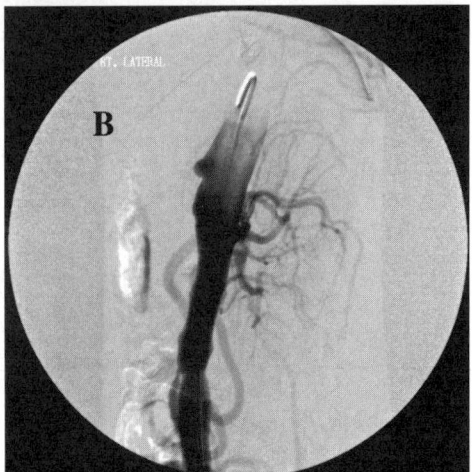

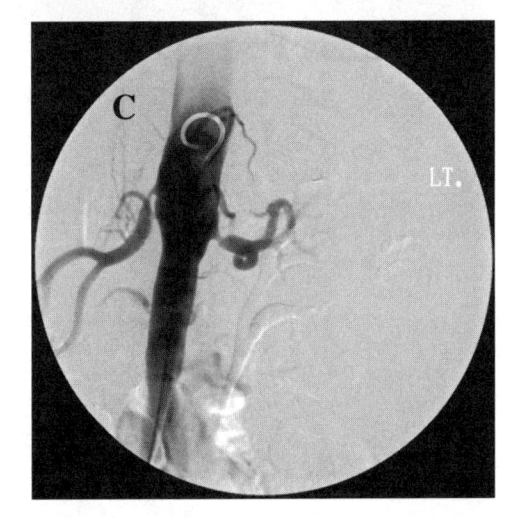

FIGURE 9. Multiple manifestations of Takayasu disease. A, Occlusion of both subclavian arteries. B and C, Occlusion of the celiac axis and superior mesenteric artery. The origins of both renal arteries are severely narrowed. The infrarenal aorta is abnormal.

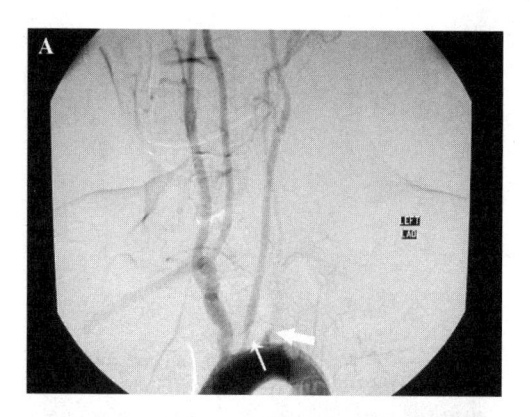

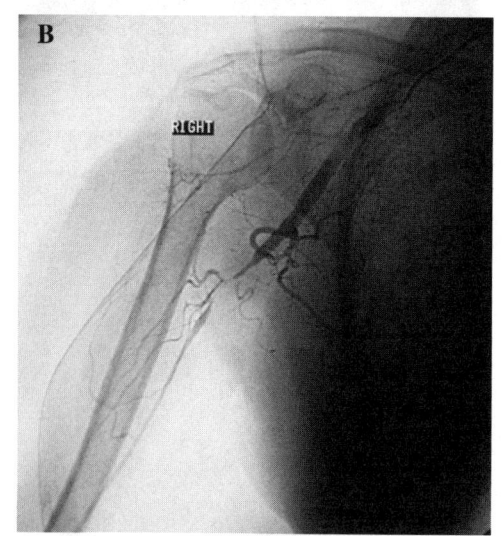

FIGURE 10. A, B, and **C,** Severe disease of the subclavian and axillary arteries typical of giant-cell arteritis.

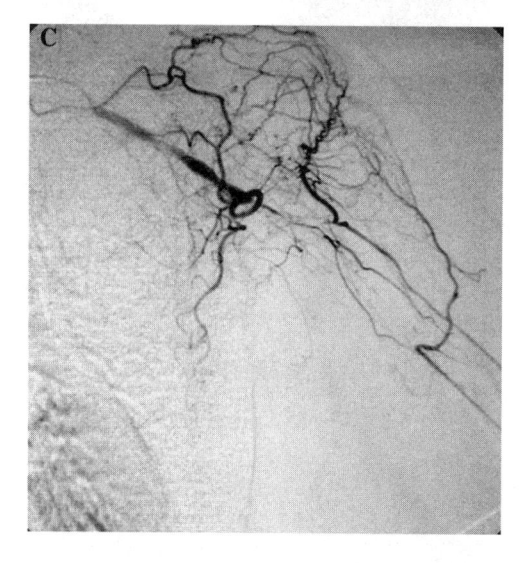

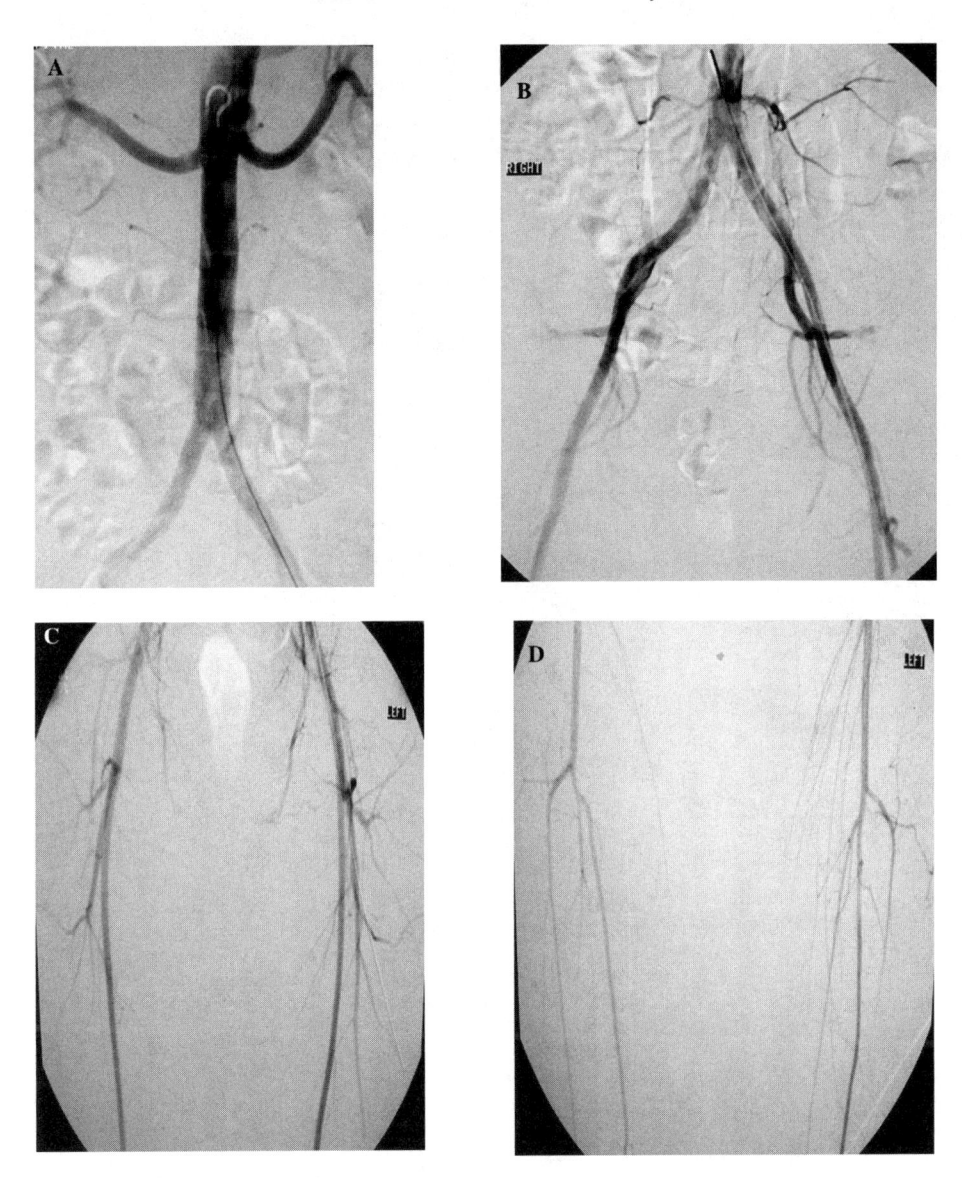

FIGURE 11. A 37-year-old man with a history of smoking two packs of cigarettes per day for the past 12 years but no history of diabetes presents with ischemic ulcers on the distal portions of the left great, second, and fifth toes and the right great toe. A, B, C, and D, Angiography of both lower extremities demonstrates absolutely normal vessels up to the level below the trifurcation. At this point are seen segmental occlusive lesions of the small- and medium-sized vessels (tibioperoneal arteries) bilaterally with formation of distinctive small-vessel collaterals around areas of occlusion known as "corkscrew collaterals" (E, right leg; F, left leg). Such arteriographic findings, coupled with the patient's history, suggest Buerger's disease. Leo Buerger of Brookline, New York, published a detailed description of the disease in which he referred to the clinical presentation of thromboangiitis obliterans as "presenile spontaneous gangrene."

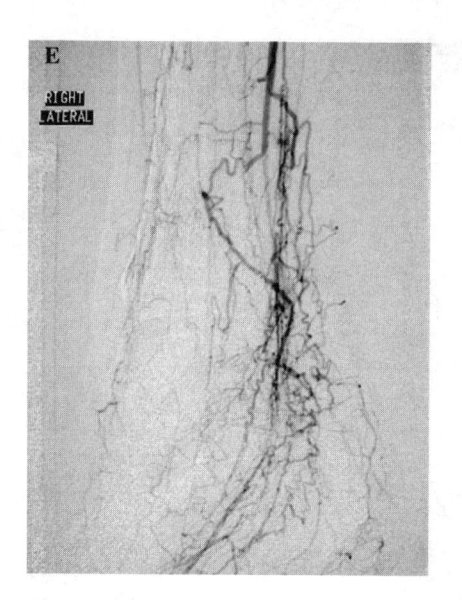

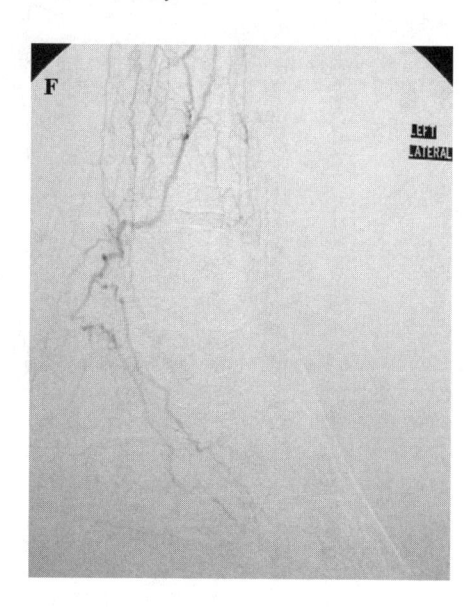

FIGURE 11. (continued)

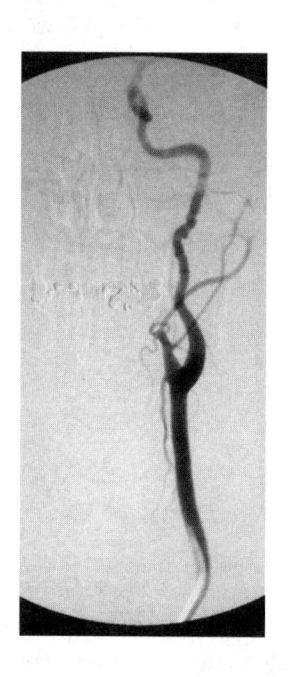

FIGURE 12. In a 55-year-old woman with new onset of transient ischemic attack, an angiogram of the carotid artery shows a "string of beads" (alternating zones of widening and narrowing) consistent with fibromuscular dysplasia (FMD). FMD involving the central nervous system has the following distribution: cervical and intracranial arteries, 85%; vertebral artery, 7%, both anterior and posterior circulation, 8%; and bilateral disease, 60–65%.

when there are areas of thinning of the wall. This type classically is described as a string or pearls on diagnostic angiography.

Type III represents adventitial dysplasia. It is the least common variant and appears to consist of a collection of fibrous tissue in the adventia that narrows the artery.

47. Define subclavian steal syndrome.

Subclavian steal syndrome (Fig. 13) describes the effects of reversal blood flow within the vertebral artery in the cerebral circulation. Patients usually present with a narrowing or occlusion

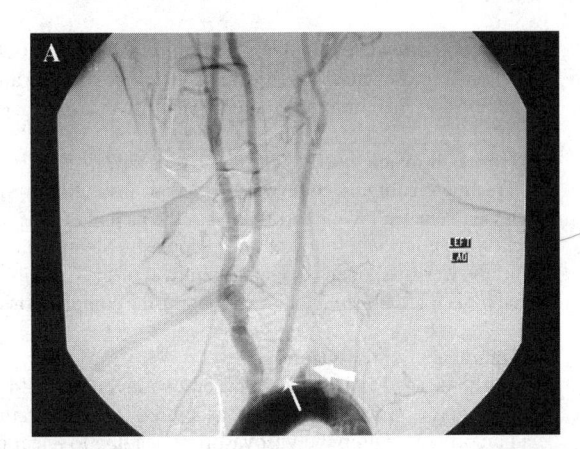

FIGURE 13. *A,* Left occipitoanterior thoracic angiogram demonstrates complete occlusion of the subclavian artery *(thick arrow)* with narrowing *(thin arrow)* at the origin of the left carotid artery. *B,* Delayed images show retrograde flow down the vertebral artery to supply the left arm. This finding is known as subclavian steal; the arm is stealing blood from the cerebral circulation.

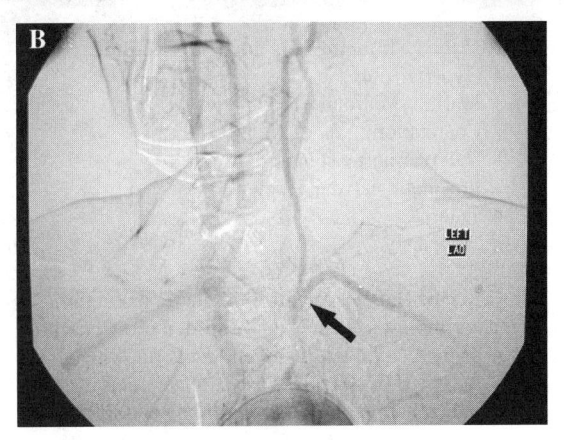

of the proximal left subclavian or brachial cephalic artery. Arm exercise leads to an increase in demand within the affected arm with subsequent reversal of flow within the vertebral arm. This syndrome can produce clinical symptoms such as dizziness, vertigo, blurred vision, diplopia, and near syncope.

48. Are occlusions of the subclavian or brachial cephalic artery causing subclavian steel syndrome amenable to recannulization?

Recannulization of the subclavian artery or brachial cephalic artery may be technically feasible. The long-term patency rates, however, have been poor. Patency rates may improve with advanced stent technology. Narrowed vessels within the subclavian or brachial cephalic arteries have shown excellent long-term patency rates.

49. Describe thoracic outlet syndrome.

Thoracic outlet syndrome allows compression of structures as they pass through the area known as the thoracic outlet. These structures include the brachial plexus, subclavian artery, and subclavian vein. They are usually compressed within the region of the interscalene triangle bounded by the anterior medial scalene muscles and the first rib.

50. What is the most common presentation of thoracic outlet syndrome?

Neurologicl symptoms are the most common symptoms of thoracic outlet syndrome, including pain and numbness of the hands and fingers.

51. Describe the vascular presentation of thoracic outlet syndrome.

Vascular presentations usually include upper extremity arm swelling due to venous compression or thrombosis. Less commonly, arterial supply can also be narrowed in thoracic outlet syndrome.

52. How is thoracic outlet syndrome treated?

Treatment is highly controversial. At our institution we perform thrombolysis for an occluded subclavian vein. Following thrombolysis, the patient is taken to the operating room, where a first-rib resection is performed, followed by angioplasty. Stenting of the subclavian veins has not been successful. Newer work is investigating removal of the first rib, followed by stenting of the vein. The overall basis for treatment includes removing the compression caused within the interscalene triangle.

53. Define aortic dissection.

Aortic dissection is a tear between two layers of the aorta. The intima is usually torn away from the media. Aortic dissection has a male-to-female ratio of 3:1. The pathology is thought to be a hemorrhage within the vasovasorum, leading to a tear or weakness of the intima.

54. List the risk factors for aortic dissection.
- Hypertension
- Marfan syndrome (Fig. 14)
- Coarctation
- Valvular aortic stenosis
- Prosthetic valve placement
- Trauma
- Pregnancy

55. Describe the classification of aortic dissection.

The simplest system is the **Stanford classification:**
- **Type A** involves the ascending aorta, which makes it a surgical situation.
- In **type B** (Fig. 15), the ascending aorta is not involved; type B is usually treated medically.

An alternate system is the **DeBakey classification:**

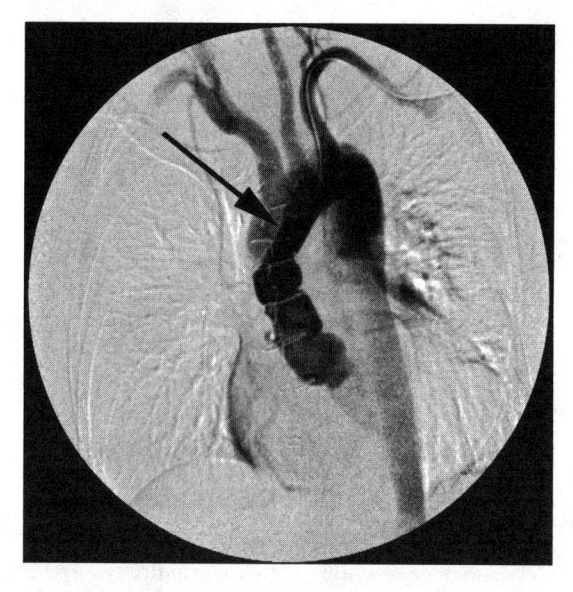

FIGURE 14. Stanford type A dissection. Arrow identifies the dissection flap. The patient previously underwent repair of the aortic valve and ascending aorta. The dissection was originally secondary to Marfan's syndrome.

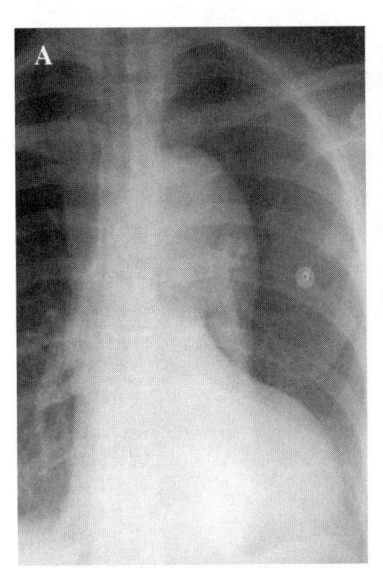

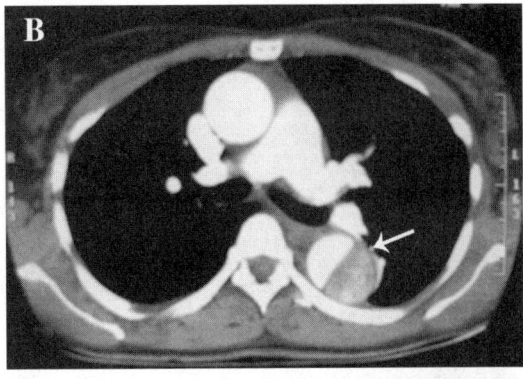

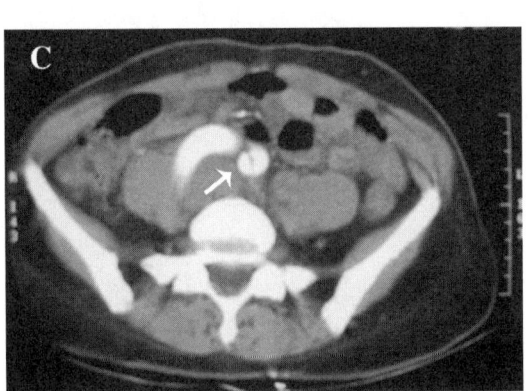

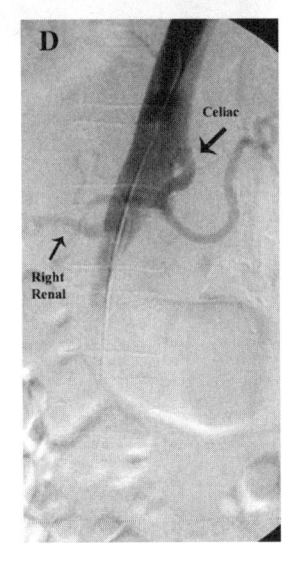

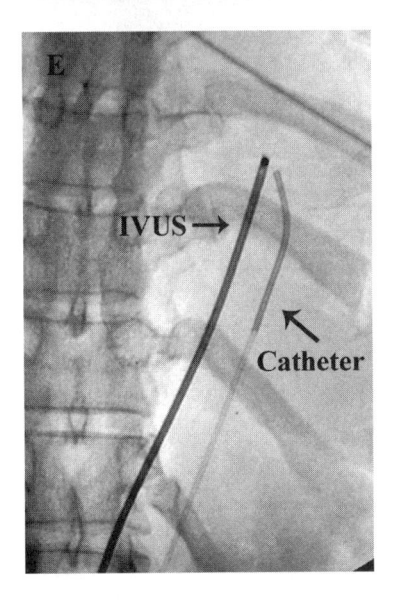

FIGURE 15. A, Initial chest x-ray in a patient with ripping back pain shows a widened aorta. **B** and **C,** CT scans show an intimal flap *(arrow),* consistent with a dissection, that extends to the iliac vessels. Because the patient's blood pressure could not be controlled, he was referred for an aortic fenestration, in which the intima is torn to equalize the pressure in the true and false lumens. An aortogram **(D)** was done, along with intravascular ultrasound **(E** and **F)**. The intravascular ultrasound clearly demonstrated the intimal flap and helped guide a wire from the true to the false lumen. After a wire is passed from the true to the false lumen, a large balloon is inflated at the level of the diaphragm and above the bifurcation **(G** and **H)**. Pressure is measured in the true and false lumens to ensure that it is equalized. This procedure is reserved for patients in whom medical treatment of a Stanford type B dissection fails or is not possible.

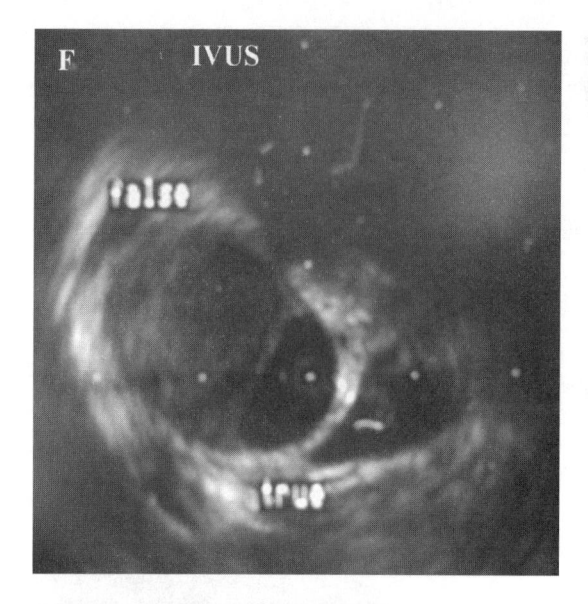

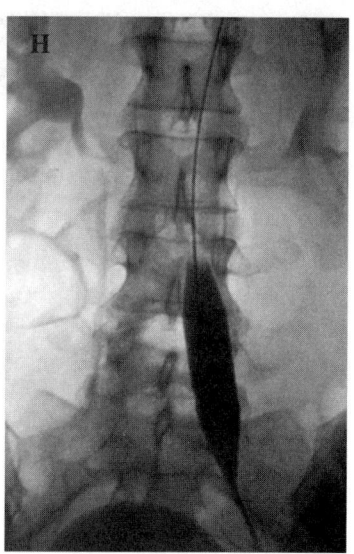

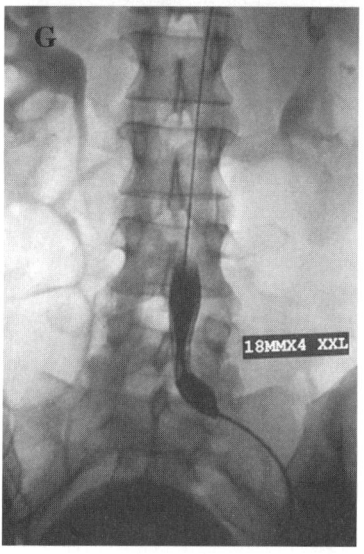

FIGURE 15. (Continued)

- **Type I** involves the entire aorta.
- **Type II** involves only the ascending aorta.
- **Type III** involves only the descending aorta past the origin of the left subclavian artery.

56. What is the best diagnostic test for an aortic dissection?
The best diagnostic test for an aortic dissection is a CT scan. An intimal flap can be viewed on a contrasted image.

57. List the clinical signs and symptoms of an aortic dissection.
- Sharp, tearing, intractable chest pain
- Murmur or bruit

- Asymmetrical peripheral pulses
- Absent femoral pulses
- Hemodynamic shock
- Neurologic deficits
- Alighieri
- Heart failure
- Recurrent arrhythmias
- Signs of pericardial tamponade

58. Are there any interventional treatments for aortic dissections?

There are no FDA-approved treatments for aortic dissection. However, ongoing studies are examining the possibility of stenting or placement of a stent graft near the origin of the dissection.

59. What is the normal size of an thoracic aorta?

Thoracic aortas usually are 2–5 cm in width.

60. List the risk factors for developing a thoracic aneurysm.

- Hypertension
- Coronary artery disease
- Vascular aneurysmal disease, including the abdomen

61. Give the mean age and male-to-female ratio of thoracic aneurysms.

Mean age: 65 years

Male-to-female ratio: approximately 3:1

62. Describe the presenting features of a thoracic aneurysm.

Thoracic aneurysms can present with sternal, back, or shoulder pain. They also can present with superior vena cava (SVC) syndrome due to venous compression or dysplasia from esophageal compression. Other findings include stridor or dyspnea from tracheal bronchial compression and possible hoarseness from compression of the recurrent laryngeal nerve.

63. Have any endovascular procedures been approved for the repair of thoracic aneurysms?

Multiple ongoing clinical trials are addressing the repair of thoracic aneurysms (Fig. 16) and hold promise for the future. A risk of paraplegia is still associated with covering the spinal arteries.

64. What is the most common site for an aortic rupture after a motor vehicle accident?

This question is difficult to answer. The most likely site for aortic trauma is at the aortic root. The majority of such patients die in the field. The most commonly seen aortic injury from a motor vehicle accident within the hospital is located at the ductus bump. The ductus forms a fixed point of the aorta. A deceleration injury may cause significant shear at this area. The third area of aortic rupture that must be evaluated is at the diaphragm. The take-home point is that the highest shear forces are at fixed points within the aorta, which include the aortic root, ductus bump, and diaphragm.

65. Are there any approved endografts for repair of aortic rupture due to trauma?

Currently there are no FDA-approved devices for the repair of aortic rupture. Multiple trials for the evaluation of repair of an aortic rupture with an endograft (Fig. 17) are ongoing. This type of repair holds significant promise.

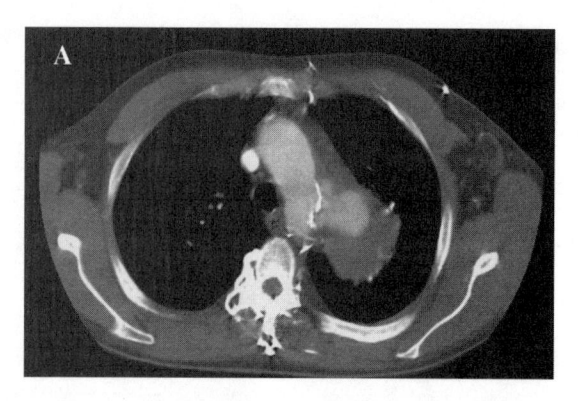

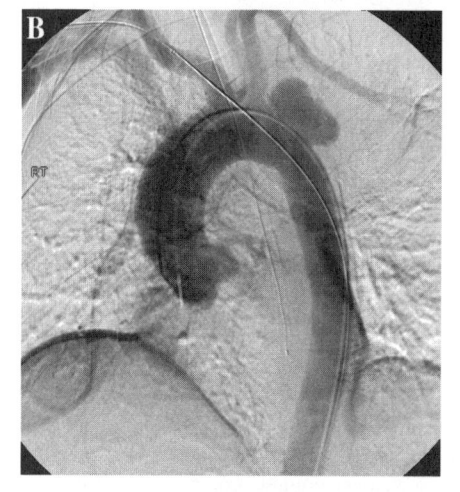

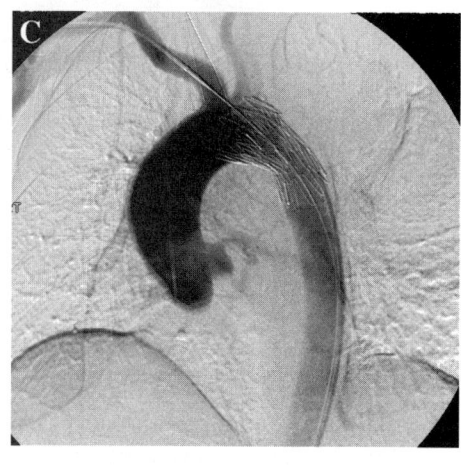

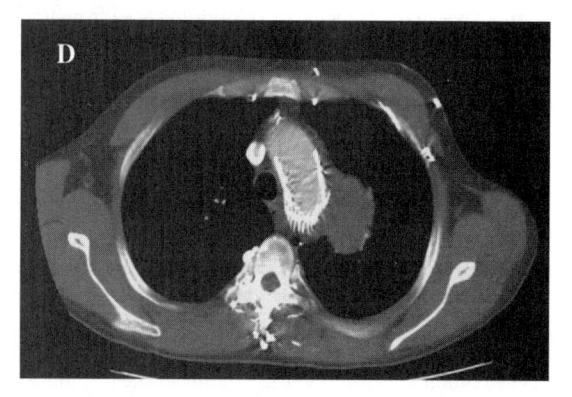

FIGURE 16. **A,** CT scan demonstrates a pseudoaneurysm of the aortic arch. **B,** Angiogram also illustrates the pseudoanerysm. **C,** A stent graft was deployed over the pseudoaneurysm. **D,** Follow-up CT demonstrates exclusion of the pseudoaneurysm.

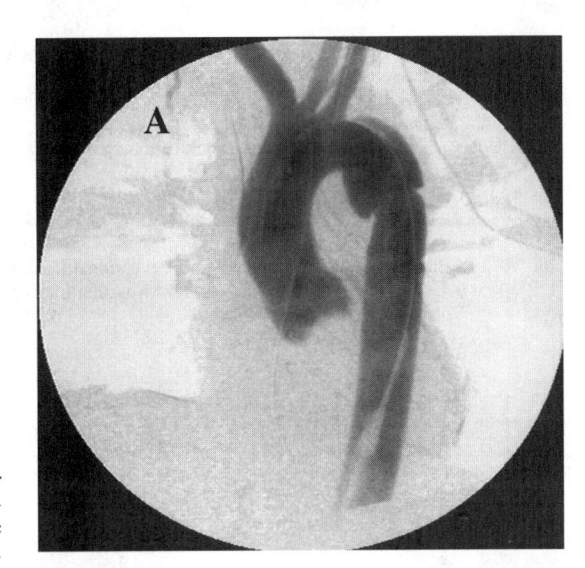

FIGURE 17. A, Left occipitoanterior angiogram of a patient involved in a motor vehicle accident shows a traumatic aortic tear just past the subclavian artery. **B,** A thoracic stent was placed (according to the institutional review board protocol), excluding the rupture. Three years after injury the patient made a complete recovery.

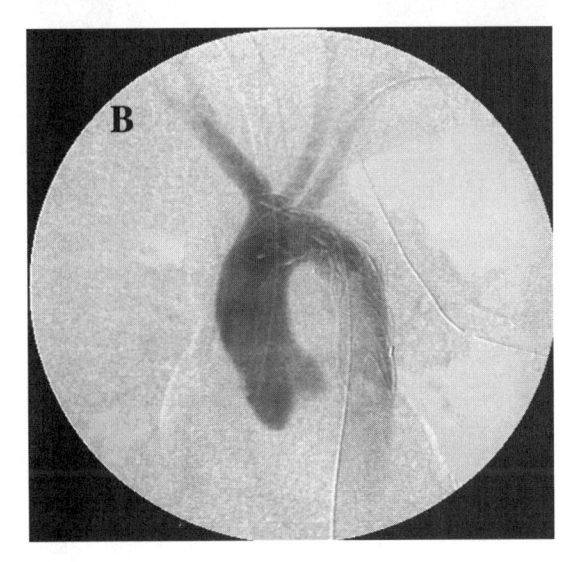

BIBLIOGRAPHY

1. Ali AT, Modrall JG, Lopez J, et al: Emerging role of endovascular grafts in complex aortoiliac occlusive disease. J Vasc Surg 38:486–491, 2003.
2. Bakal CW, et al (eds): Vascular and Interventional Radiology: Principles and Practice. New York, Thieme, 2002.
3. Baum S, Abrams HL (eds): Abrams' Angiography, 4th ed. Philadelphia, Lippincott Williams & Wilkins, 1996.
4. Brewster DC, Cronenwett JL, Hallett JW Jr, et al, for the Joint Council of the American Association for Vascular Surgery and Society for Vascular Surgery: Guidelines for the treatment of abdominal aortic aneurysms. Report of a subcommittee of the Joint Council of the American Association for Vascular Surgery and Society for Vascular Surgery. J Vasc Surg 37:1106–1117, 2003.
5. Buth J, Harris PL, Van Marrewijk C, Fransen G: Endoleaks during follow-up after endovascular repair of abdominal aortic aneurysm: Are they all dangerous? JCardiovasc Surg (Torino) 44:559–566, 2003.

6. Buth J, Harris PL, van Marrewijk C, Fransen G: The significance and management of different types of endoleaks. Semin Vasc Surg 16(2):95–102, 2003.
7. Greenberg R, Khwaja J, Haulon S, Fulton G: Aortic dissections: New perspectives and treatment paradigms. Eur J Vasc Endovasc Surg 26:579–586, 2003.
8. Kandarpa K, Aruny JE (eds): Handbook of Interventional Radiologic Procedures, 3rd ed. Philadelphia, Lippincott Williams & Wilkins, 2001.
9. Mouanoutoua M, Maddikunta R, Allaqaband S, et al: Endovascular intervention of aortoiliac occlusive disease in high-risk patients using the kissing stents technique: Long-term results. Catheter Cardiovasc Interv 60:320–326, 2003.
10. Valji K, Bralow L (edsd): Vascular and Interventional Radiology. Philadelphia, W.B. Saunders, 1999.
11. White RA, Fogarty TJ (eds): Peripheral Endovascular Interventions. New York, Springer Verlag, 1999.

11. PERIPHERAL VASCULAR DISEASE: DIAGNOSIS AND INTERVENTION

Bulent Arslan, MD

1. What are the types of vascular diseases?
Vascular diseases can be due to multiple pathologies, including atherosclerosis, trauma, vasculitidies, neoplasia, thromboembolic disease, and infection. This chapter focuses on atherosclerotic and thromboembolic pathologies.

2. Define peripheral vascular disease (PVD).
PVD is defined as disorders of the circulatory system to the extremities, viscera, and head. This chapter focuses on the lower extremities. Upper extremity, carotid, and visceral disorders are discussed elsewhere.

3. Explain the role of the interventional radiologist in diagnosis and treatment of PVD.
With the advancement of interventional techniques, the role of the interventional radiologist in management of PVD is increasing. Many interventional radiologists actively participate in patient care with clinical follow-ups and hospital admissions. Patient care is crucial if interventional radiologists want to continue providing vascular treatment.

4. How common is PVD?
Approximately 10 million patients in the United States are affected by PVD. Fifty percent are asymptomatic, 35–40 % are symptomatic but untreated, and only 10–15% are being treated .

5. What are the risk factors for PVD?
Smoking is the single most important preventable risk factor. Age, hypercholesterolemia, hypertension, diabetes, obesity, and sedentary lifestyle are other important risk factors. Elevated homocysteine levels in plasma have been shown to have a strong association with PVD, especially in patients under the age of 50 .

6. Describe the relationship of PVD with age.
Fewer than 5% of patients are younger than 60 years. More than 20% of the population over the age of 75 years has PVD, and 10% of the population over the age of 70 years suffers from lifestyle-limiting intermittent claudication secondary to PVD.

7. What are the symptoms and signs of PVD?
Patients can be asymptomatic (an estimated 50%) or present with claudication, rest pain, nonhealing ulcers, or gangrene, which may eventually lead to limb loss.

8. How does PVD affect life expectancy?
According to an article published in the *New England Journal of Medicine* in 1991, life expectancy is reduced by 10 years in patients with PVD. Seventy-five percent of the deaths are caused by cardiovascular events.

9. What are the steps in diagnosis of PVD?
Patient history, physical examination, laboratory evaluation, noninvasive vascular studies, and eventually angiography.

10. What information should be obtained in patient history?

Risk factors such as hypercholesterolemia, diabetes, early cardiac deaths in family, and degree of symptoms (claudication, rest pain, and nonhealing ulcers) should be identified.

11. Define claudication. How can it be differentiated from other causes of lower extremity pain?

Claudication is defined as pain in the calves or buttocks due to exercise. Claudication is most commonly confused with neurogenic pain due to nerve root compression. Predictable pain with exercise and relief by rest are important factors to differentiate claudication from other sources of leg pain.

12. What tests can be used in the diagnosis of PVD?

Ankle/brachial index (ABI), duplex ultrasound, magnetic resonance angiography (MRA), computed tomographic angiography (CTA), and conventional angiography.

13. Define ABI. What is its significance?

ABI = systolic ankle pressure/systolic brachial pressure. During the test, blood pressure cuffs are placed on both arms as well as ankles. The higher brachial pressure measurement is used for calculation. The higher of the dorsalis pedis and plantaris tibialis is used for ankle pressure.

14. When should conventional angiography used in PVD?

Whenever treatment is planned, either interventional or surgical. If a patient has at least lifestyle-limiting claudication and noninvasive tests are suggestive of PVD, a conventional angiogram should be planned. Consent should also be obtained for possible interventions. If the disease can be treated by angioplasty and/or stenting, the patient can go home the next morning without the need for surgery.

15. Describe the technique for performing a lower extremity angiogram.

1. Whenever feasible, a common femoral access should be obtained. If both femoral arteries are occlusive, an axillary approach is an alternative.
2. Modified Seldinger technique can be used with an 18-gauge puncture needle to advance a 0.035 guidewire into the femoral artery. Alternatively, in patients with high risk for bleeding a micropuncture access system can be used.
3. After advancing the guidewire, a 5-French sheath is placed into the artery.
4. Through this sheath over the existing guidewire a pigtail catheter is advanced into the aorta to the level of the renal arteries to start with an abdominal aortic angiogram. We prefer an Omni-Flush catheter, which allows us to gain access to the contralateral iliac system with the help of a guidewire.
5. Subsequently the catheter is pulled back to the distal aorta to obtain pelvic angiograms in anteroposterior (AP), right anterior oblique (RAO), and left anterior oblique (LAO) views.
6. If bilateral lower extremity angiogram is needed, you can continue imaging down to the level of the feet in a stepwise fashion.

16. Describe the total amount and injection rate of contrast agent used for lower extremity angiography.

- An aortic injection should be 10–20 ml/sec for a total of 20–40 ml.
- A pelvic injection should be 5–10 ml/sec for a total of 10–15 ml.
- Lower extremity injections should be adjusted according to catheter position and distance of the imaged segment to the catheter.
- During imaging of the superficial femoral artery, if the catheter is positioned at the distal aorta to obtain bilateral lower extremity angiogram, 5 ml/sec for a total of 15 ml and 1/3 ml increase, as needed for distal arteries, should be adequate.
- If the catheter is positioned in the external iliac artery, 3–5 ml/sec for a total of 6–15 ml, depending on the location of the imaged segment, should suffice.

These values should be adjusted according to patient weight and kidney function.

17. What access problems may you encounter during angiogram?

Difficulty in gaining access into the artery and not being able to advance the wire after gaining access into the artery, usually due to a diseased/calcified artery.

18. How should you manage the above problems?

To overcome this problem, the first step includes initial examination of the pulse in both groins and selecting the side with the better pulse. Use of anatomic landmarks under fluoroscopy or ultrasound guidance also helps. If all attempts fail, the next step is to search for another access site. Either contralateral groin or axillary approach (preferably left) can be tried. Brachial and radial approaches are less desirable; they are more commonly favored by invasive cardiologists.

19. What questions should be answered before performing an angiogram?

The following issues should be evaluated in advance to prevent problems immediately before and during the procedure:

- Is the study indicated? Evaluate noninvasive studies that were (should have been) performed.
- Is there a treatment plan? Access site should be chosen accordingly.
- Is the patient's renal function normal?
- Are coagulation studies normal?
- Does the patient have diabetes, hypertension, or contrast allergy?
- Is the patient capable of giving informed consent?

20. Describe management of problems related to contrast administration.

For a minor reaction patients can be pretreated with three doses of 50 mg of prednisone every 8 hours before the procedure and with 50 mg of benadryl 1 hour before the procedure. If the study is emergent and iodinated contrast is definitely needed, 100 mg of Solu-Medrol can be administered intravenously before the procedure. Patients with history of anaphylactic reaction should not receive iodinated contrast. Either carbon dioxide or Gadolinium should be used.

In patients with elevated creatinine (1.5–2.0), we prefer administering Mucomyst, 600 mg twice daily for 2 days, starting the day before the procedure. In addition, hydration with intravenous fluids (as much as the patient can safely tolerate) may help. If creatinine is higher than 2.0, the use of alternative contrast agents may be wise (Fig. 1).

21. Describe management of problems related to coagulation before procedures requiring arterial access.

International normalized ratio (INR) and platelets are of major concern. If INR is greater than 1.5, vitamin K (if the procedure is not urgent) or fresh frozen plasma (if the procedure is relatively urgent) can be administered to correct the INR. If the platelet count is less than 50000, platelets can be administered just before or during the procedure.

22. Identify the six types of atherosclerotic peripheral vascular disease.

Type I (initial), type II (fatty streak), and type III (intermediate) lesions are not clinically recognizable. Advanced lesions are type IV (atheroma), type V (fibrotic) and type VI (complicated).

23. What are the treatment options for PVD?

Medical treatment with lifestyle adjustment, interventional procedures, and surgical procedures.

24. Describe medical treatment of atherosclerotic PVD.

Exercise protocol and smoking cessation are mainstays of medical treatment. Considering the significant death rate from cardiovascular disorders (75%), with 10 years reduced life expectancy, aspirin therapy may be beneficial. Cilostazol (Pletal) is a phosphodiesterase III inhibitor that improves clandication by improving collateral flow.

Control of blood glucose level in diabetes, cholesterol levels in hyperlipidemia, and blood pressure in hypertension is highly important. Although these measures may help, atherosclerosis

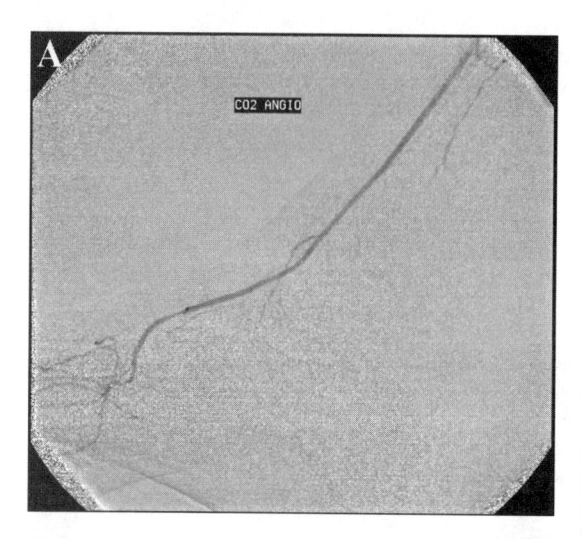

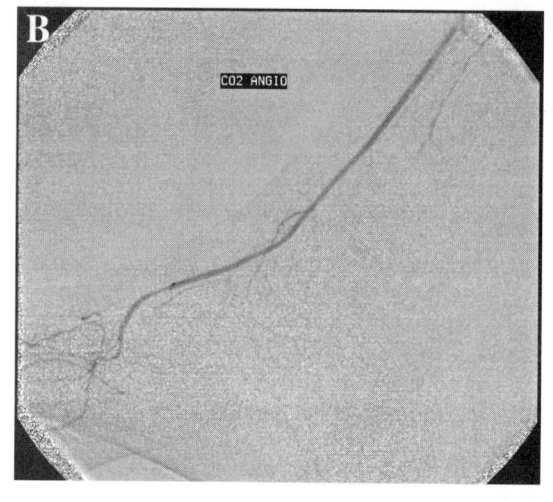

FIGURE 1. In patients with abnormal levels of blood urea nitrogen and creatinine, alternative contrast agents should be considered. Two options are carbon dioxide and gadolinium. **A** and **B**, Two views from a run-off in which carbon dioxide was used as the contrast agent.

is a progressive disease and the best medical therapy may provide minimal improvement and delay of the intervention. For this reason, continuous follow-up with noninvasive studies is crucial.

25. What interventional procedures can be used in treatment of PVD?
Angioplasty, cryoplasty, stent placement, atherectomy, and thrombolysis (Fig. 2).

26. According to the Standards Committee of the Society for Internventional Radiology, what categories of lesions are appropriate for percutaneous angioplasty?
- For **category 1** lesions, balloon angioplasty alone is the procedure of choice. Treatment of these lesions results in a high technical success rate and generally in complete relief of symptoms or normalization of pressure gradients.
- **Category 2** lesions are well suited for angioplasty. Treatment results in complete relief of or significant improvement in symptoms, pulses, or pressure gradients. This category includes lesions treated with percutaneous procedures that will be followed by surgical bypass to treat multilevel vascular disease.
- **Category 3** lesions are amenable to percutaneous therapy, but because of disease extent, location, or severity, percutaneous treatment has a moderate chance of initial technical suc-

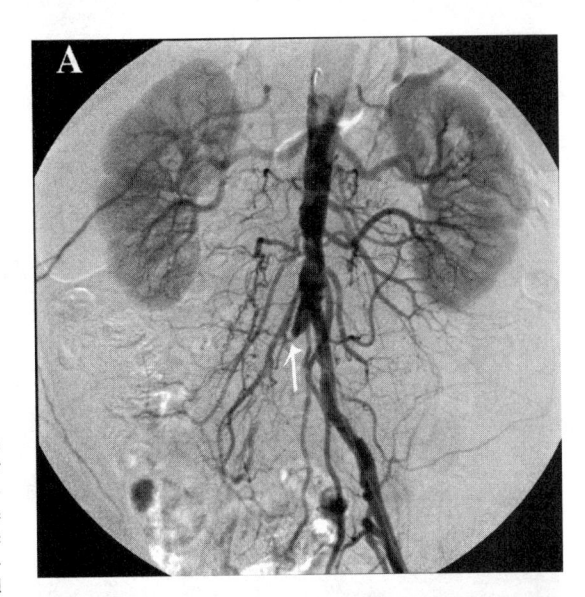

FIGURE 2. A 65-year-old man with long-standing buttock and right lower extremity claudication. **A,** Abdominal-pelvic angiogram demonstrates complete occlusion of the right common iliac artery *(arrow).* **B,** The right common iliac artery was successfully recanalized with an endovascular stent. At present this type of lesion is appropriately treated only with stent placement, although newer technology, such as cryoplasty, may change this concept. Cryoplasty cools the vessel before it is dilated. Early results with this technique show promise.

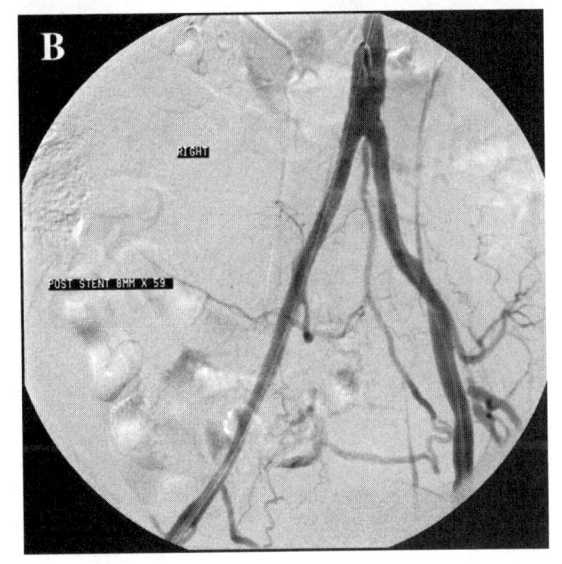

cess or long-term benefit compared with surgical bypass. However, percutaneous transluminal angioplasty (PTA) may be performed, generally because of patient risk factors or lack of suitable bypass material.
- **Category 4** lesions are found with extensive vascular disease. Percutaneous therapy has a limited role because of a low technical success rate or poor long-term benefit. In very high-risk patients or when no surgical procedure is applicable, PTA may have some role.

27. **Describe categories of lesions for infrarenal aortic angioplasty.**
    - **Category 1** lesions involve less than 2-cm stenosis of the infrarenal abdominal aorta, with minimal atherosclerotic disease of the aorta.
    - **Category 2** lesions involve 2- to 4-cm stenosis of the infrarenal abdominal aorta, with mild atherosclerotic disease of the aorta.

- **Category 3** lesions involve (1) greater than 4-cm stenosis of the infrarenal abdominal aorta, (b) aortic stenosis with atheroembolic disease (blue toe syndrome), or (c) 2- to 4-cm stenosis of the infrarenal abdominal aorta, with moderate-to-severe atherosclerosis of the aorta otherwise.
- **Category 4** lesions are aortic occlusions and aortic stenosis associated with an abdominal aortic aneurysm.

28. What are the indications for infrarenal aortic stenting?

Treatment of aortic stenosis may be performed in patients with claudication of the legs or buttocks (Fig. 3). Many male patients may also have impotence. Patients with atheroembolic symp-

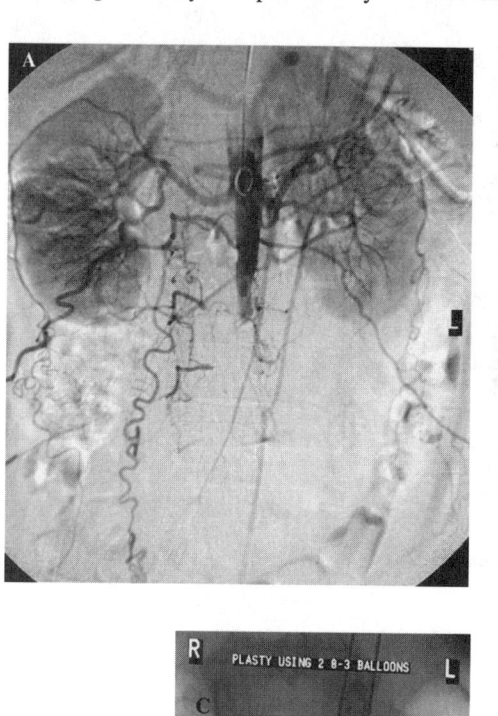

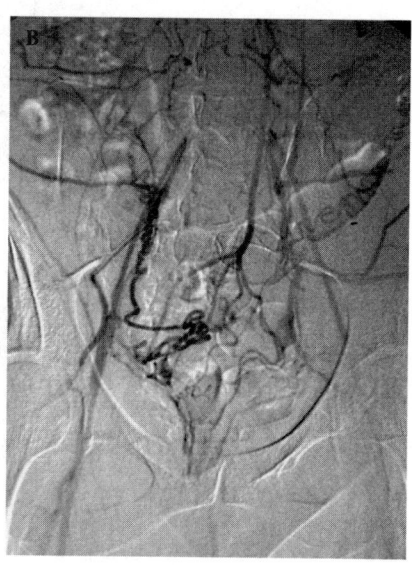

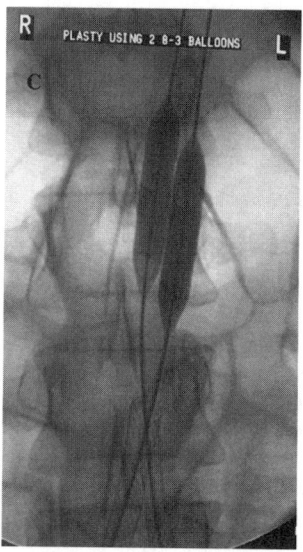

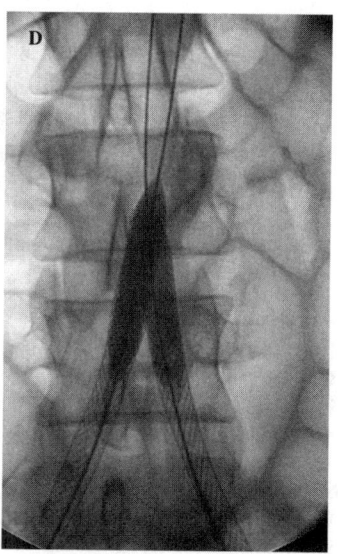

FIGURE 3. (continued)

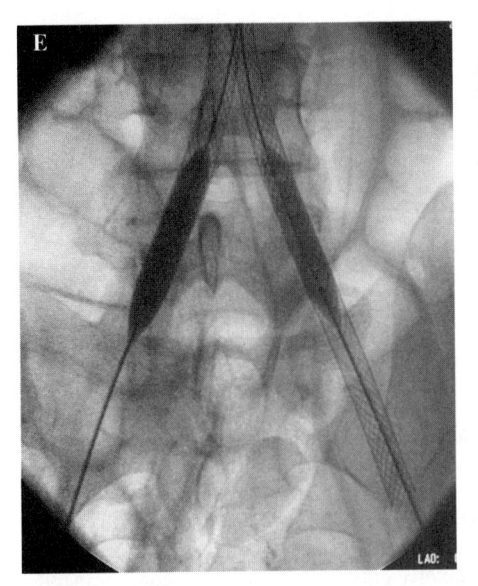

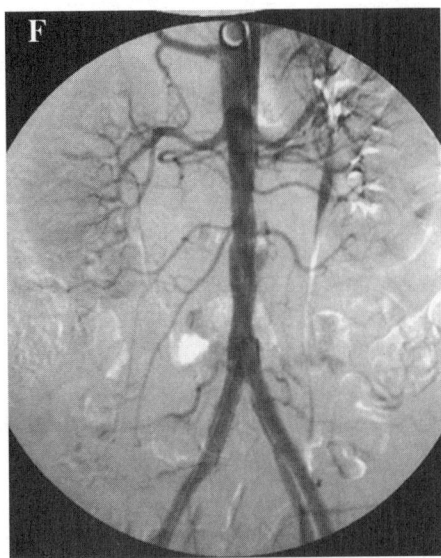

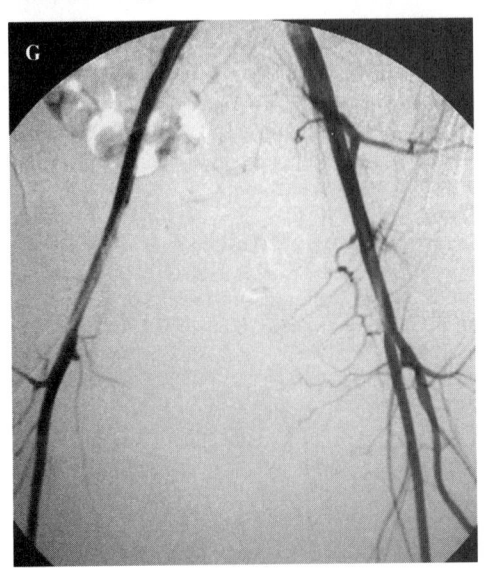

FIGURE 3. The combination of buttock claudication, erectile dysfunction, and faint Doppler femoral pulses is termed Leriche syndrome, named for the surgeon who first described the condition in 1923. Leriche syndrome results from either preocclusive stenosis or complete occlusion of the infrarenal aorta due to severe aortic atherosclerosis. Diagnostic aortograms performed in a patient who was a poor surgical candidate revealed infrarenal aortic occlusion (**A**) with reconstitution of bilateral common iliac arteries (**B**). Access was obtained with the help of ultrasound in left axillary artery and bilateral common iliac arteries, and aortoiliac reconstruction was performed with percutaneous transluminal angioplasty. Stents were placed in the aorta (**C**) and bilateral iliac arteries (**D** and **E**). The final angiograms (**F** and **G**) demonstrated good results.

toms (blue toe syndrome) may also benefit, but the data about percutaneous therapy in this group are limited. Recently available covered stents may have the added advantage of compressing the plaque between the stent wall and aortic wall, making the deployment safer.

29. What are the 1-year and 5-year patency rates for infrarenal aortic angioplasty?

Excellent results have been obtained in small number of patients. According to SCVIR, Peripheral Vascular Interventions Syllabus, the 1-year patency rate is 95% and the 5-year patency rate is 80%.

30. Describe categories of lesions for iliac angioplasty.
- **Category 1** lesions involve stenosis less than 3 cm in length; lesions are concentric and noncalcified.

- **Category 2** lesions involve stenosis of 3–5 cm in length or calcified or eccentric stenosis less than 3 cm in length.
- **Category 3** lesions involve stenosis pf 5–10 cm in length or chronic occlusions less than 5 cm in length after thrombolytic therapy.
- **Category 4** lesions are (1) stenosis greater than 10 cm in length, (2) chronic occlusions greater than 5 cm in length after thrombolytic therapy, (3) extensive bilateral aortoiliac atherosclerotic disease, or (4) iliac stenosis in patients with abdominal aortic aneurysm or other lesions requiring aortic or iliac surgery.

31. What is the 5-year patency rate for iliac angioplasty?

The 5-year patency rates for iliac PTA are 80–90%, approaching the patency rates of surgical bypass. With careful selection of patients with category 1 and category 2 lesions, the technical success rate is above 90–95%.

32. Describe categories of lesions for femoropopliteal angioplasty.

- **Category 1** lesions involve single stenosis or occlusions, up to 3 cm in length, that are not at the origin of the superficial femoral artery or the distal portion of the popliteal artery.
- **Category 2** lesions involve (1) single stenosis or occlusions, 3–10 cm in length, not involving the distal popliteal artery; (2) heavily calcified stenosis up to 3 cm in length; (3) multiple lesions, each less than 3 cm, that involve either stenosis or occlusions; or (4) single or multiple lesions in cases with no continuous tibial runoff to improve inflow for distal surgical bypass.
- **Category 3** lesions involve (*1*) single lesions, 3–10 cm in length, involving the distal popliteal artery; (2) multiple focal lesions, each 3–5 cm, that may be heavily calcified; or (*3*) single lesions, either stenosis or occlusions, with a length greater than 10 cm.
- **Category 4** lesions are complete occlusions of the common and/or superficial femoral artery or complete popliteal and proximal trifurcation occlusions.

33. What is considered clinical success for femoropopliteal interventions?

Clinical success in the femoropopliteal segment is defined as relief of or substantial improvement in symptoms, increase in the ankle-brachial index of at least 0.15, and/or normalization of the popliteal pulse, thigh/calf pulse volume recording or Doppler pressure (Fig. 4).

34. What are the indications for infrapopliteal angioplasty?

With the introduction of new techniques (Fig. 4) and equipment, infrapopliteal procedures are more commonly performed. Severe claudication that prevents minimal ambulation may be an acceptable indication, particularly if more than one tibial vessel is to be treated. Mild-to-moderate claudication generally is not an indication for treatment of these vessels; treatment at other levels generally relieves the symptoms, and the risk of occlusion is unacceptably high for this group of patients.

35. Explain the difference between primary stenting and secondary stenting.

Primary stenting refers to the initial intention to stent a lesion, as with a balloon mounted stent or deployment of a self-expanding stent through a lesion, without attempting an angioplasty. Secondary stenting refers to cases in which a stent is used after failure of an initial attempt at angioplasty or the condition is complicated by a dissection.

36. What are the current indications for iliac stenting?

Failed angioplasties and treatment of dissections after an angioplasty.

37. List the factors that are important in stent selection.

Obviously not all stents will be ideal. Stent selection according to the type and location of disease is an important factor in outcome. Leung et al. list the following factors as important:

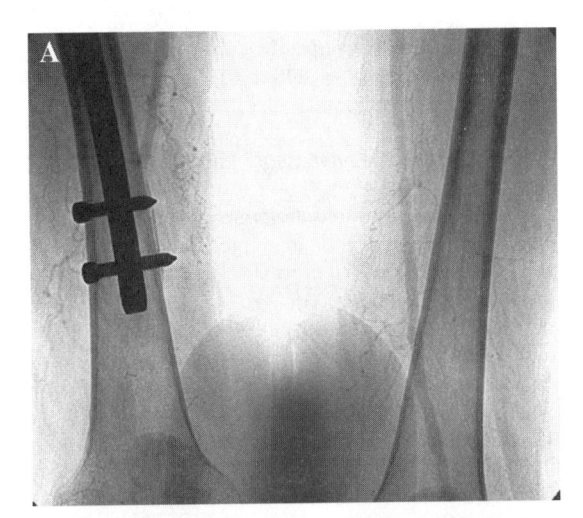

FIGURE 4. Newer dilatation techniques include cryoplasty. **A,** Initial angiogram demonstrates occlusion of the superior femoral artery. **B,** A wire was manipulated through the occlusion. **C,** Crysoplasty was done using a 6-mm balloon. Initial results show promise compared with the patency rates of angioplasty. Cryoplasty, which cools the blood vessel during dilatation, is thought to create a more organized dilatation and to stop apoptosis.

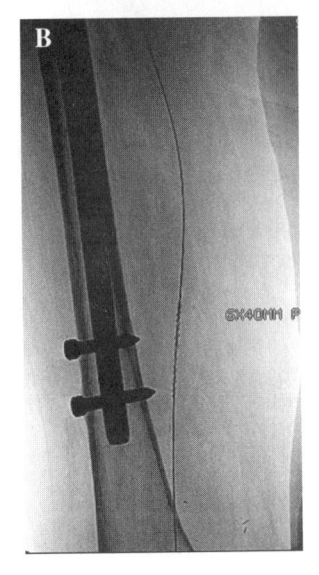

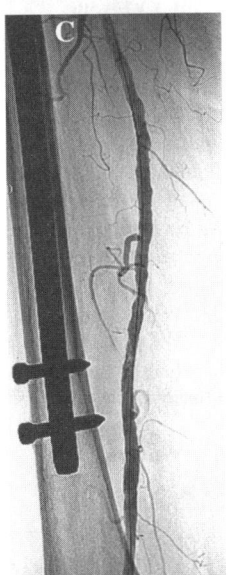

- High radial force/hoop strength to resist recoil
- Minimal or no induction of intimal hyperplasia or restenosis
- Longitudinal flexibility to negotiate tortuosity
- High radiopacity
- Radial elasticity or crush resistance
- Ability to conform to the vessel
- Low profile and high expansion ratio
- Minimal or no foreshortening for precise placement
- Easy deployment
- Maintenance of side branch patency
- MR imaging compatibility
- Durability
- Low price

38. List the major groups of stents.

Balloon-expandable, self-expandable, and covered stents. Very few of these stents are approved by FDA for intravascular use.

39. Summarize the advantages and disadvantages of balloon-expandable vs. self-expandable stents.

Balloon-expandable stents are mounted over a balloon and deployed by inflation of the balloon. Their deployment is more precise due to minimal foreshortening, and they are rigid with good radial strength that prevents elastic recoil of the artery. If compressed, however, they have no elasticity to reopen.

Self-expandable stents, most of which are made of Nitinol (except the Wallstent, which is made of steel) have good elasticity. Foreshortening is more of a problem, especially with Wallstent. Self-expandable Nitinol stents have good initial patency results in the femoropopliteal system.

40. What is the "kissing balloon technique"?

This technique is commonly used for proximal common iliac artery angioplasty. It involves simultaneous inflation of balloons during angioplasty to prevent embolization of plaque to the contralateral site.

41. Describe the surgical treatment options for peripheral arterial occlusive disease of lower extremities.

Bypass surgery can be performed with prosthetic grafts or autologous vein grafts. Bypasses above the superior femoral artery are performed by prosthetic grafts. These grafts may be aorta-femoral, aorta-iliac, axillary-femoral, or femoral-femoral. Femoral to popliteal bypass grafts are usually performed with an autologous vein due to their increased patency. If available, the greater saphenous vein on the same side is reversed and anastomosed to the femoral artery above the lesion and to the popliteal artery below the lesion. Reversal eliminates the need for stripping of the valves.

42. What are the findings of acute embolic peripheral vascular occlusion vs. chronic occlusion?

In acute embolic occlusion (Fig. 5) no collateral vessels are seen. Usually there is a sharp cut-off of the blood flow. The meniscus sign is helpful when present. Chronic occlusion is associated with significant collateral formation. Calcification of the arteries may also give a clue.

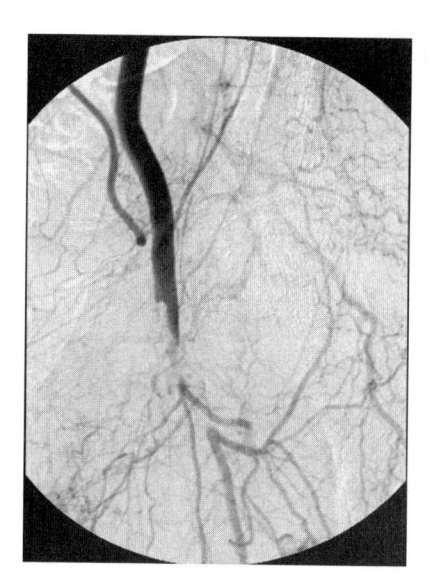

FIGURE 5. Embolus to the common femoral artery. The most common origin of the embolus is the heart. Emboli tend to lodge at bifurcations (femoral artery/trifurcation/first branch of the superior mesenteric artery). Treatment options include embolectomy and thrombolysis. Surgical embolectomy is the therapy of choice in patients with severe ischemia.

43. List the signs and symptoms of acute arterial occlusion.
The five Ps: **p**ain, **p**allor, **p**ulselessness, **p**aresthesias, and **p**aralysis

44. Summarize the suggested standards for reports dealing with lower extremity ischemia.
According to the Ad-hoc Committee on Reporting Standards of the Society of Vascular Surgery/North American Chapter and the International Society for Cardiovascular Surgery, ischemia is categorized in three groups:

1. A **viable limb** is characterized by intact capillary refill, normal motor and sensory function, and the presence of arterial and venous Doppler signals.

2. The **threatened limb** requires urgent intervention to achieve limb salvage. Capillary refill is slow, and there may be mild motor and/or sensory abnormalities. Distal arterial Doppler signals are usually inaudible, but venous signals are present.

3. **Irreversible ischemia** is characterized by absent capillary refill, marked motor abnormality or frank paralysis, significant sensory loss or anesthesia, and inaudible arterial and venous signals.

45. What are the treatment options for acute embolic occlusion of lower extremity arteries?
Interventional therapy involves thrombolysis with a thrombolytic agent. This therapy can be performed with a pulse spray technique or by slow infusion through an infusion catheter over 12–24 hours. Thrombectomy devices are also available. An alternative approach is surgical thrombectomy, in which cut-down and direct exposure of the artery are required. Vascular surgeons may also use a Fogarty balloon to remove the thrombus.

46. What are the commonly used thrombolytic agents?
Urokinase, tissue plasminogen activator (TPA), and tenecteplase (TNK). In addition to treatment of acute thrombosis, thrombolytic agents can also be used in treatment of chronic iliac occlusions (Figs. 6 and 7) before performing angioplasty and/or stenting (Figs. 8 and 9).

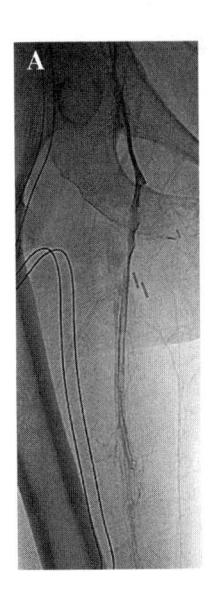

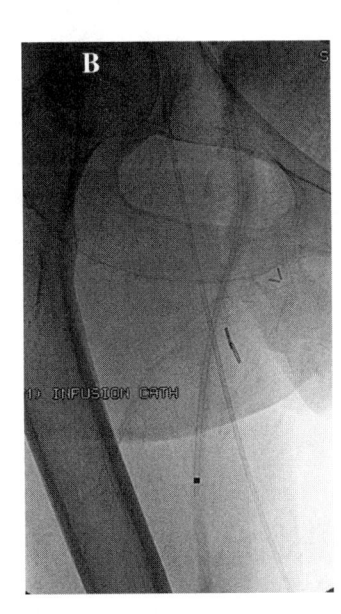

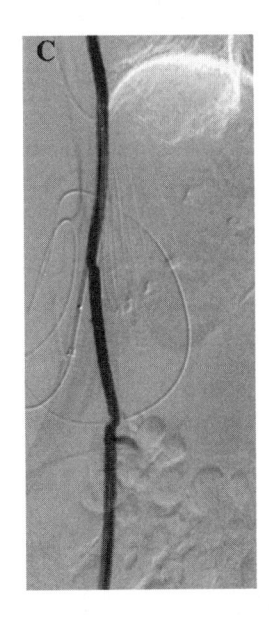

FIGURE 6. A, Occluded axillary-femoral and femoral-popliteal bypass grafts. **B,** Therapy with tissue plasminogen activator was begun using a crossed catheter technique. **C,** Within 24 hours the graft was open.

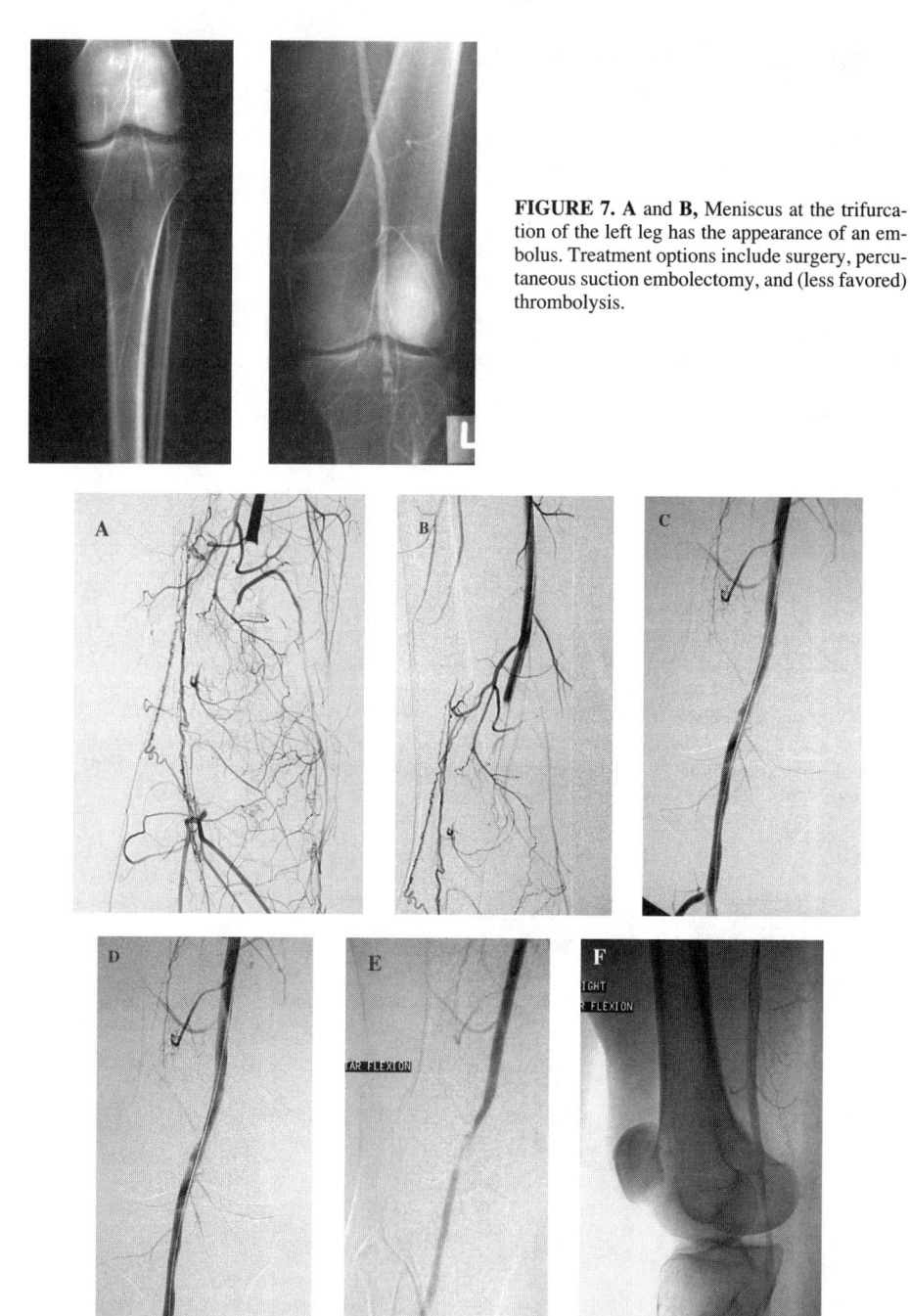

FIGURE 7. **A** and **B,** Meniscus at the trifurcation of the left leg has the appearance of an embolus. Treatment options include surgery, percutaneous suction embolectomy, and (less favored) thrombolysis.

FIGURE 8. A 30-year-old man presented with acute right leg pain. Two weeks earlier he had begun a new exercise program. The right leg was cool with diminished pulses. **A,** Angiogram demonstrates thrombus in the popliteal artery. **B,** An infusion wire was passed and thrombolysis was initiated. **C,** Within 12 hours the vessel was open. **D,** When the patient's leg was in neutral position, distal flow was normal. **E** and **F,** Flexion of the leg leads to narrowing of the popliteal artery. This finding is characteristic of popliteal entrapment syndrome.

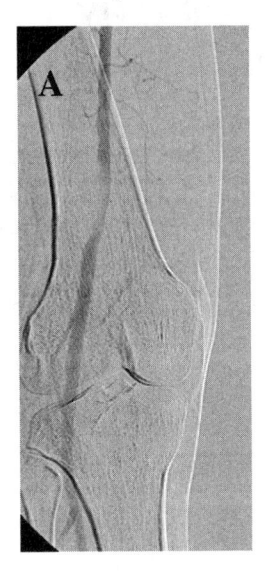

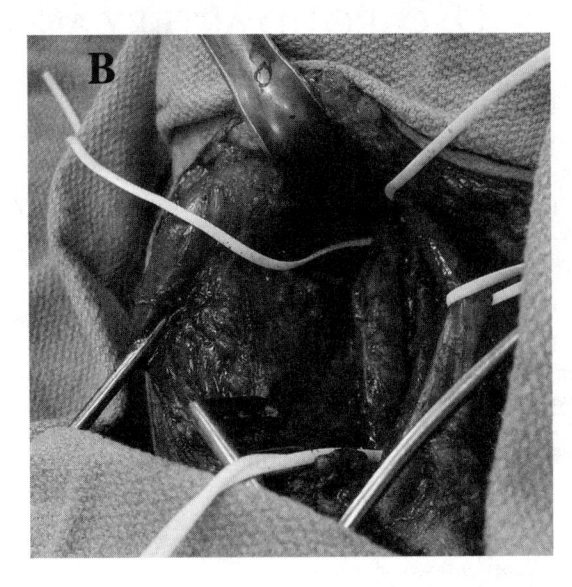

FIGURE 9. A, External compression of the right popliteal artery. **B,** Surgery confirmed the diagnosis of cystic adventitial disease of the popliteal artery. A yellow gelatinous material was found within the adventitia. The differential diagnosis included popliteal entrapment syndrome.

BIBLIOGRAPHY

1. Brattstrom L, Israelsson B, Norrving B, et al: Impaired homocysteine metabolism in early-onset cerebral and peripheral occlusive arterial disease. Atherosclerosis 81:51–60, 1990.
2. Clarke R, Daly L, Robinson K, et al: Hyperhomocysteinemia: An independent risk factor for vascular disease. N Engl J Med 324:1149–1155, 1991.
3. Criqui MH, Fronek A, Barrett-Connor E, et al: The prevalence of peripheral arterial disease in a defined population Circulation 71:510–515, 1985.
4. Kinney TB, Rose SC: Intraarterial pressure measurements during angiographic evaluation of peripheral vascular disease: Techniques, interpretation, applications, and limitations. Am J Roentgenol Vol 166:277–284, YEAR?
5. Leung DA, Spinosa DJ, Hagspiel KD, et al: Selection of stents for treating iliac arterial occlusive disease. Vasc Interv Radiol 14(2 Pt 1):137–152, 2003.
6. Palmaz JC, Laborde JC, Rivera FJ, et al: Stenting of the iliac arteries with the Palmaz stent: Experience from a multicenter trial. Cardiovasc Intervent Radiol 15:291–297, 1992.
7. Perler BA, Becker GJ: Vascular Intervention: A Clinical Approach. New York, Thieme, 1998.
8. Richter GM, Roeren T, Brado M, et al: Further update of the randomized trial: Iliac stent placement versus PTA-morphology, clinical success rates, and failure analysis. Presented at the 18th Annual Scientific Meeting of the SCVIR, New Orleans, March 1993.
9. Rutherford RB, Flanigan DP, Gupta SK, et al: Suggested standards for reports dealing with lower extremity ischemia. J Vasc Surg 4:80–94, 1986.
10. Society of Interventional Radiology Standards of Practice Committee: Guidelines for Percutaneous Transluminal Angioplasty. J Vasc Interv Radiol 14:S209-S217. 2003.
11. Stary HC, Blankenhorn DH, Chandler AB, et al: A definition of the intima of human arteries and of its atherosclerosis prone regions. A report from the Committee on Vascular Lesions of the Council on Arteriosclerosis, American Heart Association. Circulation 85:391–405, 1992.
12. Stary HC, Chandler AB, Dinsmore RE, et al: A definition of advanced types of atherosclerotic lesions and a histological classification of atherosclerosis. A report from the Committee on Vascular Lesions of the Council on Arteriosclerosis, American Heart Association. Arterioscl Thromb Vasc Biol 15:1512–1531, 1995.

12. CAROTID ARTERY ANGIOGRAPHY AND INTERVENTION

Wael E. A. Saad, MBBCh

Carotid artery angioplasty and stenting are not currently a Medicare- or FDA-approved procedure. This chapter describes off-label uses of stents and cerebral protection devices. These procedures involve a very high risk. We advise against performing them without permission and adequate training.

1. Who first described a case linking stroke and extracranial carotid artery disease?

In 1856 Savory described a case of extracranial internal carotid artery (ICA) occlusion and bilateral subclavian artery occlusion with hemiplegia. In 1914 Ramsey Hunt correlated the relationship between partial carotid artery occlusion and what he termed "cerebral intermittent claudication."

2. Who first did carotid angiography to diagnosis artery occlusion?

Moniz in 1927.

3. Name the branches of the external carotid.
- Superior thyroidal artery
- Ascending pharyngeal artery
- Lingual artery
- Facial artery (external maxillary artery)
- Occipital artery
- Postauricular artery
- Superficial temporal artery
- (Internal) maxillary artery (largest branch)

4. List the anatomic portions of the internal carotid artery.
- Cervical portion
- Petrosal portion
- Cavernous portion

5. Describe the origin of the common carotid arteries.
- The right branch originates from the bifurcation of the innominate artery.
- The left branch usually arises from the aortic arch directly between the take-off of the innominate artery (proximally) and the left subclavian artery (distally).

6. What is a bovine arch?

The bovine arch is an aortic arch in which the common carotid arteries arise from one common trunk.

7. What are the branches of the common carotid arteries?

Usually the common carotid artery gives no branches; in rare cases, however, it may give the following:
- Superior thyroid artery
- Ascending pharyngeal artery
- Inferior thyroid artery
- Least common, vertebral artery

8. From what does the middle meningeal artery arise?

The maxillary artery, which is the largest branch of the external carotid artery.

9. What is the implication of aortic arch atheromata (> 4 mm) on the incidence of stroke?
In an autopsy study of 500 patients, Amererco found that 26% of stroke patients had aortic arch atheromata

10. Summarize the impact of stroke on the community.
- It is the third leading cause of death in the United States.
- It is the number-one cause of disability in the United States.
- It is the most feared medical condition in the United States.

11. What is the most common cause of stroke?
At least 70% of stroke cases are attributed to brachiocephalic atherosclerotic disease (which includes common carotid and internal carotid atherosclerotic disease).

12. What is unique about brachiocephalic atherosclerotic disease compared with the rest of the vascular pathology in the human body?
Brachiocephalic atherosclerotic disease is embolic in nature and less commonly leads to stenosis or occlusion.

13. Explain the significance of the pathologic features of plaque.
Regardless of the size of the plaque and significance of carotid stenosis, the following are important:

EMBOLOGENIC	NONEMBOLOGENIC
TIA, RIND	Asymptomatic
10% annual risk for major stroke	1% annual risk
Irregular, ulcerated lesions	Smooth lesions on angiography
Intramural hemorrhage with ulcerations and necrosis	Less hemorrhagic, less friable, fibrous plaque

TIA = transient ischemic attack, RIND = reversible ischemic neurologic deficit.

14. What is the stroke rate for asymptomatic stenosis?
- 70–99% stenosis: stroke risk, 5.7% (1.9% annual risk)
- 50–70% stenosis: stroke risk, 3.6%

15. What is more important than the degree of stenosis in determining the rate of major stroke?
Symptomatic carotid lesions (transient ischemic attacks).

16. Is there a benefit in performing carotid endarteretomy (CEA) in patients with asymptomatic carotid lesions?
Of four major trials comparing medical therapy with CEA, three showed a lower rate of stroke with medical therapy than the rate of myocardial infarction and transient ischemic attacks with CEA (i.e., CEA was not beneficial).

17. What did the Asymptomatic Carotid Atherosclerosis Study (ACAS) show?
The ACAS showed that the natural stroke risk/rate for asymptomatic stenosis > 60% was 2.2% annually; with CEA, the rate decreased to 1.0% annually. This 1.2% annual reduction in stroke occurred in minor strokes and not in major strokes

18. Summarize the significance of ulcerated plaques.
- Ulcerated plaques have a superimposed risk of cerebrovascular accident (CVA) on top of the degree of stenosis.

- An incremental increase of stenosis from 75% to 95% with ulcerated plaques increases the 2-year stroke rate from 26.3% (with 75% stenosis) to 73.2% (with 95% stenosis). However, the incremental increase of stenosis from 75% to 95% in nonulcerated plaques had an invariable 2-year stroke rate of 21.0%.

19. What is the significance of the echo-texture of plaque by ultrasound?
Sterpetti et.al. found that echolucent/hetrogenous plaques were associated with a considerably higher rate of stroke than were echogenic plaques.

20. Which is wider—the external or internal carotid artery?
The relative width is age-dependent. Children have a relatively wider internal carotid artery. In the elderly the two arteries are almost equal in diameter at their origins, but the external carotid artery rapidly tapers off due to multiple branches

21. Name two features of the internal carotid artery that are not favorable for endoluminal interventions based on experience of other arterial interventions in other parts of the body.
1. The internal carotid artery is cone-shaped, being wide proximally and narrower distally. This shape poses some difficulty with stent deployment and apposition with the carotid wall.
2. The internal carotid artery is an end-artery leading to the brain, which is an unforgiving organ for embolic material that may be dislodged during endoluminal maneuvers/procedures.

22. Do calcified plaques have an increased risk for stroke?
No. However, circumferential carotid artery plaque responds poorly to angioplasty and may pose difficulty in stent apposition.

23. What is the etiology of stroke?
- Atheroembolic (internal carotid artery, common carotid artery, aortic arch): 80%
- Cardioembolic (left atrium vs. system with patent foramen ovale)
- Intracerebral (subarachnoid hemorrhage, atherosclerotic disease of intracerebral artery)

24. List the modifiable risk factors for stroke.
- Cardiac disease
- Diabetes mellitus
- Hypertension
- Hypercholesterolemia
- Smoking
- Physical inactivity
- Excessive alcohol

25. What is the medical therapy for stroke prevention?
Antiplatelet medication (aspirin, ticlopidine, clopidogrel).

26. Describe the mechanism of action of ticlotpidine and clopidogrel.
Both drugs reduce platelet aggregation, which is mediated by adenosine diphosphate (ADP).

27. Summarize the key results of the North American Symptomatic Carotid Endartrectomy Trial (NASCET).
- Nascet showed a 2-year ipsilateral stroke risk of 9% vs. 26% in patients with 70–99% stenosis who underwent CEA vs. medical therapy
- The periprocedural complication rates (including major and minor strokes, death, or transient ischemic attack) for patients with 70–99% stenosis were 5.8% in the surgical arm and 3.3% in the medical arm.

28. What are the 30-day periprocedural complication rates for carotid angioplasty and stenting (CAS)?

According to the Global Carotid Artery Stent Registry of more than 4800 cases, the periprocedural complication rate is 4.77%:
- Minor stroke: 2.45%
- Major stroke: 1.48%
- Mortality rate: 0.84%

29. What is the gold standard for treating carotid artery atherosclerotic stenosis?

CEA is the gold-standard procedure: It is one of the most successful vascular surgeries.

30. What are the relative indications for CAS?

- Cases in which neck dissection to expose the carotid artery for CEA is difficult
  Prior CEA
  Prior neck dissection (e.g., radical neck dissection)
  Radiation therapy to the neck
- High surgical risk candidates with comorbidities
- Poorly accessible lesions, high up in the skull base (high bifurcation) at the stem of the common carotid artery

31. List in order the technical steps for CAS.

1. Diagnostic angiography (aortic arch and four-vessel angiography, including intracerebral) (Fig. 1)
2. Carotid guiding sheath placement
3. Predilation of the stenosis
4. Stent deployment (Fig. 2)
5. Post-stent dilation

32. How is the long carotid guiding sheath placed?

A stiff exchange, 0.035-inch wire is placed ("parked") in the ipsilateral external carotid artery (a safe artery)—not the internal carotid artery. The 7-French sheath is then advanced over the wire. The sheath tip is placed in the common carotid artery.

FIGURE 1. A patient who underwent carotid surgery presented with recurrent stenosis (**A**). A stent (**B**) was placed across the narrowing with an excellent angiographic result. Stenting was done in a clinical trial with distal embolic protection device.

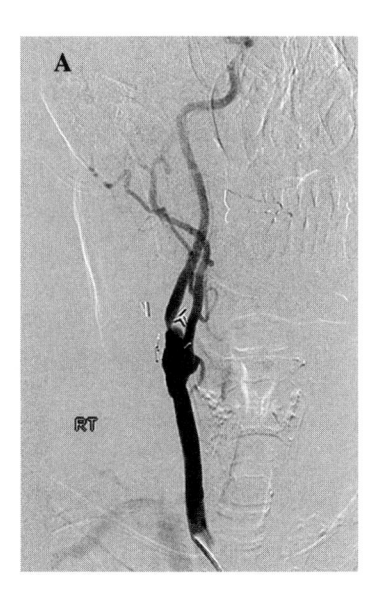

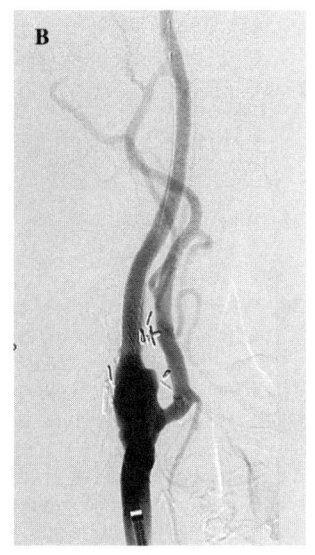

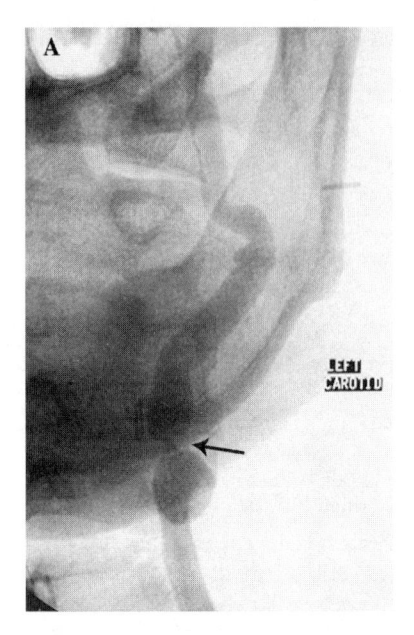

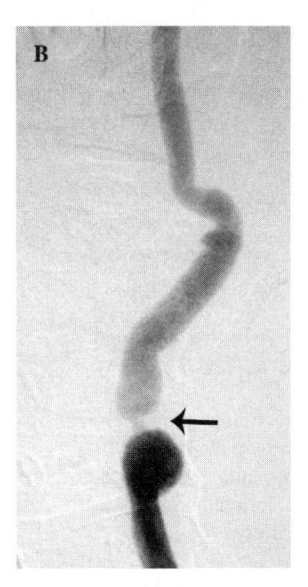

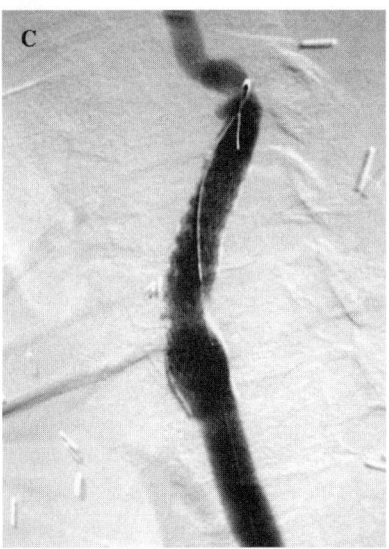

FIGURE 2. Ultrasound revealed recurrent carotid artery stenosis after carotid endarterectomy in a 75-year-old man. Angiogram demonstrated severe stenosis (**A** and **B**), which was treated with excellent results (**C**).

33. What kind of problems can be encountered during the carotid sheath advancement?
- Inability to advance the sheath, especially at the origin of the common carotid artery, due to the angle of the take-off with the arch.
- Placing the sheath in the common carotid artery occasionally displaces the bifurcation upward, which can create kinks in the internal carotid artery, especially if the artery is tortuous.

34. Describe the role of predilation with a balloon prior to stenting.
Predilation opens a significant stenosis so that an undeployed stent can pass the lesion with ease and without friction and thus reduce the risk of fragmentation and embolization. The stent should never be forced across a stenosis.

Carotid Artery Angiography and Intervention

35. If the stent cannot be passed across the lesion with ease, what should be done?

Initial predilation balloon angioplasty is usually done with a 4-mm balloon. If this procedure is not enough, a 5-mm balloon should be used. If the 5-mm balloon is not sufficient, a short balloon-expandable stent is placed to make way for the more definitive self-expanding stent, which is placed across it.

36. How do you avoid stenting across the take-off of the external carotid artery?

You don't avoid it. The stent is frequently pulled across the external carotid artery. It usually does not close the ostium significantly, and the external carotid artery has many collaterals. If its opening is significantly closed, the external carotid artery can be approached through the stent mesh and reopened with a 2-mm balloon over an 0.014 guidewire.

37. What is the technical success rate for CAS?

The technical success rate has been reported as high as 98–99%.

38. Where should the tip of the guidewire be when the definitive stent is deployed?

The tip of the guidewire should be at the level of the skull base but not beyond the petrous portion of the carotid.

39. What kind of problems can be seen by angiography in the internal carotid artery distal to the deployed stent?
- Kinking of the distal internal carotid artery. This problem resolves when the wire and sheath are pulled back.
- Spasm of the distal internal carotid artery. This problem is not uncommon and is due to mechanical irritation of the distal internal carotid artery. It is remedied with 100–200 µg of nitroglycerine through the access sheath.

40. What kind of cardiovascular problems can be encountered in the periprocedural period?

Bradycardia and even transient asystole may occur with balloon dilation and stent deployment of mechanical pressure on baroreceptors. If bradycardia is significant and prolonged, atropine can be given.

41. What causes the transient cognitive and neurologic deficits during the procedure and within the first 48 hours after the procedure?
- Transient cerebral ischemia, which occurs with balloon angioplasty and resolves with deflation of the balloon.
- Contrast encephalopathy, which is due to the increased contrast dose on the ipsilateral cerebral hemisphere.
- Luxury perfusion, which is more common is hypertensive patients with a calcified critical lesion (> 90% stenosis) of the internal carotid artery. Patients recover within 24 hours.

42. Describe the carotid dissections that can occur after CAS. How are they managed?
- **More common:** dissection distal to the deployed stent. This is a serious dissection that can potentially propagate more distally into the intracranial carotid. Therapy is with flexible stent deployment.
- **Less common:** dissection proximal to the deployed stent. This dissection cannot propagate distally if an adequately deployed stent is in place. (Treatment is conservative.)

43. What factors increase the risk of dissection during carotid artery intervention procedure?
- Increased carotid tortuosity and kinking
- Post-stent dilatation with the balloon dilated across the distal end of the stent with high inflation pressure
- Forcing stiff balloons and stiff-ended stent delivery system
- Stenting with a flimsy guidewire with little support

44. What kind of stent should be used in CAS? Why?

Self-expanding stents should be used. They have a continuous radial force that causes the stent to re-expand when compressed externally. Since the carotid arteries are superficial and covered by a thin layer of skin and the stents are vulnerable to extrinsic compression, balloon-expanding stents may become kinked and will not recoil.

45. What is the most significant complication of carotid stenting?

Distal embolization to the brain. Therefore, it is essential to monitor the neurologic status of the patient at every step of the procedure (Figs. 3–6).

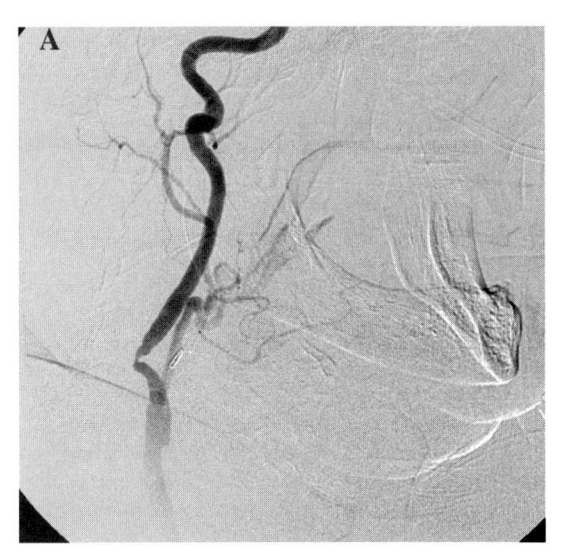

FIGURE 3. A, Recurrent stenosis of the carotid artery 2 years after surgery. **B,** A cerebral protection device (Boston Scientific, Natick, MA) was placed *(arrow)*. Currently no cerebral protection device has been approved by the Food and Drug Administration. **C,** In the present patient, the stent was placed with good angiographic results. The completion angiogram was done before the device was removed.

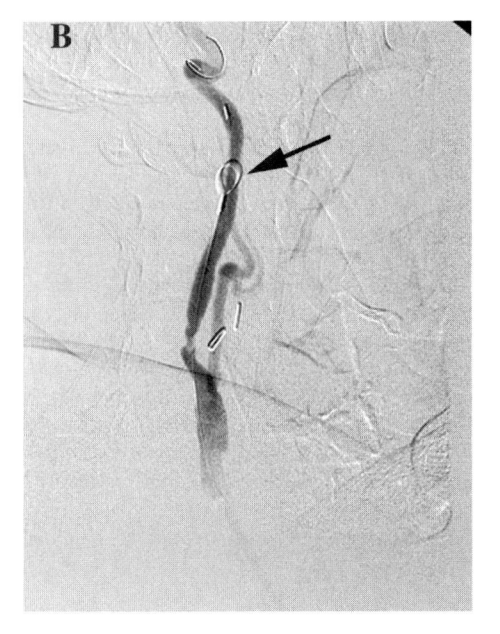

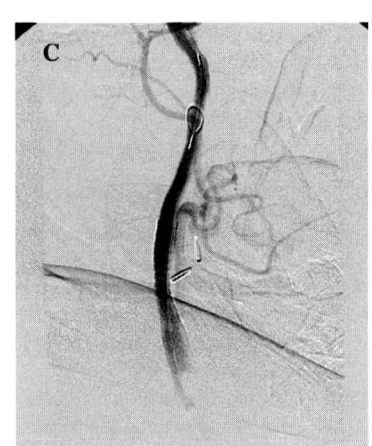

Carotid Artery Angiography and Intervention

FIGURE 4. EPI filterwire EX is currently in clinical trials as a cerebral protection device. It is currently approved by the Food and Drug Administration for use in the coronary system. The theory behind all cerebral protection devices is to capture embolic material during wire manipulation, stent deployment, and balloon dilatation to avoid stroke. (Courtesy of Boston Scientific Corporation.)

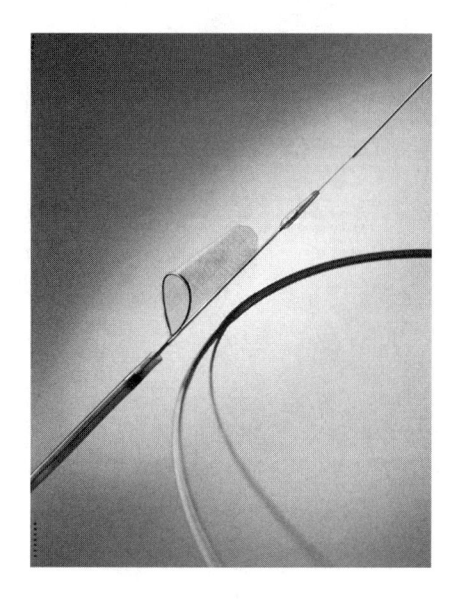

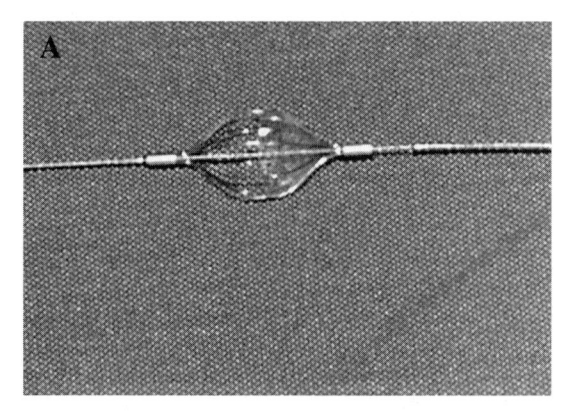

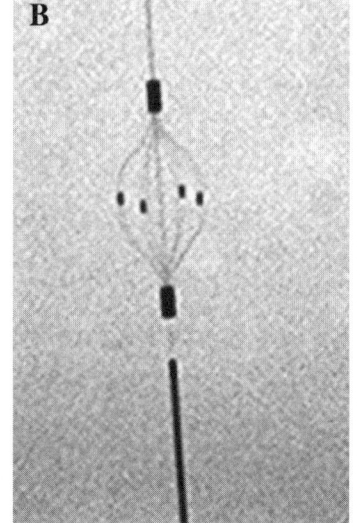

FIGURE 5. Photograph (**A**) and x-ray (**B**) of the Angioguard (Cortis, Cincinnati, OH) cerebral protection device. This device is currently in clinical trials.

46. List the indications for CAS.
- Symptomatic atherosclerotic carotid disease
- Carotid artery dissection
- Carotid artery pseudoaneurysm exclusion
- True carotid artery aneurysm

47. How frequent is stent thrombosis in CAS?
Stent thrombosis in CAS is rare (< 1/600).

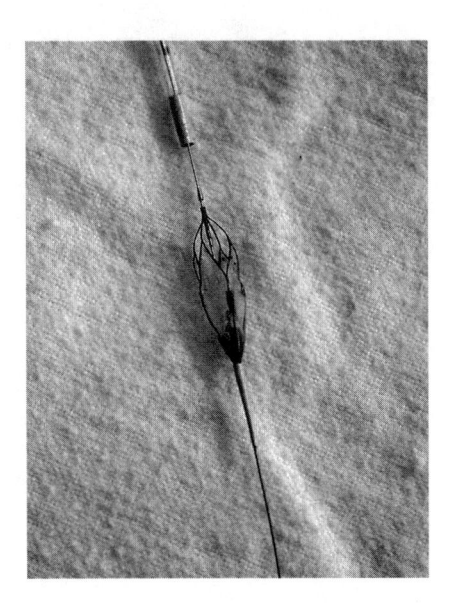

FIGURE 6. The Accunet (Guidant, Indianapolis, IN) protection device was used in the Carotid Revascularization Endarterectomy versus Stenting Trial (CREST). This lesion was stented 2 years after surgery. The lesion was smooth and thought to be at low risk for embolization. Note the debris within the protection device.

48. What is the nature of materials that embolize to the brain?
Fragments caught in a filter were examined by microscope and found to be thrombus/fibrin, plaque (cholesterol), and aggregated blood cells (white blood cells and red blood cells).

49. List the methods of neuroembolic protection.
- Distal occlusion (balloon)
- Proximal occlusion (balloon)
- Distal filters

50. Name the features of an ideal neuroembolic protection device.
- Must be reliable
- Must make the procedure unobtrusive
- Must add minimal complexity and minimal time to the procedure
- Must be easy to use with no added risks to the patient

51. How do distal occlusion devices work?
They occlude the internal carotid artery distal to the stenosis and cause stasis of blood flow, thus preventing embolic material from going to the brain. Once the CAS is performed, the blood with the embolic material is aspirated. Some people advocate additional flushing of the remaining embolic material into the external carotid artery. The balloon is then deflated and blood flow is restored.

52. Describe the mechanism of distal filter neuroembolic protection.
The filter is placed distal to the lesion and on the guidewire. The filter catches the embolic material without impeding the antegrade flow. After CAS, the filter is closed and removed inside the sheath.

53. Name some distal neuroembolic protection filters under clinical trial.
- MedNova Neuroshield (MedNova Inc., Ireland)
- EPI filter wire (Boston Scientific)
- Angioguard filter
- Sci-Med Sentinel

- ArteriA Bate floating catheter
- E-Trgs Filter
- Scion Filter

54. What are the most common sites for true carotid artery aneurysms?
Most common site: common carotid artery, especially near the bifurcation (fusiform aneurysm).
Second most common site: mid-to-distal internal carotid artery (saccular aneurysm).

55. List causes of carotid aneurysms.
- Atherosclerotic disease
- Prior carotid or neck surgery
- Trauma
- Syphilis

BIBLIOGRAPHY

1. Connors JJ III: The nature of cervical carotid stenosis. Techn Vasc Intervent Radiol 3(2):62–64, 2000.
2. Gray WA: Procedural techniques of carotid stenting. Techn Vasc Intervent Radiol 3(2):86–91, 2000.
3. Ohki T, Marin ML, Lyon RT, et al: Human ex-vivo carotid artery bifurcation stenting: Correlation of lesion characteristics with embolic potential. J Vasc Surg 27:463–471, 1998.
4. Roubin GS: Carotid stenting: Clinical approach. J Vasc Intervent Radiol 11:326–331, 2000.
5. Sterpetti AV, Schultz RD, Feldhaus RJ, et al: Ultrasonographic features of carotid plaque and the risk of subsequent neurological deficits. Surgery 104:652–660, 1998.
6. Taylor DW: Clinical advisory: Carotid endartrectomy for patients with asymptomatic internal carotid artery stenosis. The Asymptomatic Carotid Atherosclerosis Study Group. Neurol Sci 129:76–77, 1995.
7. Taylor DW, Barnett HJM: Beneficial effect of carotid endartrectomy in symptomatic patients with high-grade stenosis. North American Symptomatic Carotid Endartrectomy Trial Collaborators. N Engl J Med 325:445–453, 1991.
8. Wholey MH, Jarmolowski CR, Wholey Mark, Eles GR: Carotid artery stent placement: Ready for prime time? J Vasc Intervent Radiol 14:1–10, 2003.
9. Williams JS: Mechanical devices used for carotid stenting. Tech Vasc Intervent Radiol 3(2);102–113, 2000.
10. Yadav JS, Roubin GS, Lyer S, et al: Elective stenting of the extracranial carotid arteries. Circulation 95:376–381, 1997.

13. BRONCHIAL ARTERY ANGIOGRAPHY AND INTERVENTION
Arun Basu, MD

1. **Bronchial arteries are nutrient arteries to which three end organs?**
   The lungs, esophagus and part of the pericardium are the three end organs of the bronchial arteries.

2. **What are the most common parent vessels of the primary bronchial arteries bilaterally?**
   Although the origin of the bronchial arteries varies, in 78% of people the **right bronchial artery** arises from either the first aortic intercostal artery (intercostobronchial artery) or a trunk shared with the left bronchial artery from the dorsa lateral aspect of the descending aorta. In 67% of cases, it courses posterior to the esophagus. The **left bronchial tree** is rooted by two arteries that arise from the descending aorta: one near the origin/trunk and the second, the inferior bronchial artery, from an inferior portion of the aorta. The three bronchial arteries originate between the levels of the fourth and sixth thoracic vertebral bodies.

3. **What is the clinical definition of massive hemoptysis?**
   250–500 ml of blood in a 24-hour period.

4. **In the setting of massive hemoptysis, what is the most common cause of mortality?**
   Asphyxiation, not exsanguination.

5. **What are the most common causes of massive hemoptysis?**
   Chronic inflammatory processes such as cavitary tuberculosis, bronchiectasis, aspergilloma (Fig. 1), and cystic fibrosis (Fig. 2) are common causes of massive hemoptysis. Less commonly massive hemoptysis may be caused by tumors or vascular malformations.

6. **Which vascular systems are most commonly involved in massive hemoptysis?**
   Massive hemoptysis largely originates from the bronchial system or recruited systemic circulation.

7. **The pulmonary arterial system is involved in massive hemoptysis in approximately what percentage of cases?**
   The pulmonary arterial system is involved in approximately less than 10% of all cases of massive hemoptysis.

8. **In approximately what percentage of cases of massive hemoptysis are nonbronchial arteries involved? Which arteries are they?**
   Approximately 35% of cases involve nonbronchial arteries, most commonly an intercostal artery, a branch of the internal mammary, subclavian (Fig. 3) or axillary artery, or a branch of the inferior phrenic artery.

9. **After identifying the source of bleeding, why must an interventionalist review the bronchial arteriogram meticulously before initiating bronchial artery embolization therapy?**
   Although the anterior spinal artery (the artery of Adamkiewicz [see Fig. 2B]) usually originates from the aorta at a lower point than the bronchial artery trunks, it is not uncommon to identify spinal radicular branches from the bronchial artery.

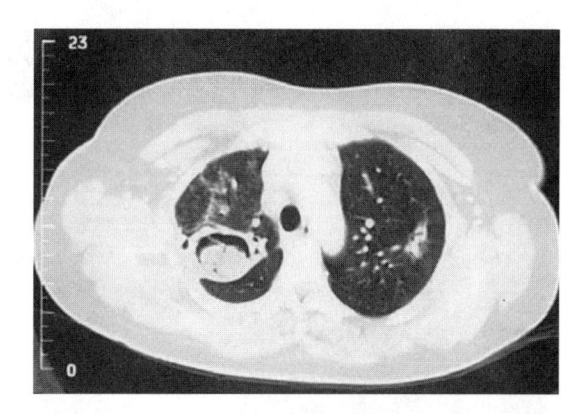

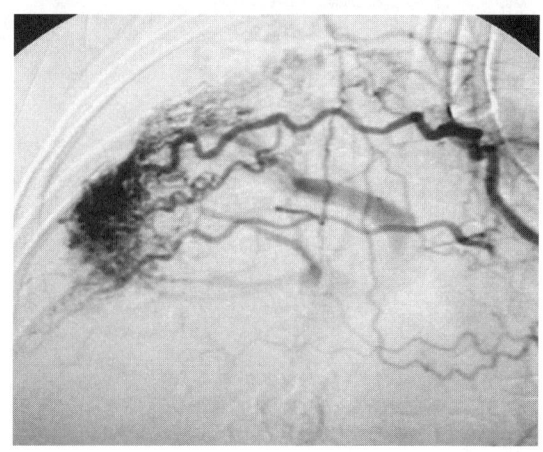

FIGURE 1. A, CT of the chest depicting aspergilloma in right upper lobe. **B,** Bronchial angiogram in the same patient showing vascular supply to the aspergilloma. **C,** Angiogram after embolization of the bronchial artery supplying the aspergilloma with polyvinyl alcohol (PVA) particles of 300–500 m and multiple coils.

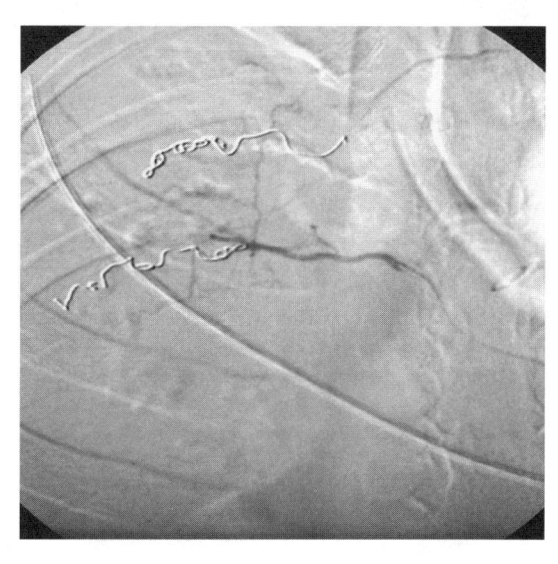

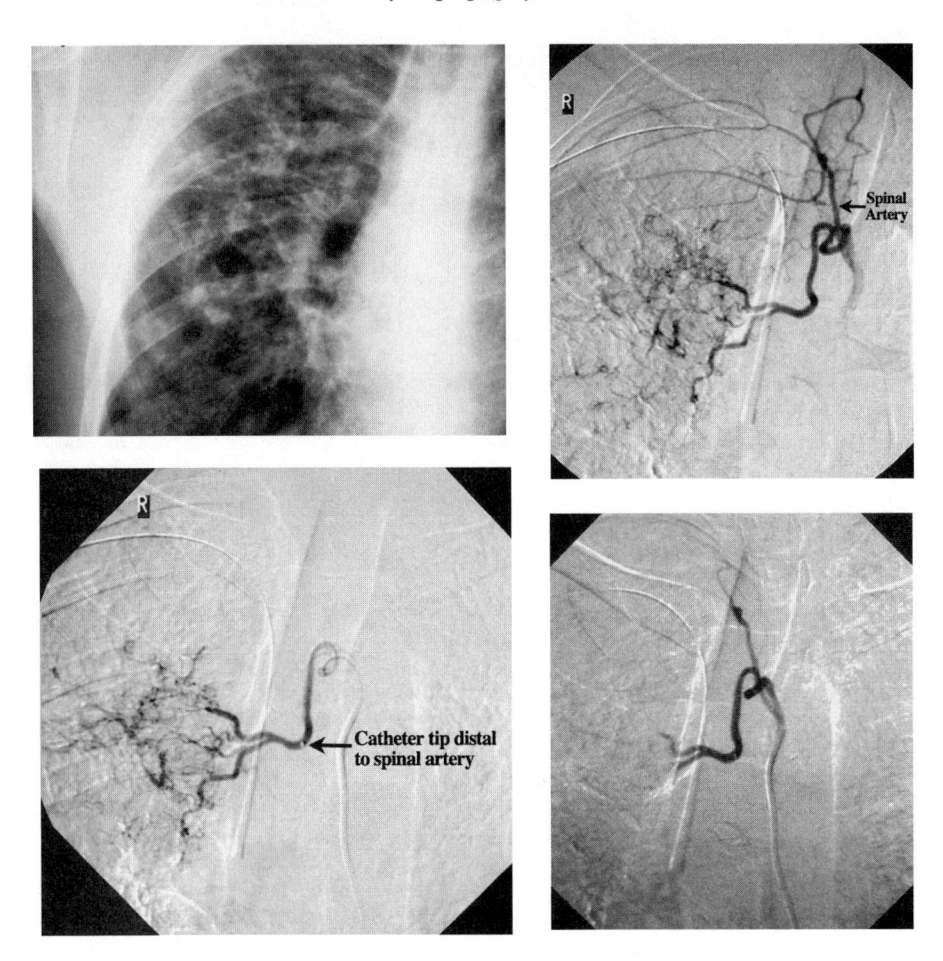

FIGURE 2. A, Chest x-ray depicting typical cystic fibrosis findings. **B,** Bronchial angiogram showing the abnormal tortuous right bronchial artery as well as the spinal artery. **C,** The catheter is advanced beyond the origin of the spinal artery prior to embolization. **D,** After embolization with 300- to 500-μ polyvinyl alcohol (PVA) particles, showing complete occlusion of the artery.

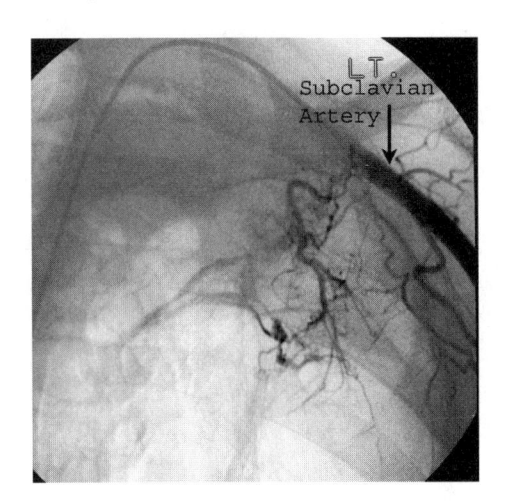

FIGURE 3. Left subclavian artery giving a branch to left upper lobe that causes the bleed in this patient.

10. What technical modification must an interventionalist perform in patients with spinal radicular branches of the hemorrhaging bronchial artery?

The interventionalist must advance the microcatheter distal to the branch take-off to avoid catastrophic morbidity associated with occlusion of arterial supply to the spinal cord (see Figs. 2B and 2C).

11. What other modalities may be used to identify the source of massive hemoptysis? How useful are they?

Bronchoscopy, radionuclide bleeding scans, and clinical history. Often the patient is able to sense which lung is the source of bleeding. Bronchoscopy and radionuclide bleeding scans are of limited utility in the setting of massive hemoptysis.

12. How often is contrast extravasation from a bronchial artery seen on angiogram in the clinical setting of hemoptysis?

In approximately 22% of cases contrast extravasation is useful in identifying an active bleed (Fig. 4).

13. What are the four most common signs on angiogram of an active bronchial arterial bleed?
1. Hypervascularity
2. Shunting from the bronchial artery to the pulmonary artery
3. Aneurysms of the bronchial artery
4. Occlusion of bronchial artery branches

14. True of false: In patients with massive hemoptysis and diffuse cystic fibrosis disease or multilobar bronchiectasis, embolization of any or all identifiable bronchial artery branches is recommended.

True. Collateral pulmonary branches will subsequently provide the lung's nutrient supply.

15. True or False: It is feasible to embolize any identifiable bronchial artery branch in the setting of massive hemoptysis with no identifiable source of bleeding.

True (see question 14).

16. In the absence of an identifiable site of bronchial artery bleeding, what vessel other than the pulmonary arteries should be angiographically evaluated for extra-bronchial arterial supply?

Bilateral subclavian arteries should be angiographically evaluated for extra-bronchial arterial supply.

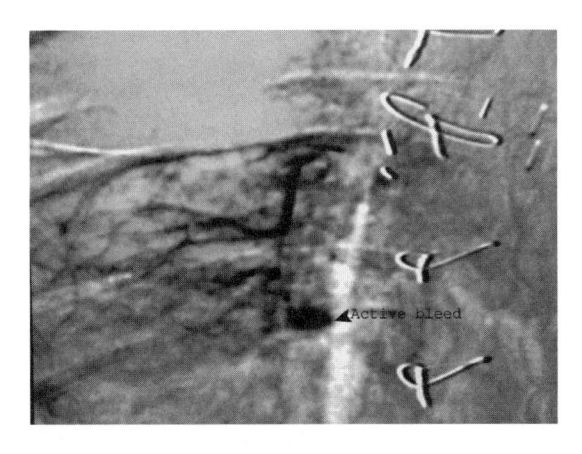

FIGURE 4. Right bronchial angiogram depicting active bleeding.

17. What agents may be used for bronchial artery occlusion?
Particulate emboli are the agents of choice. Particles of polyvinyl alcohol and gelform should range in size from 300 μ to 500 μ. Because gelfoam particles are at least partially resorbed in 30 days time, polyvinyl alcohol provides a longer-term occlusion. As absolute alcohol, boiling contrast or particulate powders cause occlusion at the smallest arterial level and lead to tissue necrosis, which can cause morbidity in the form of bronchial, esophageal, or spinal infarcts. Coils are often used for focal larger vessels; after their use, collateral formation soon follows.

18. Early rebleeding occurs in what percentage of patients? How is rebleeding managed?
About 15% of patients experience rebleeding. In this setting embolization revision should be performed along with an exhaustive search for systemic collaterals, contributing pulmonary artery branches, and additional bronchial arteries.

19. What percentage of patients experience late rebleeding? How are they managed?
About 20% of patients experience late rebleeding. Such patients may be managed by bronchial artery embolization revision. Medical management of the specific inflammatory etiology has been proved to be the most effective factor in minimizing this morbidity.

20. True or False: Patients with aspergillomas have a 50% risk of rebleeding.
True.

21. True or False: The first-line treatment choice for refractory medically managed massive hemoptysis is bronchial artery embolization followed by surgical intervention.
True.

22. What other possible therapeutic interventions may involve bronchial artery arteriography?
Delivery of chemotherapy to pulmonary masses is another application for therapeutic intervention. Viral vectors for gene therapy in genetic disorders such as cystic fibrosis are in trial for arterial delivery following vascular endothelial growth factor and post-delivery subtotal occlusion to enhance vascular permeability.

23. True or False: Bronchial artery embolization can be used in the setting of massive hemoptysis in patients with cystic fibrosis.
True.

24. Name two other sources of bleeding from the bronchial system.
Arteriovenous malformations (Fig. 5) and Rasmussen aneurysms are much less common sources of bleeding in the bronchial system.

25. What is a common angiographic finding in the bronchial arterial system of patients with chronic pulmonary disease?
Hypertrophy of the bronchial arteries with subsequent communication to the pulmonary artery system is a common finding.

26. What is the normal diameter of a bronchial artery?
Three millimeters is the normal diameter of a bronchial artery.

27. What will selective intubation of the nonhemorrhaging bronchus or balloon occlusion of the bronchus of the hemorrhaging lung accomplish?
Asphyxiation due to aspiration of blood may be prevented.

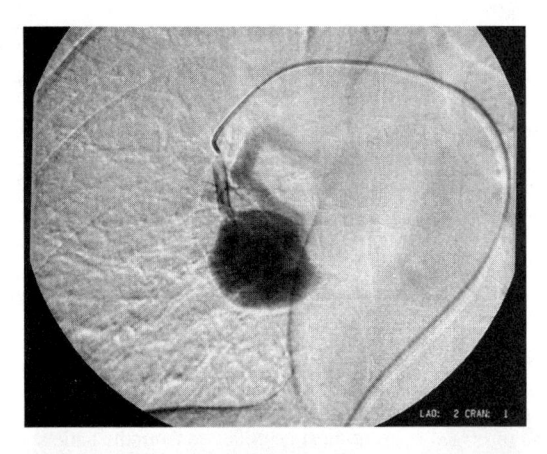

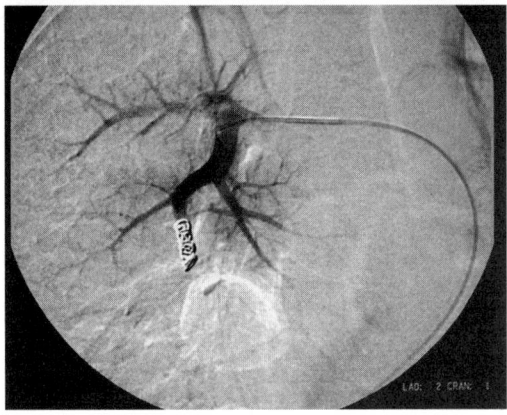

FIGURE 5. A, Right lower lobe pulmonary arteriovenous malformation (AVM). **B,** After embolization of AVM with multiple coils.

28. In the setting of massive hemoptysis with localized bronchial bleeding, is hypertrophy of a bronchial artery evidence enough to proceed with embolization in the absence of other contraindications?
Yes.

29. True or false: Bronchial artery embolization does not infarct lung tissue because the lung has a second circulatory system, the pulmonary arteries.
False. In sheep and dog models, occlusion of the bronchial artery system led to some pulmonary infarction; however, this complication was noted to be small because pulmonary collaterals eased its effects.

30. What is the most common complication associated with bronchial artery embolization?
Chest pain occurs in nearly 10% of patients. The pain lasts only a few hours after the procedure.

31. True of False: Bronchial artery embolization cannot be used in the setting of HIV pulmonary disease.
False. The HIV population has in fact dramatically increased the pool of patients who benefit from such interventions.

32. Who conducted the first recorded bronchial artery embolization procedures?
Lubchenko of Moscow in the 1970s and Ulflacker of Brazil in the 1980s.

33. What are the most commonly done preprocedure investigations?
Imaging includes a chest radiograph, computed tomography (CT) of the chest, or possibly high-resolution CT. In some settings bronchoscopy is performed. Platelets, complete blood count, and coagulation factors are often assessed. The acid-fast bacillus (AFB) test is usually also performed.

34. True or false: A massive localized dye injection to arteries feeding the spinal cord can result in paralysis.
True.

35. Describe the preprocedure protocol.
Written and verbal informed consent must be obtained from the patient or guardian. The patient's airway must be adequately managed. Intravenous access must be gained. The patient's blood type must be typed and cross-matched. Procedure monitoring, such as oxygen saturation, blood pressure and heart rate, must be maintained. Often a baseline neurologic exam may be prudent to help evaluate any postprocedure neurologic morbidity.

BIBLIOGRAPHY

1. Bakhai A., Sheridan DJ, Coutelle CC: Bronchial artery delivery of viral vectors for gene delivery in cystic fibrosis: Superior to airway delivery? BMC Pulm Med 2:2, 2002.
2. Bergman RA, Thompson SA, Afifi AK, Saadeh FA: Compendium of Human Anatomic Variation: Catalog, Atlas and World Literature. Baltimore, Urban & Schwarzenberg, 1988.
3. Cauldwell EA, Siekert RG, Lininger RE, Anson BJ: The bronchial arteries. An anatomic study of 150 human cadavers. Surg Gynecol Obstet 86:395–412, 1948.
4. Cohen AM, Doershuk CF, Stern RC: Bronchial artery embolization to control hemoptysis in cystic fibrosis. Radiology 175:401–405, 1990.
5. Ivanick MJ, Thorwarth W, Donohue J, et al: Infarction of the left mainstem bronchus: A complication of bronchial artery embolization. AJR 141:535–537, 1983.
6. Katoh O, Kishikawa T, Yamada H, et al: Recurrent bleeding after arterial embolization in patients with hemoptysis. Chest 97:541–546, 1990.
7. Keller FS, Rosch J, Loflin TG, et al: Nonbronchial systemic collateral arteries: Significance in percutaneous embolotherapy for hemoptysis. Radiology 164:687–692, 1987.
8. Liebow AA: Patterns of origin and distribution of the major bronchial arteries in man. Am J Anat 117:19–32, 1965.
9. Michalewski K: Topography of the bronchial branches of the aorta. Folia Morphol Warsaw 28:417–441, 1969.
10. Pinet F, Froment JC: Angiography and embolization of systemic thoracic arteries. In Abrams HL (ed): Abrams Angiography, vol. 1, 3rd ed. Little Brown & Company, Boston, 1983, pp 845–867.
11. Rabkin JE, Astafiev VI, Gothman LN, Grigorjev YG: Transcatheter embolization in the management of pulmonary hemorrhage. Radiology 1987;163:361–365, 1987.
12. Stoll JF, Bettman MA: Bronchial artery embolization to control hemoptysis: A review. Cardiovasc Intervent Radiol 11:263–269, 1988.
13. Tobin CE: The bronchial arteries and their connections with other vessels in the human lung. Surg Gynecol Obstet 95:741–750, 1952.
14. Uflacker R, Kaemmerer A, Picon PD, et al: Bronchial artery embolization in the management of hemoptysis: Technical aspects and long term results Radiology 157:637–644, 1985.

14. RENOVASCULAR DISEASE AND INTERVENTION

Kalpesh C. Patel, MD

1. **List the clinical, anatomic, and physiologic indications for renal artery intervention.**
   Clinical indications
   - Hypertension that is severe or difficult to control
   - Recent-onset or progressive moderate to severe renal dysfunction
   - Recurrent pulmonary edema

   Anatomic indications
   - Stenosis > 60% in diameter
   - Post-stenotic dilatation
   - Collateral circulation
   - Decreased renal size: length difference ≥ 1.5 cm or decrease in renal length ≥ 1 cm

   Physiologic indications
   - Positive radionuclide scan
   - Renal vein renin assay
   - Duplex ultrasound (including resistive index)
   - Transstenotic pressure gradient: 10% peak systolic arterial pressure or 5% mean arterial pressure

2. **Summarize the normal renal vascular anatomy.**
   Aorta > renal artery > anterior and posterior division > segmental arteries > interlobar arteries > arcuate arteries.
   - 65%: single vessel
   - 35%: aberrant vascular supply (common in malrotated and horseshoe kidney)

3. **What arterial variants may arise from the renal arteries?**
   - Gonadal arteries arise from renal arteries in 20% of cases.
   - Inferior phrenic artery occasionally arises from the renal artery.
   - Inferior adrenal arteries often arise from the renal artery.

4. **Define renal artery stenosis (RAS).**
   RAS is defined as narrowing of the main renal artery or one of its branches. Stenoses less than 50% are usually insignificant, whereas those greater than 70% are quite often significant.

5. **Give the incidence and prevalence of RAS.**
   Renal vascular disease accounts for less than 1% of all cases of hypertension in people who have moderately increased blood pressure. But in certain high-risk groups, renal vascular disease may be the cause of 10% to 40 % of all hypertension. RAS due to fibromuscular dyspalsia (FMD) occurs almost exclusively in women aged 30–40 years and rarely affects African Americans or Asians.

6. **List the risk factors for atherosclerotic RAS.**
   - Carotid artery disease
   - Coronary artery disease
   - Diabetes mellitus
   - Hypertension
   - Obesity

- Old age
- Peripheral vascular disease (vascular disease in the extremities, e.g., the legs)
- Smoking
- Familial history of FMD-related RAS

7. List the noninvasive screening tests for RAS and their respective sensitivities and specificities.
- Duplex ultrasound: sensitivity, 89%; specificity, 97%
- Renal nuclear scintigraphy with captopril: sensitivity, 84%; specificity, 92%
- Renal computed tomographic angiography (CTA): sensitivity, 92%; specificity, 83%
- Renal magnetic resonance angiography (MRA; Fig. 1): sensitivity, 98%; specificity, 100%

8. List the two most common causes of RAS.
Atherosclerosis (70%; Fig. 2) and fibromuscular dyspalsia (25%; Fig. 3).

9. In what percentage of patients is RAS the cause of hypertension?
5%

10. List the diagnostic and therapeutic indications for renal angiography.
Diagnostic indications
- Renovascular hypertension
- Tumors (Fig. 4)
- Transplant

Therapeutic indications
- Percutaneous transluminal angioplastpy (PTA) or stent placement secondary to renovascular hypertension or embolization

11. What findings suggest that RAS is hemodynamically significant?
- Luminal stenosis greater than 50%
- Post-stenotic dilatation

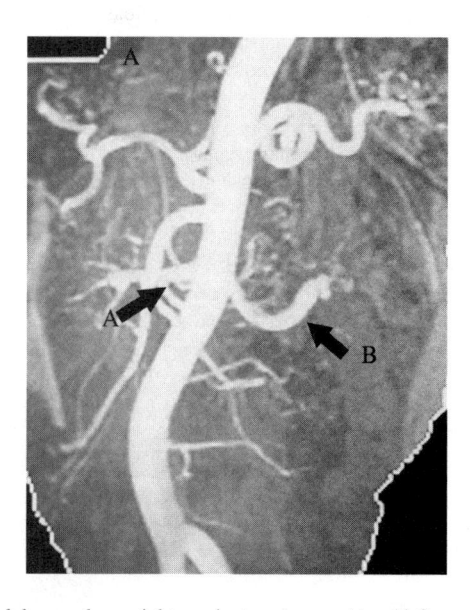

FIGURE 1. MRA of the abdomen shows right renal artery *(arrow A)* and left renal artery *(arrow B)*.

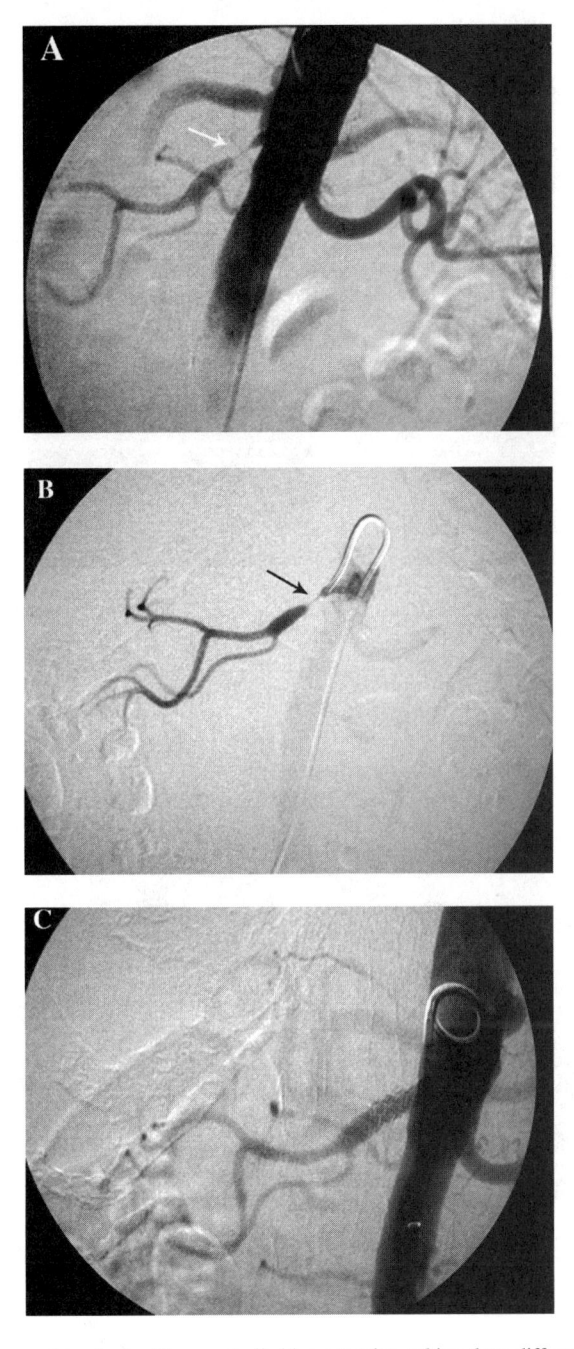

FIGURE 2. A 49-year-old patient with uncontrolled hypertension, taking three different medications, presents for a renal angiogram. Abdominal aortogram (**A**) and selective right angiogram (**B**) demonstrated preocclusive stenosis. The stenosis was treated with percutaneous transluminal angioplasty and stenting with excellent results (**C**). The patient's blood pressure was 209/98 mmHg before the procedure but immediately dropped to 160/93 mmHg after the procedure.

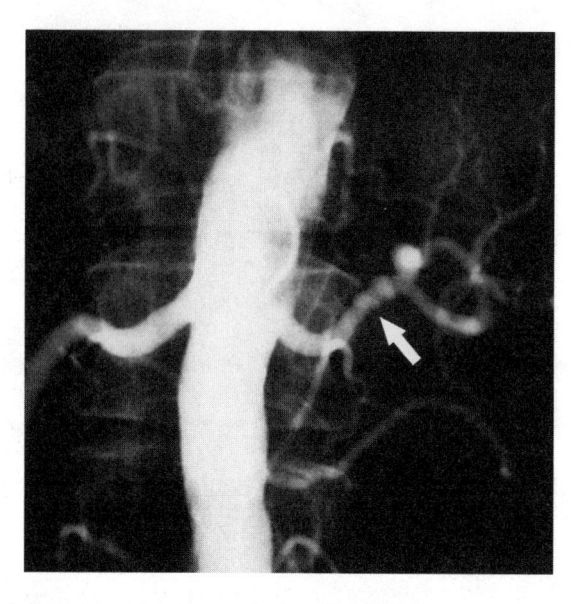

FIGURE 3. Abdominal aortogram demonstrates "string of beads" appearance of the left renal artery consistent with fibromuscular dysplasia *(arrow)*.

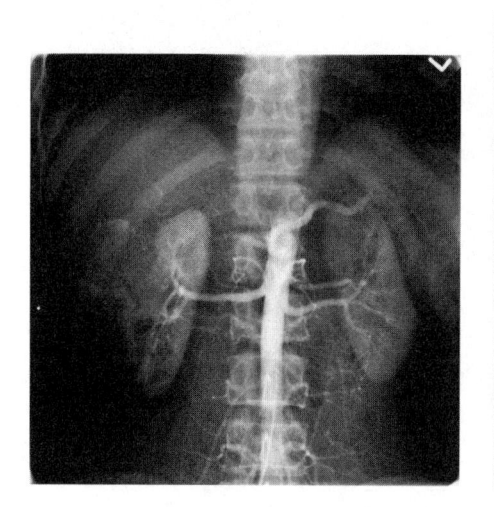

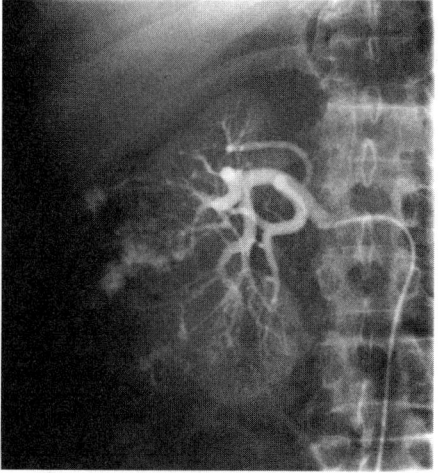

FIGURE 4. Two patients (**A** and **B**) with neovascularity consistent with a tumor.

- Peak systolic pressure gradient > 15%
- Presence of collaterals

12. Describe a typical ostial lesion.

A typical ostial lesion may be concentric or eccentric, smooth or irregular. Lesions are often bilateral and occur in the proximal 2 cm of the renal arteries (Fig. 5).

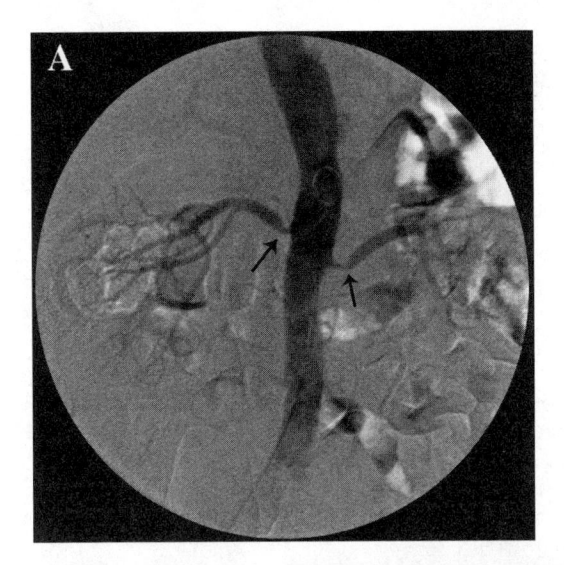

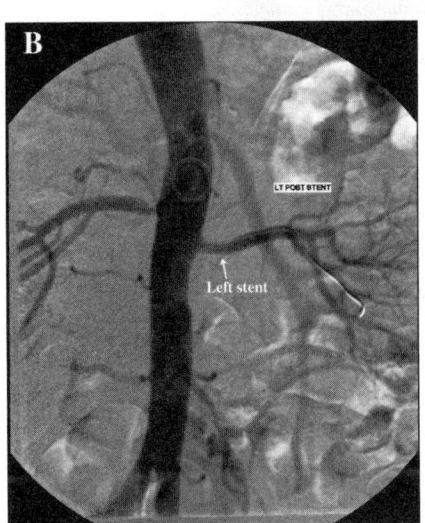

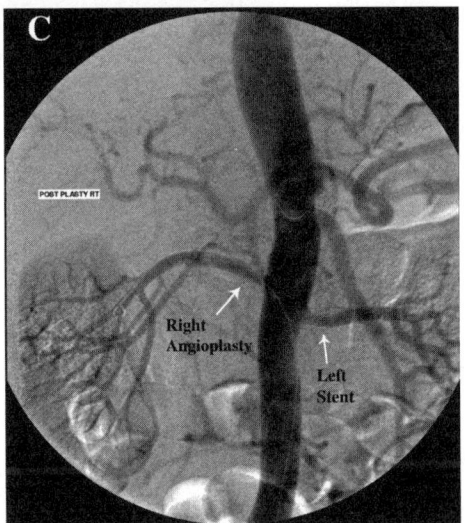

FIGURE 5. A, Abdominal angiogram in a patient with renal hypertension demonstrating bilateral proximal renal artery stenosis (arrows). **B,** Angiogram shows good results after placement of a stent in the left renal artery. **C,** Final angiogram after left renal stent and right percutaneous transluminal angioplasty demonstrates good results.

13. **List the absolute and relative contraindications for renal angioplasty.**
    Absolute contraindications
    - Medically unstable patient
    - Insignificant stenosis

    Relative contraindications
    - Long segment occlusion of the renal arteries
    - Aortic atherosclerotic plaque extending into the proximal renal artery
    - Extensively diseased aorta leading to the possibility of embolization

14. **What types of catheters are used most commonly for renal angiography?**
    - Shepherd's crook catheter
    - Omni selective catheter
    - C2 catheter

15. **What method is used to gain femoral access for renal angiography?**
    Seldinger technique.

16. **Describe the procedure for renal angioplasty.**
    1. Determine whether the procedure is truly indicated.
    2. Gain arterial access using the Seldinger technique.
    3. Place 7-French sheath in common femoral artery.
    4. Administer 3,000 units of heparin intravenously.
    5. Obtain diagnostic aortogram with pigtail or tennis racquet catheter
    6. Select main renal artery using SOS-Omni selective catheter.
    7. Place Wholey guidewire into distal renal artery and advance catheter over lesion.
    8. Predilate main artery with 4- or 5-mm balloon, usually 2 cm long.
    9. Advance preselected stent over wire into renal artery and position to appropriate location.
    10. Inflate balloon to deploy stent.
    11. Obtain renal arteriogram by injection through guiding catheter.

17. **What is the technical success rate for the procedure?**
    80–90%.

18. **What is the therapeutic success rate?**
    For FMD, 90–100%; for atherosclerosis, 80%.

19. **What is the most important factor determining recurrence of stenosis?**
    Postangioplasty residual diameter stenosis of 30% or greater.

20. **List the common complications of the angioplasty with their incidence.**
    - Local thrombus (1%)
    - Arterial rupture (1–2%; Fig. 6)
    - Angioplasty related nonocclusive dissection (2–4%)
    - Guidewire dissection (4%)
    - Renal failure (1.5- 6.0%)
    - Nephrectomy (1%)
    - Segmental renal infarction and perinephric hematoma (3%; Fig. 7)

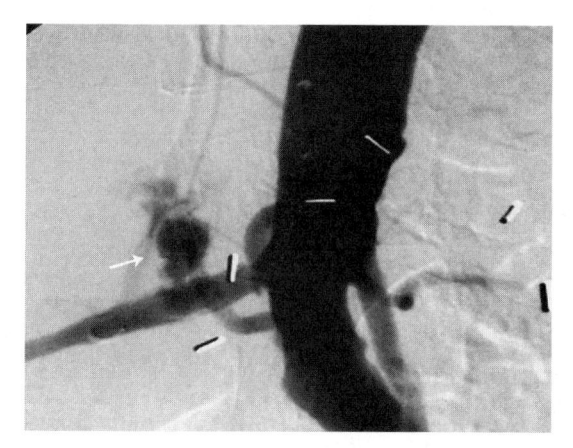

FIGURE 6. A patient with right renal artery stenosis underwent percutaneous transluminal angioplasty followed by active extravasations. A stent was placed, but the above angiogram shows no improvement. The patient was then taken to the operating room, where he was successfully treated.

Renovascular Disease and Intervention   105

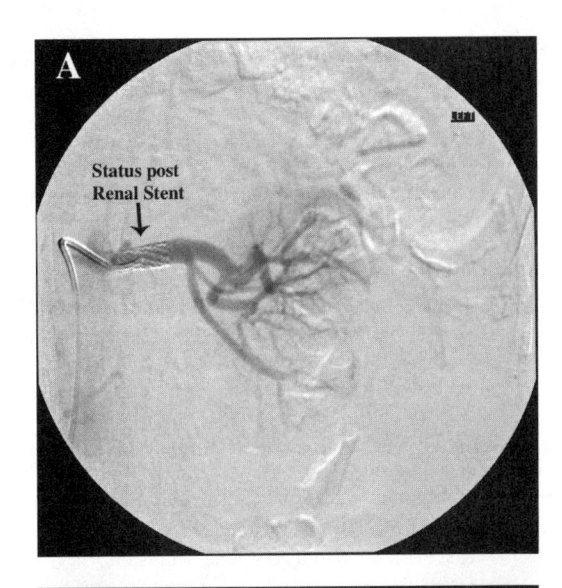

FIGURE 7. A, Angiogram demonstrates status after deployment of left renal stent *(arrow).* **B,** Selective angiogram shows renal parenchymal defect *(arrows).* **C,** CT obtained shows the stent *(black arrow)* as well as perinephric hemorrhage *(white arrow).* This complication results from passage of the guidewire distally into the renal parenchyma during stent placement.

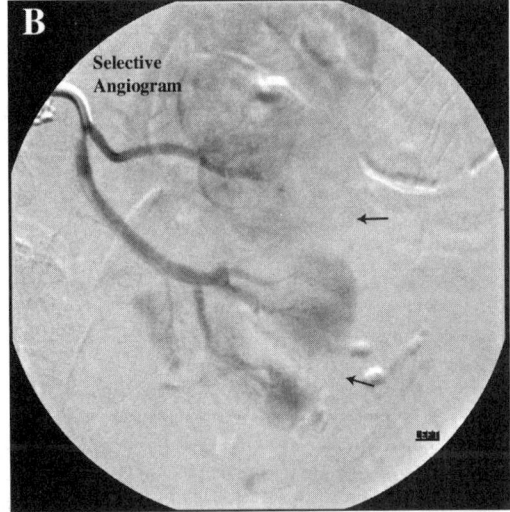

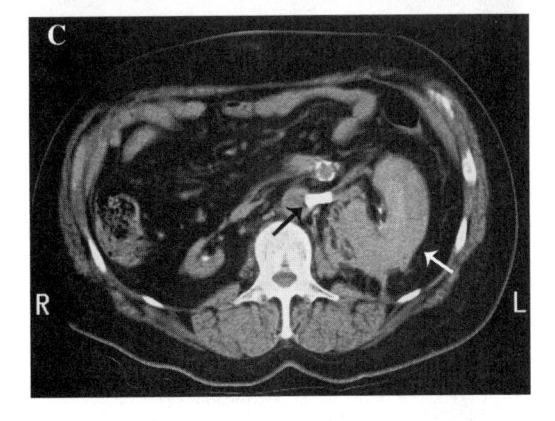

21. **List the indications for renal artery stenting.**
    - Recurrent stenosis after angioplasty
    - Ostial renal artery stenosis.
    - Postoperative stenosis (renal artery bypass and transplant renal arteries)
    - Highly eccentric renal artery stenosis.
    - Acute failure of percutaneous transluminal renal angioplasty (PTRA)
    - Renal artery size of 4–8 mm
    - Disease limited to main renal artery.

22. **List the contraindications for renal artery stenting.**
    Relative: branch vessel disease with lesion length exceeding 2 cm.
    Absolute: kidney size less than 6 cm, small renal artery size (< 4 mm), diffuse intrarenal vascular disease, noncompliant lesion, vessel rupture during PTA.

23. **What type of stent is most commonly used for renal artery stenosis?**
    Balloon expandable.

24. **List the indications for stent placement.**
    - Recanalization of a complete occlusion
    - Ostial stenosis
    - Suboptimal PTRA outcome (residual stenosis, dissection)
    - Early restenosis after PTRA

25. **What is the most common cause of restenosis after stent placement?**
    Restenosis after stent implantation is usually caused by neointimal hyperplasia (Fig. 8).

26. **List the types of complications with renal artery stenting.**
    Catheter-related complications
    - Flow-limiting dissection
    - Guidewire vessel perforation
    - Femoral pseudoaneurysm
    - Groin hematoma requiring surgery, transfusion, or prolonged hospitalization

    Stenting-related complications
    - Distal malpositioning of the stent with > 50% residual stenosis
    - Protrusion of the stent into the aorta by > 2 mm
    - Stent dislodgement with nontarget vessel deployment or requiring surgical removal.

    Related to either catherization or stenting
    - Atheroembolization: livido reticularis, eosinophilia, and/or decreased renal function
    - Spasm
    - Thrombosis

27. **What is the most common cause of renovascular hypertension in children and young adults?**
    FMD of the renal artery.

28. **Describe the typical appearance of FMD in a renal angiogram.**
    "String of beads" = alternating areas of stenosis (weblike constrictions) (Fig. 9).

29. **What is the treatment of choice for FMD?**
    Transluminal balloon angioplasty (90% success rate with low restenosis rate) (Fig. 10).

30. **Define polyarteritis nodosa (PAN).**
    PAN is defined as systemic necrotizing vasculitis of small and medium-sized muscular arteries characterized by necrotizing granulomas of all wall layers.

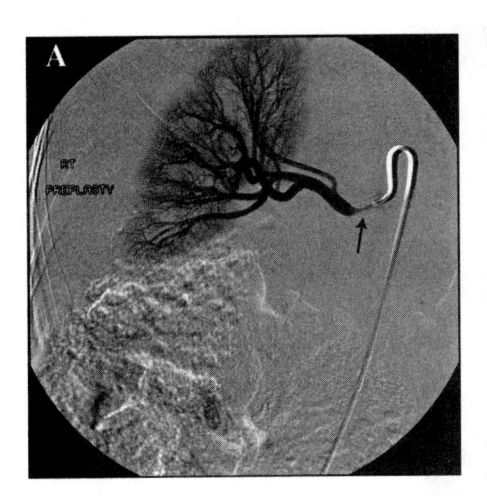

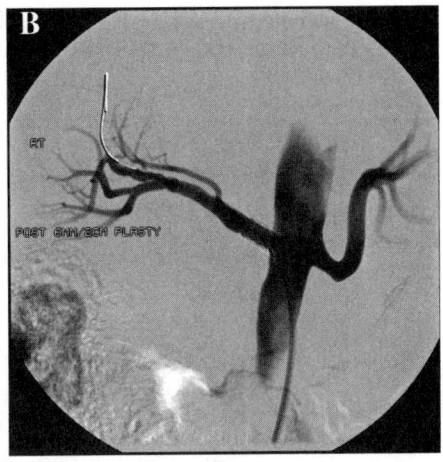

FIGURE 8. A 50-year-old man with a diagnosis of renal hypertension, successfully treated in the past, presented with recurrent hypertension. Renal artery ultrasound suggested stent stenosis. **A,** Selective right renal angiogram demonstrates stent restenosis *(arrow).* **B,** Angiogram after successful angioplasty.

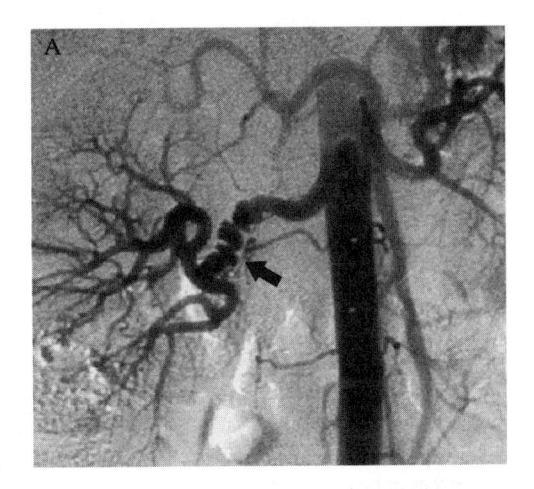

FIGURE 9. Abdominal aortograms (**A** and **B**) demonstrate "string of beads" *(arrow in A)* appearance of the right renal artery in two different patients with fibromuscular dysplasia.

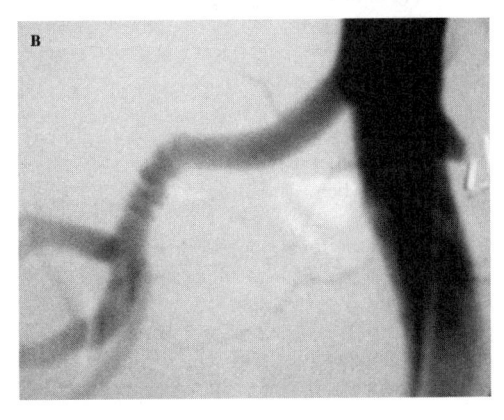

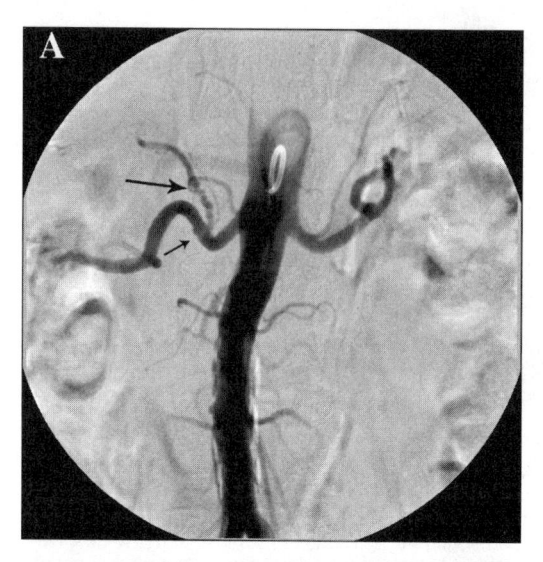

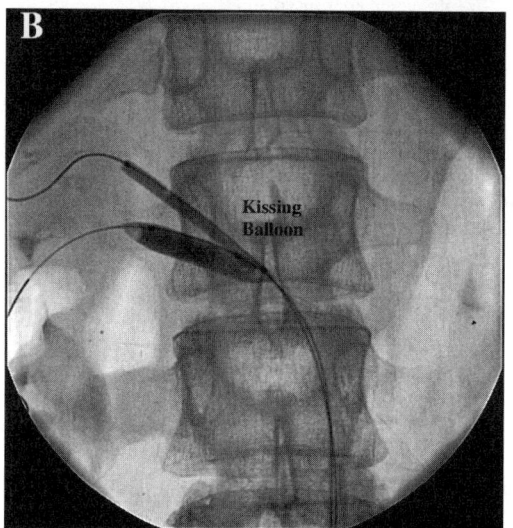

FIGURE 10. A 35-year-old woman with hypertension presents for evaluation to rule out fibromuscular dysplasia (FMD). **A,** Abdominal angiogram demonstrates "bead of pearl" appearance of the right renal artery and accessory branch, consistent with fibromuscular hyperplasia *(arrows)*. **B,** Due to FMD changes at the branch point, a kissing balloon technique was used for angioplasty to protect the arteries. **C,** Final image demonstrates good results after angioplasty.

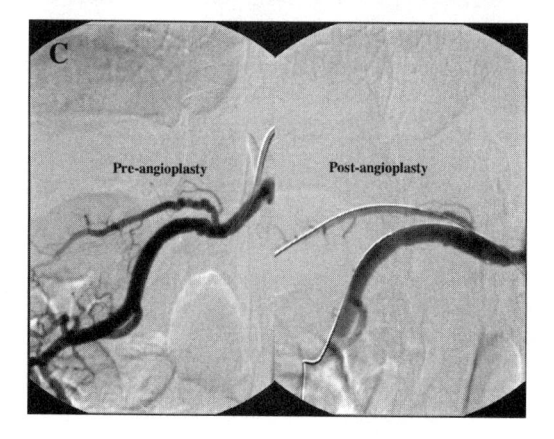

31. What is the most frequently affected organ in PAN?
Kidney (85%)

32. List the findings of PAN.
- Multiple small intrarenal aneurysms (interlobar, arcuate, interlobular arteries) (Fig. 11)
- Aneurysms may disappear (thrombosis) or appear in new locations
- Arterial narrowing + thrombosis (chronic stage/ healing stage)
- Multiple small cortical infarcts

33. Describe the findings of PAN on angiography.
- 1- to 5-mm saccular aneurysms of small and medium-sized arteries in 60–75% as a result of necrosis of internal elastic lamina (hallmark)
- Luminal irregularities + stenosis of arteries
- Arterial occlusions + small tissue infarctions

34. Does therapeutic angiography play a role in PAN?
No. PAN is treated with steroids.

35. What is TRAS?
Transplant renal artery stenosis.

36. Why is the recognition of TRAS important?
TRAS occurs in 3–12.5% of transplant patients and is an increasingly recognized cause of potentially curable allograft dysfunction and refractory hypertension (Fig. 12).

37. Describe the "kissing balloon" technique. When is it indicated?
The kissing balloon technique is used in the angioplasty suite to place two balloons in adjacent arteries. The balloons are inflated simultaneously to keep both arteries open. This technique is indicated when a lesion must be dilated near a bifurcation of a vessel.

38. What is the restenosis rate for TRAS?
20%. However, despite the high restenosis rate, there is only a 22% rate of graft loss during 3-year follow-up, attesting to the durability of repeat interventions.

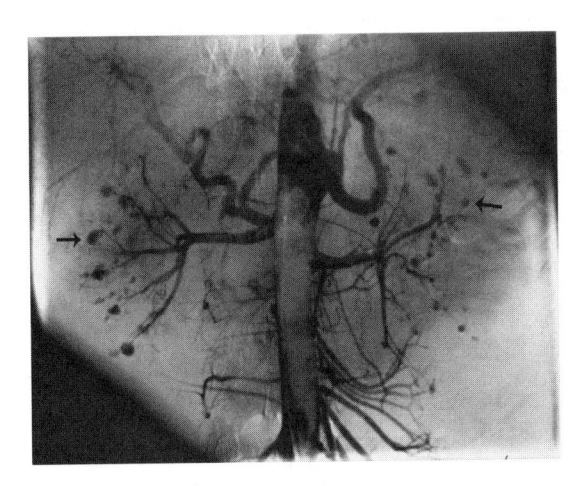

FIGURE 11. Abdominal aortogram demonstrates multiple small intrarenal ansurysms *(arrows)* consistent with polyarteritis nodosa in a 35-year-old man with painless hematuria and a history of hepatitis B.

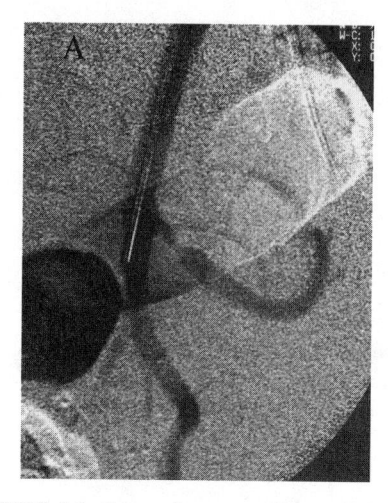

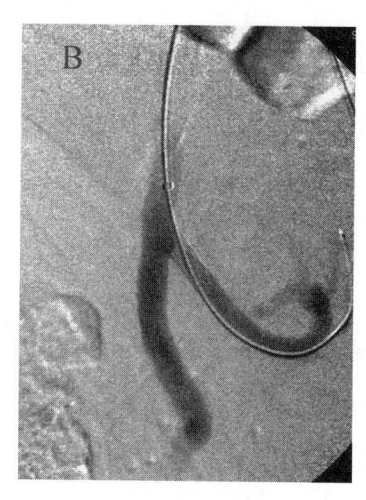

FIGURE 12. Selective renal artery angiogram of right pelvic renal transplant demonstrates severe stenosis (**A**). This was treated with a balloon-expandable stent (**B**). (Courtesy of Daniel Brown, MD, Mallinckrodt Institute, St. Louis, MO)

39. What causes cute renal artery occlusion?
- Embolic: atherosclerotic plaque, platelet thrombus, classic thrombus
- In situ thrombosis, with underlying anatomic abnormality or hypercoaguable condition
- Iatrogenic: after angioplasty or stent placement

40. Explain the difference between "protected" and "unprotected" kidneys.
Protected kidney: If thrombosis occurs in association with a severe preexistent stenosis, the kidney may be protected from ischemia by sufficient existing collateral vessels to preserve the majority of the renal parenchyma.

Unprotected kidney: normal kidney with an acute thrombus.

41. Which type of kidney has a higher probability of renal damage with an acute thrombus?
The unprotected kidney. Of interest, underlying medical disease actually serves as a protective mechanism to the kidney. Not usually the case!

42. What are the predictive factors for optimal results of renal artery thrombolysis?
- Acute or subacute in situ thrombosis with persistent collaterals
- Partial occlusions
- Acute iatrogenic thrombosis without anatomic obstruction
- Acute emboli treated within 3 hours

43. What are the predictive factors for poor results of renal artery thrombolysis?
- Chronic thrombosis
- Acute emboli without preexistent collaterals
- Total occlusions
- Acute iatrogenic thrombosis with anatomic obstruction
- Acute or subacute emboli treated after 3 hours

44. List the indications for renal artery embolization.
- Control of active hemorrhage (i.e., trauma)
- Obliteration of abnormal arteriovenous communications (e.g., arteriovenous fistula [AVF], arteriovenous malformation [AVM]) (Fig. 13)

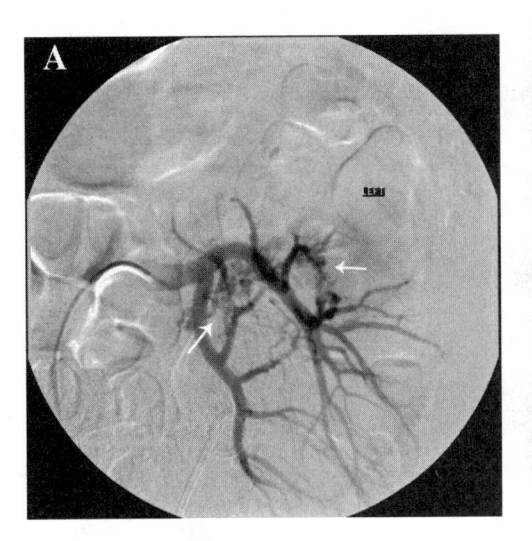

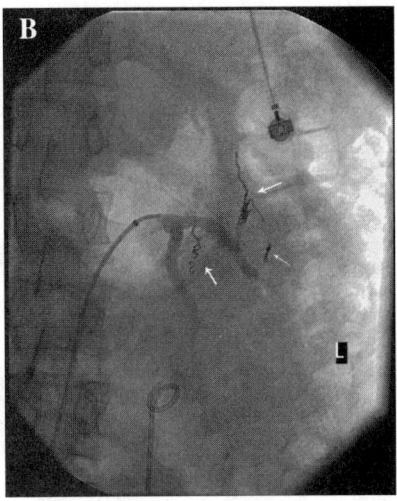

FIGURE 13. A 35-year-old woman involved in a motor vehicle accident 7 years ago presented with left foot drop. She was 34 weeks into her pregnancy when she developed massive hematuria and underwent premature delivery. A nephroureteral stent was placed, and she was referred for a renal angiogram. **A,** Left renal angiogram shows multiple small, tortuous arteries with early draining veins—findings consistent with arteriovenous malformation (AVM). **B,** The patient underwent successful coil embolization. The AVM was probably congenital rather than due to the trauma of the motor vehicle accident, especially since the patient denied any abdominal trauma. In addition, multiple AVMs were present. They became more pronounced during pregnancy because of pregnancy-induced hyperemia.

- Devascularization of tumors
- Embolization of aneurysms and pseduoaneurysms
- Parenchymal ablation

45. Categorize the agents used for embolization.
   Solids: coils, gelfoam, pledgets, detachable balloons.
   Particulates: polyvinyl acetate (PVA).
   Liquids: dehydrated alcohol.

46. List the conditions in which each of the above agents is used.
   Solid agents: AVF, AVM, pseudoanuerysms, and bleeding sites; precise site-specific agents are required.
   Particulates and liquids: tumor embolization and parenchymal ablation; site-specific agents are not required.

47. List the immediate complications in renal artery embolization.
   - Catheter related: dissection, perforation, and groin hematomas
   - Nontarget embolization (Fig. 14)

48. List the delayed complications in renal artery embolization.
   - Contrast-induced nephrotoxicity
   - Postembolization syndrome: fever, pain, leukocytosis
   - Soft tissue necrosis

49. Does transcatheter embolization have a role in traumatic occlusion of the renal arteries?
   Possibly—if there is segmental bleeding that may be embolized.

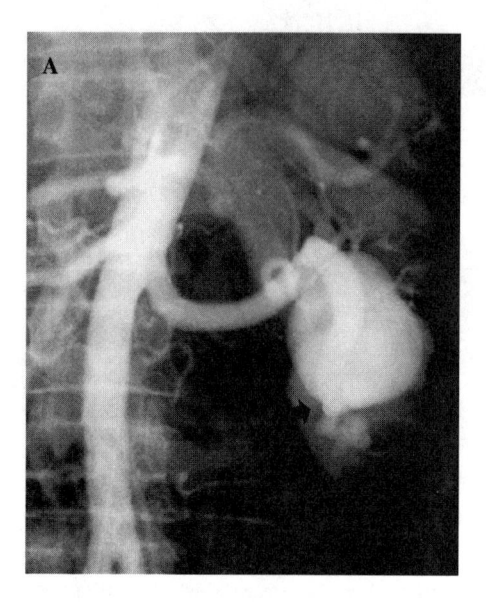

FIGURE 14. A 64-year-old woman was evaluated for hematuria. She was normotensive with normal renal function tests. Aortography and selective left renal arteriography demonstrated an arteriovenous malformation (AVM) of the left kidney (**A, B,** and **C**). The patient was successfully treated with embolization. A 5-French catheter was advanced into the dilated lower pole artery; then a coaxial 3-French catheter (**D**) was advanced into the peripheral aspect of the artery. Several large 0.018-inch coils (14 mm x 10 mm) were deployed in the distal artery. The coils failed to engage the artery and instead passed through the arterial communication into the large venous varix (**E**). Several large coils were then deposited more proximally in the feeding vessel. Follow-up arteriography demonstrated occlusion of the malformation with preserved renal parenchymal flow into the upper and mid poles of the left kidney (**F**). Often only one enlarged feeding artery drains into one or several large varix-like structures. Congenital AVMs may have multiple feeding arteries, whereas acquired arteriovenous fistulas have a single arteriovenous communication.

50. What is the most common cause of renal AVF?
Renal biopsy.

51. Why is an initial abdominal aortogram essential in the preembolization of renal arteries?
It enables identification of accessory renal arteries as well as intercostal, lumbar, and retroperitoneal collaterals, which may provide parasitized arterial flow to a renal tumor.

BIBLIOGRAPHY

1. Beaujeux R, Saussine C, Al-Fakir A, et al: Superselective endovascular treatment of renal vascular lesions. J Urol 153:14–17, 1995.
2. Blum U, Billmann P, Krause T, et al: Effect of low dose thrombolysis on clinical outcome in acute renal artery thromboembolism. Ann Vasc Surgery 7:549–554, 1993.
3. Dahnert W: Radiology Review Manual, 3rd ed. Baltimore, Williams & Wilkins, 1996.
4. Fervenza FC, Lafayette RA, Alfrey EJ, Petersen J: Renal artery stenosis in kidney transplants. Am J Kid Dis 31:142–148, 1998.
5. Fisher RG, Ben-Menachem Y: Angiography and embolization in renal trauma, in Baum S (ed): Abrams Angiography, 4th ed, vol 2 Philadelphia, Lippincott, 1997.
6. Gay SB, Woodcock RJ Jr: Radiology Recall. Philadelphia, Lippincott, 2000.
7. O'Neil EA, Hansen KJ, Canzanello BJ, et al: Prevalence of ischemic nephropathy in patients with renal insufficiency. Am Surg 58:485–490, 1992.
8. Pohl MA, Novick AC: Natural history of atherosclerotic and fibrous renal artery disease: Clinical implications. Am J Kidney Dis 5:120–130, 1985.
9. Rogers P, Roberts A, Schloesser P, Wong W: Pocket Radiologist: Interventional Top 100 Procedures. Salt Lake City, Amersts, 2003.
10. Rundback JH, Katsen BT, Semba CP: Techniques in Vascular and Interventional Radiology. Philadelphia, W.B. Saunders, 1999.
11. Weissleder R, Rieumont MJ, Wittenberg J: Primer of Diagnostic Imaging, 2nd ed. St. Louis, Mosby, 1997.

15. MESENTERIC ANGIOGRAPHY AND INTERVENTION

Wael E. A. Saad, MBBCh, and William Kuo, MD

1. **Describe the arteriographic characteristics of hepatocellullar carcinoma.**
   - Dilated hepatic artery
   - Highly vascular
   - Prominent neovascularity and arteriovenous shunting.
   - Portal vein invasion
   - Cirrhosis with irregular peripheral hepatic arteries

2. **Describe the arteriographic characteristics of benign hepatic masses.**
   Hemangioma (Fig. 1)
   - Normal, nondilated hepatic arteries
   - No neovascularity or arteriovenous shunting
   - Early peripheral ring enhancement
   - Well-defined vascular space, which is prominent in the mid-to-late arterial phase
   - Delayed washout

   Adenoma
   - Hepatic artery branches stretched around mass, feeding tumor at the periphery
   - 50% of cases exhibit high vascularity
   - Displaces but does not invade the portal vein

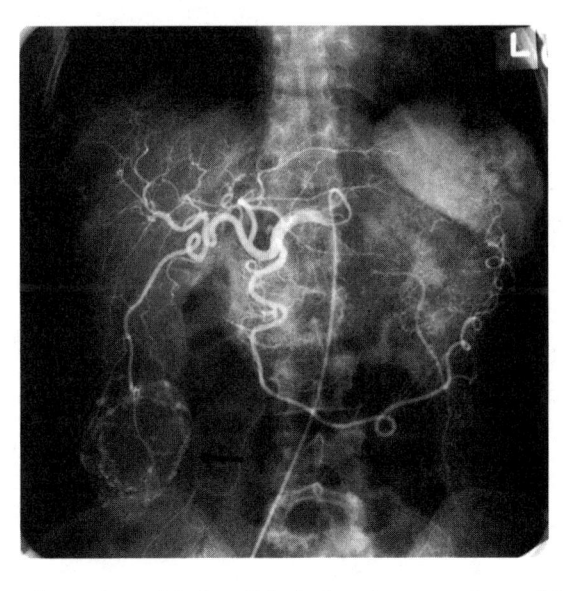

FIGURE 1. Cavernous hemangioma of the liver. Selective hepatic artery angiogram (historical gold standard for this disorder) demonstrates dilated, irregular punctate vascular lakes starting at the periphery in a ring-shaped configuration consistent with the diagnosis. Hemangioma is the most common benign liver tumor (76%) and the second most common of all liver tumors after metastases. The overall incidence is 1–4%. The combination of a large cavernous hemangioma of the liver with thrombocytopenia due to platelet sequestration within the hemangioma is called Kasabach-Merrit syndrome.

Focal nodular hyperplasia (FNH)
- Hepatic artery branch penetrates toward center of mass and branches out in a "spoke-wheel" pattern
- No neovascularity.
- Lucent ring (avascular ring) may or may not be present around periphery of mass

3. Describe the presentations of visceral aneurysms.

Most are asymptomatic and are found incidentally by radiographic imaging. They are being found more frequently in the era of cross-sectional imaging (computed tomography, ultrasound, magnetic resonance imaging). When symptomatic, 25% present emergently (bleeding) and are associated with a 9% mortality rate.

4. List, in order of frequency, the sites of visceral aneurysms.
- Splenic artery (60%)
- Hepatic artery (20%)
- Superior mesenteric artery (SMA)
- Celiac axis
- Gastric and gastro-epiploic arteries
- Pancreaticoduodenal arteries
- Gastroduodenal artery (GDA)

5. List the causes and conditions associated with true visceral aneurysms.
- Atherosclerosis
- Medial degeneration
- Fibrous dysplasia
- Infections
- Inflammation/vasculitis
- Trauma.
- Pregnancy (also increases the risk of rupture)

6. List the causes and conditions associated with pseudoaneurysms.
- Trauma
- Postoperative status
- Infection
- Inflammation (e.g., pancreatitis)

7. When should visceral aneurysm be treated?

True visceral aneurysms are treated according to the risk of rupture. Visceral aneurysms are usually treated when their size exceeds 1.5–2.5 cm in diameter (2.0 cm is the cut-off for splenic artery aneurysms) (Fig. 2). An alternative cut-off sizing method is an aneurysm that is at least twice the diameter of the parent artery.

Pseudoaneurysms are inherently unstable (they may be considered as contained ruptures), are associated with bleeding (intermittent or indolent/continuous), and are usually treated regardless of size.

8. What are the reasons for performing an abdominal aortogram and/or a regional angiogram before treating visceral aneurysms?

To get the lay-of-the-land:
- To check for concomitant/coexisting aneurysms
- To identify major feeding vessels from major aortic branches
- To eliminate confusion caused by guidwire and/or catheter-induced spasm

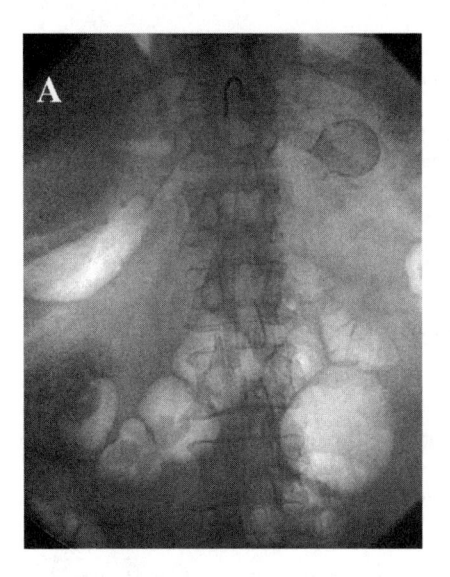

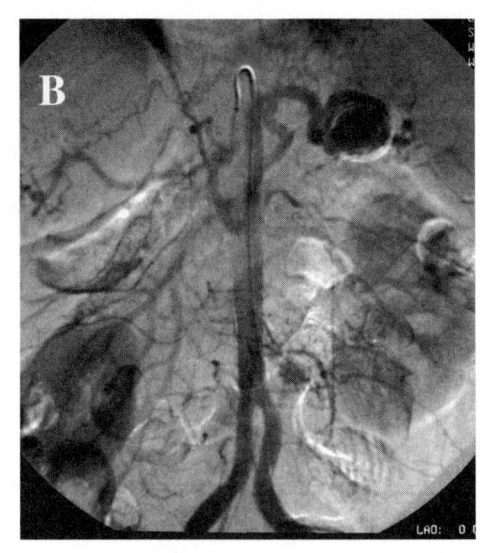

FIGURE 2. **A,** Plain film demonstrates a calcification in the area of the splenic artery. **B,** Selective celiac angiogram shows filling of a pseudoaneurysm. The therapy of choice is endovascular embolization (proximal and distal to the aneurysm).

9. What are the reasons for performing diagnostic selective and super-selective angiography at multiple projections before treating visceral aneurysms?

To improve angiographic diagnostic sensitivity and plan endoluminal treatment strategy:
- Some aneurysms may be seen only by selective angiography
- Proper determination of the size of the aneurysm neck (in cases of saccular aneurysms)
- Determination of collateral flow and importance (vitality) of involved artery (parent artery)
- Determination of the number of feeding vessels as well as efferent vessels

10. What does "evaluating the importance and vitality" of an artery mean? Why is it important to do so?

Importance and vitality are evaluated when the parent artery giving off the aneurysm is an end-artery and its sacrifice is being contemplated. If it is not a vital artery and embolizing the parent artery itself will not do significant or irreversible harm, the artery is deemed not important and not vital or dispensable.

For example, embolizing a segmental branch of the renal artery is considered acceptable. However, before embolizing a major hepatic artery, the portal vein must be patent by angiography to ensure adequate blood supply to the liver after sacrificing the hepatic artery.

11. In cases of saccular aneurysms, when should the nonvital parent artery be embolized at sites both proximal and distal to the aneurysm?

Embolization at sites both proximal and distal to an aneurysm is essential in arteries that have significant collateralization because aneurysms can be supplied (and continue to grow) by retrograde flow through the involved artery.

12. Give examples of arteries with significant collateralization.
- GDA
- Splenic artery
- Intrahepatic hepatic artery

(In short, upper GI arteries)

13. When and why is the diameter of the neck of a saccular aneurysm important to evaluate?

Evaluation of the diameter of neck of a saccular aneurysm is important when the involved artery (parent artery) is vital and its lumen should be preserved. Evaluating the neck diameter of a saccular aneurysm is more of a relative measurement (relative to the maximum aneurysm diameter) and less of an absolute measurement.

A narrow vs. a wide aneurysm neck determines the safest method to treat the aneurysm endoluminally. Wide aneurysm necks increase the risk of distal embolization by escape of the embolic material from the aneurysm into the parent artery.

14. List the endoluminal options for treating saccular visceral aneurysms.

Nonvital parent artery: coil embolization of the parent artery: Consider proximal and distal embolization in high collateral arteries.

Vital parent artery
- Narrow neck: Simple catheter-directed embolization of the aneurysm itself.
- Wide neck: (1) covered stent (stent-graft) across the aneurysm to exclude it form the parent artery flow or (2) transcatheter aneurysm embolization with embolic material-trapping methods.

15. How can embolic material be trapped during embolization of a wide-neck saccular aneurysm in an attempt to preserve the lumen of a vital parent artery?

1. By placing a bare stent (metal mesh) across the aneurysm neck and embolizing the aneurysm with a catheter through the interstices (mesh) of the stent.

2. By temporarily inflating a balloon across the neck of an aneurysm every time a coil is deployed (via catheter) in the aneurysm.

16. When is direct percutaneous embolization used?

Direct needle access (20-gauge needle) with image guidance allows embolization with coils, thrombin, or a combination of both. This method is used when the aneurysm is not endoluminally accessible, especially when occlusion of the parent artery is not a viable option.

17. Summarize the differences between intra- and extrahepatic pseudoaneurysms of the hepatic artery in liver transplant recipients.

	INTRAHEPATIC PSEUDOANEURYSMS	EXTRAHEPATIC PSEUDOANEURYSMS
Prevalence	31%	69%
Common site	Right hepatic lobe	Surgical anastomoses
Etiology	Percutaneous liver biopsies	Surgical/technical problems
	Percutaneous biliary drains	Postoperative infection/ subhepatic collections
Hepatic artery thrombosis (HAT)	Usually not associated with HAT	44% are associated with HAT
Mortality	50%	78%
Retransplantation	Not necessary if prevented from progressing.	Eventually required

18. Describe the types of vascular shunting that can occur within the liver in patients with heriditary hemorrhagic telangectasia (HHT).

- Hepatic artery to hepatic vein
- Hepatic artery to portal vein
- Portal vein to hepatic vein
- Hepatic vein to hepatic vein (not a true [functional] shunt and difficult to visualize angiographically)

19. Which type of shunting in HHT is associated with poor outcome after hepatic artery embolization?

Portal vein to hepatic vein shunting is associated with postembolization parenchymal necrosis and poor outcome after endovascular therapy.

20. Discuss the results of endoluminal embolization of intrahepatic arteriovenous malformations (AVMs) in patients with HHT.

Like many AVMs throughout the body (pulmonary AVMs are a major exception), intrahepatic AVMs carry high morbidity (25%) and mortality (17%) rates with or without various forms of management. The rate of emergent liver transplantation is 8–9%.

21. List the causes of upper gastrointestinal (UGI) bleeding.
- Peptic ulcer disease (most common cause before the advent of H2 blockers, when approximately 40% of UGI bleeds were due to duodenal peptic ulcers alone)
- Mallory-Weiss tear
- Gastroesophageal varices
- Portal hypertensive gastropathy
- Gastritis
- AVMs
- Aortoenteric fistulas
- Dieulafoy's disease
- Visceral pseudoaneurysms
- Hematobilia
- Tumors (benign or malignant)

22. What is the first-line diagnostic evaluation for UGI bleeding? Why?
Esophagogastroduodenoscopy (EGD) for the following reasons:
- EGD allows diagnosis of the site and etiology of bleeding.
- EGD evaluates for coexisting causes of bleeding.
- Tissue samples can be obtained to rule out malignancy.
- Emergent endoscopic therapy can be performed at least to temporize/stabilize the patient.
- Even when unsuccessful at treating the bleeding, EGD localizes and characterizes it to help in surgical planning and management and/or direct the interventional radiologist to the appropriate vascular territory.

23. Give two examples of pathologic causes and sites (confirmed by endoscopy) for UGI hemorrhage in which embolization of particular arteries is helpful, regardless of whether extravasation is observed by angiography.
- Mallory-Weiss tear: left gastric artery
- Ulcer in the posterior wall of the duodenal bulb: GDA (Fig. 3)

24. List the endovascular options in treating UGI bleeding and compare their results.
- Catheter-directed vasopressin infusion
- Catheter-directed embolization

The initial results of both methods of treatment are comparable. However, vasopressin is associated with a 20% recurrence rate, reducing its overall success rate to 52% compared with embolization. In addition, vasopressin is contraindicated in patients with coronary artery disease, hypertension, and other cardiovascular systemic disease.

25. List the embolic materials that can be used in UGI bleeding and characterize their duration of action.
- Metal coils (Gianturco spring coils-Cook): permanent
- Ivalon /PVA: permanent
- Cyano-acrylate (glue): Most likely permanent

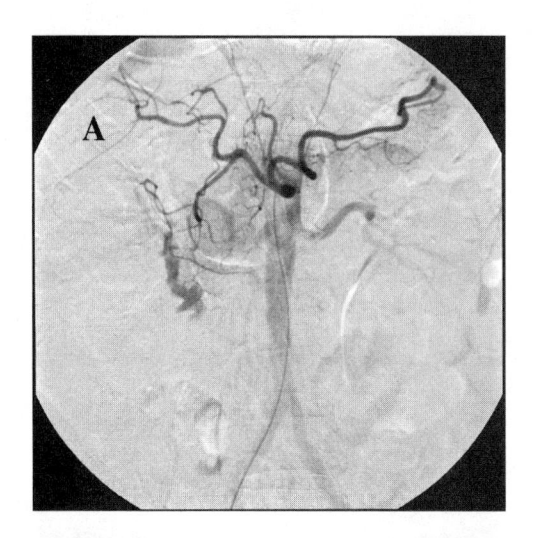

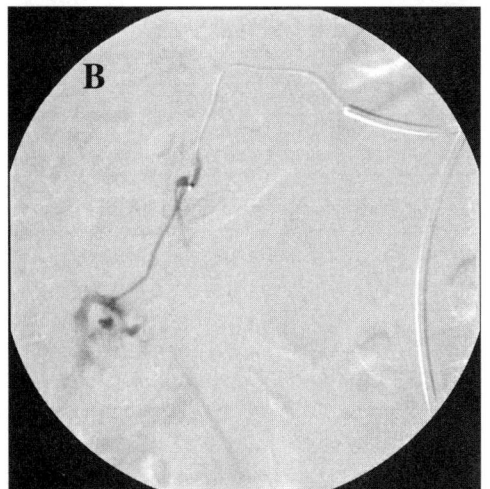

FIGURE 3. A, Initial angiogram from the celiac axis shows contrast extravasation into the duodenum. **B,** Selective view shows a similar finding. **C,** After embolization there is no further extravasation. Endoscopy illustrated a duodenal ulcer.

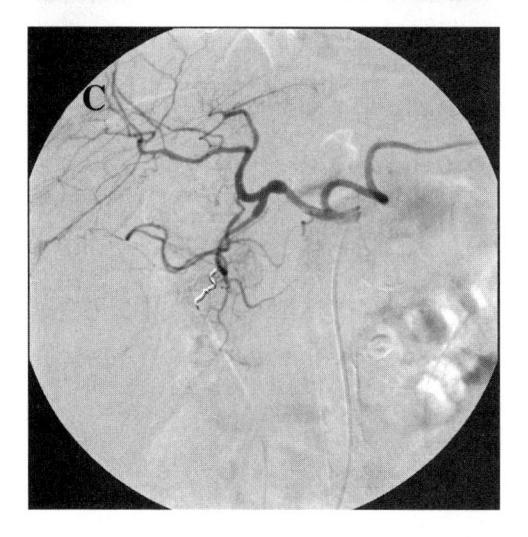

- Detachable balloons: permanent
- Gelfoam: temporary (2–4 weeks); can be permanent if it causes a local inflammatory reaction
- Autologous blood clot: temporary (hours)

26. Describe the collateral pathways reconstituting a GDA bleed.

If the GDA is embolized proximally only (from the common hepatic artery off the celiac axis), there are two major collateral pathways that reconstitute flow (and thus bleeding) in the GDA:
- Splenic artery to left gastroepiploic artery, then retrograde through the right gastroepiploic artery into the GDA
- Via the inferior pancreaticoduodenal artery (first branch of SMA)

27. Ideally, how should the GDA be embolized to ensure the best outcome (cessation of bleeding)?

Because of the pattern of collateralization it is important to "bridge" a bleeding site off the GDA (if technically feasible). In other words, the GDA should be embolized in its entirety from proximal to distal (from a celiac approach) or vice versa (from an SMA approach).

28. What major arteriograms should be obtained during a diagnostic and/or therapeutic work-up of a UGI bleed?

Both a celiac axis and an SMA angiogram should be obtained to evaluate the collateral pathways between the two major vessels. The collaterals themselves may be the sites of bleeding, and, depending on flow dynamics, one of the major angiograms may show the hemorrhage better than the other. Another reason is to evaluate the collaterals to plan for a definitive embolization.

29. What is a Dieulafoy lesion or erosion?

It is an abnormal cirsoid aneurysmal artery that protrudes through a small mucosal defect, typically along the lesser curvature and within 6 cm of the gastroesophageal junction. It is a well-described cause of UGI bleeding. The left gastric artery is the primary artery involved and should be investigated angiographically.

30. Summarize the results of UGI embolization.
- Approximately 40% of UGI bleeds are identified by angiography.
- The technical success rate is 97%.
- The clinical success rate is 59%.
- More than 50% of failures occur within 24 hours after the embolization.
- Successful embolization allows surgery to be avoided in 50% of cases.
- The hospital mortality rate (not procedure-related mortality) is 37–38%.
- The mortality rate is reduced by 45% compared with surgical mortality (83%).
- Concomitant coagulopathy reduces the success rate by 40% and significantly increases the mortality rate.

31. Give the diffrential diagnosis of microaneurysms in the splanchnic vessels.

The top three causes are as follows:
- Polyarteritis nodosa (PAN)
- Systemic lupus erythromatosus (SLE)
- Substance abuse vasculitis (e.g., "speed kidney" due to amphetamine abuse)

Less common causes include neurofibromatosis (NF), Wegener's granulomatosis, Kawasaki's disease, FMD, and septic emboli (micromycotic aneurysms).

32. Describe the angiographic features of PAN.

Angiographic findings are seen in 80% of patients (Fig. 4). Their distribution may be summarized as follows:
- Hepatic artery: 60%
- Renal artery: 47%
- Mesenteric artery: 38%

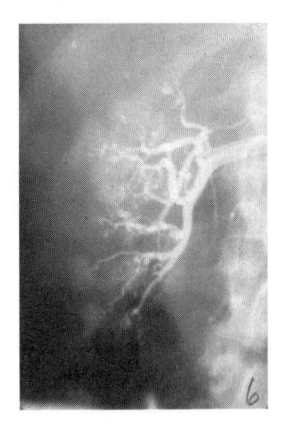

FIGURE 4. A 35-year-old man with a history of hepatitis B presented with painless hematuria. Abdominal aortogram demonstrated multiple small intrarenal aneurysms *(arrows)* consistent with polyarteritis nodosa (PAN). All organs may be involved in PAN, although the kidney (85% of cases) is the most frequently affected organ, followed by the heart (65%), liver (50%), pancreas, bowel, and central nervous system (cerebrovascular accident, seizure). Angiography has a 61% sensitivity rate and a 80% true-positive rate for the diagnosis of PAN. With steroid treatment the 5-year survival rate is 50%.

Angiographic features include predilection for mid-to-small size arterial bifurcations:
- Saccular microaneurysms (1–5 mm in diameter)
- Small vessel segmental stenoses
- Small vessel thrombosis / occlusion

33. Give the etiologic classification of acute mesenteric ischemia.
1. Arterial occlusive disease
   - Embolus (cardiac or aortic): 50% (Fig. 5)
   - Thrombosis on top of atherosclerotic disease: 20% (Fig. 6)
   - Dissection (aortic and/or mesenteric): rare
2. Arterial nonocclusive disease (low-flow states such as hypovolemia and hypotension): 20%
3. Mesenteric venous thrombosis: 10%

34. Give the etiologic classification of chronic mesenteric ischemia.
All cases of chronic mesenteric ischemia are due to arterial occlusive disease:
- Atherosclerosis
- Chronic dissection
- Vasculitis/FMD

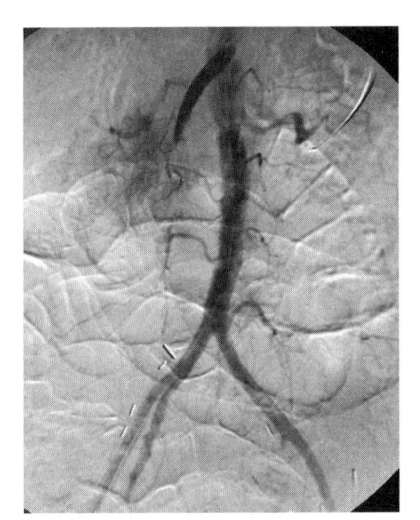

FIGURE 5. Single view from a selective angiogram of the superior mesenteric artery (SMA) demonstrates cutoff of the SMA at the first branch point. This finding is characteristic of colonic ischemia due to an embolus.

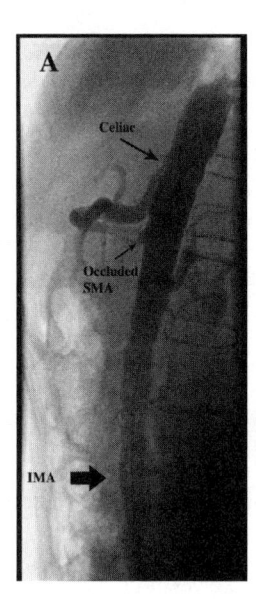

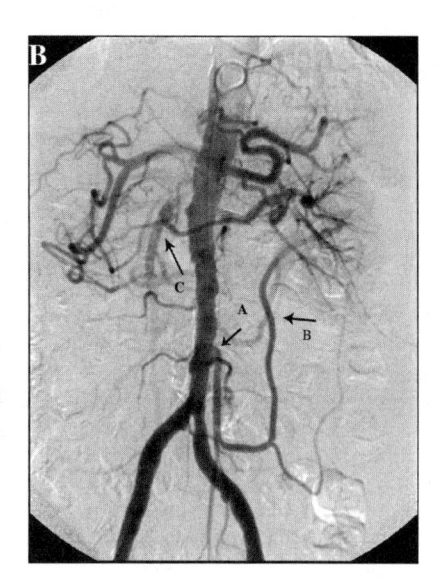

FIGURE 6. A 65-year-old male smoker with hypertension and diabetes presented with long-standing postprandial pain. **A,** Angiogram of the lateral abdominal aorta demonstrated severe stenosis at the origin of the celiac artery, occluded superior mesenteric artery (SMA), and patent inferior mesenteric artery (IMA). **B,** Anteroposterior (AP) view of the abdominal aorta angiogram demonstrates multiple findings. *Arrow A* points to the origin of the IMA, which gives rise to a tortuous, dilated meandering artery *(arrow B)*. This finding on an AP view is a sign of chronic mesenteric ischemia. The meandering artery reconstitutes the SMA just distal to its occlusion to supply the SMA distribution *(arrow C)*. Other findings include occluded right renal artery and stent in the left renal artery.

- Median arcuate syndrome
- Abdominal aortic coarctation or aneurysm

35. Describe the classic clinical scenario of a patient suffering from acute mesenteric ischemia.
- Sudden generalized abdominal pain (may be subacute or intermittent)
- Pain out of proportion to exam.
- Melena (bad sign)
- 80% mortality rate

36. When mesenteric ischemia is a concern, what angiographic image should be acquired first?
Alateral aortogram to evaluate the patency of the origins of the celiac axis and the SMA. The SMA is the usual culprit. An anteroposterior aortogram should be obtained next to evaluate for aortic disease as well as concomitant renal artery emboli. Remember that 50% of acute ischemia is due to emboli.

37. Describe the classic angiographic findings of an embolus causing acute mesenteric ischemia.
Contrast outlines a convex filling defect (meniscus) that partially or completely occludes the SMA just beyond its first branch (inferior pancreaticoduodenal artery). This site of embolic impaction is seen in 85% of embolic cases.

38. How can an embolus in the SMA be treated endoluminally?
By catheter-directed thrombolysis (successful in anecdotal cases) or by suction embolectomy via a large catheter. The majority of interventionalists recommend strongly against endoluminal

intervention in this setting. The classic teaching is that patients with acute mesenteric ischemia should be surgically explored for nonviable bowel resection and surgical embolectomy. The value of preoperative angiography is to help identify the site of obstruction for the surgeon to bring a fast, effective and minimal revascularization.

39. What angiographic features are associated with nonocclusive mesenteric ischemia?
Angiographic features include vasoconstriction/spasm of the SMA and its branches with interposed areas of normal caliber artery segments. The problem may resolve with transcatheter administration of vasodilators (a diagnostic and therapeutic test).

40. Describe the symptoms associated with chronic mesenteric ischemia.
The classic symptom is chronic pain with indolent onset. Pain starts approximately $1^1/_2$ hours after eating and resolves approximately 2–3 hours later (abdominal angina). As a result, patients avoid eating large meals (fear of eating) and lose weight. At least two of the three mesenteric vessels (celiac, SMA, or IMA) must be significantly stenosed or occluded to cause these symptoms.

41. Describe the median arcuate ligament syndrome and its angiographic features.
In this syndrome, which tends to occur in young, thin female patients, the celiac artery is compressed by the median arcuate ligament of the diaphragm. A notch-like impression is seen on the superior surface of the celiac axis on expiration (exhaling) and resolves on deep inspiration (inhaling).

42. Summarize the results of percutaneous angioplasty and stenting of mesenteric vessels in chronic mesenteric ischemia.
- Technical success rate: 80–96% (Fig. 7)
- Major complication rate: 8–16%
- Immediate clinical success rate: 80–88%
- Long-term clinical success rate: 67–83%
- 6- and 18-month primary patency of successfully treated vessels: 92% and 74%, respectively.

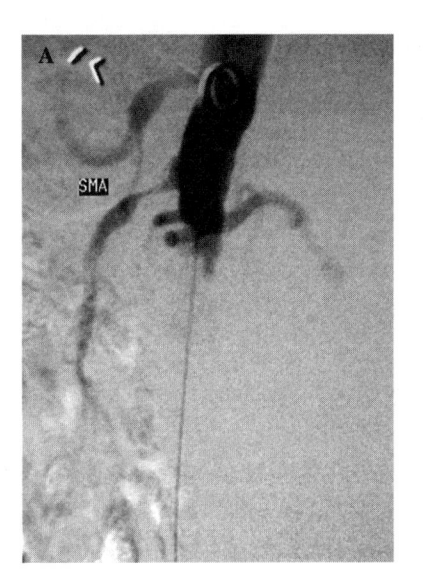

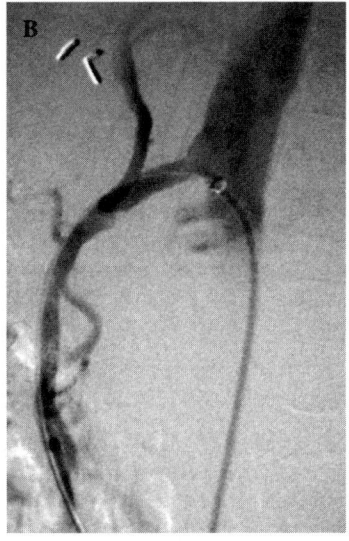

FIGURE 7. A patient with weight loss and clinical suspicion for chronic mesenteric ischemia underwent a CT scan, which demonstrated stenosis of the superior mesenteric artery (SMA). **A,** Lateral abdominal aortic angiogram demonstrated severe stenosis at the origin of the SMA. **B,** The stenosis was successfully treated with percutaneous transluminal angioplasty and stent.

BIBLIOGRAPHY

1. Arata MA, Cope C: Principles used in the management of visceral aneurysms. Tech Vasc Intervent Radiol 3(3):124–129, 2000.
2. Carr SC, Pearce WH, Vogelzang RL, et al: Current management of visceral artery aneurysms. Surgery 120:627–633, 1996.
3. Kaufman JA: Visceral arteries. In: Kaufman JA, Lee MJ (eds): The Requisites: Vascular and Interventional Radiology. St. Louis, Mosby, 2004, pp 286–322.
4. LaBerge JM, Wall SD: Abdominal aortography, visceral and renal arteriography. In LaBerge JM, Gordon RL, Kerlan RK Jr, Wilson MW (eds): Interventional Radiology Essentials. Philadelphia, Lippincott Williams & Wilkins, 2000, pp 45–62.
5. Lang EV, Picus D, Marx MV, et al: Massive upper gastrointestinal hemorrhage with normal findings on arteriography: Value of prophylactic embolization of the left gastric artery. Am J Roentgenol 158:547–549, 1992.
6. Marshall MM, Muiesan P, Srinivasan P, et al: Hepatic artery pseudoaneurysms following liver transplantation: Incidence, presenting features and management. Clin Radiol 56(7):579–587, 2001.
7. Matsumoto AH, Angle JF, Spinosa DJ: Percutaneous transluminal angioplasty and stenting in the treatment of chronic mesenteric ischemia: Results and long-term follow-up. J Am Coll Surg 194(1 Suppl):S22-S31, 2002.
8. Matsumoto AH, Tegtmeyer CJ, Fitzcharles ET, et al: Percutaneous transluminal angioplasty of visceral arterial stenoses: results and long-term clinical follow-up. JVasc Intervent Radiol 6(2):165–174, 1995.
9. Reilly HF, al-Kawas FH: Dieulafoy's lesion: Diagnosis and management. Dig Dis Sci 36:1702–1707, 1991.
10. Saluja S, White RI Jr: Hereditary hemorrhagic telangiectasia of the liver: Hyperperfusion with relative ischemia—Poverty amidst plenty. Radiology 230:25–27, 2004.
11. Sarafuddin MJ, Olson CH, Sun S, et al: Endovascular treatment of celiac and mesenteric arteries stenoses: Applications and results. J Vasc Surg 38(4):692–688, 2003.
12. Sheeran SR, Murphy TP, Khwaja A, et al: Stent placement for treatment of mesenteric artery stenoses or occlusions. J Vasc Intervent Radiol 10(7):861–867, 1999.
13. Venbrux AC: Upper gastrointestinal bleeding: Diagnostic evaluation and management. In Haskal ZJ, Kerlan RK, Teratola SO (eds): SCVIR Syllabus: Thoracic and Visceral Vascular Interventions. Fairfax, VA, Society of Interventional Radiology 1996, pp 235–246.
14. Weintraub JL, Haskal ZJ: Embolotherapy of upper gastrointestinal hemorrhage. Tech Vasc Interv Radiol 3(3):162–170, 2000.
15. Whiting JH Jr, Korzenik JR, Miller FJ Jr, et al: Fatal outcome after embolotherapy for hepatic arteriovenous malformations of the liver in two patients with hereditary hemorrhagic telangiectasia. J Vasc Intervent Radiol 11: 855–858, 2000.

16. UTERINE ARTERY EMBOLIZATION FOR FIBROIDS

Nikhil C. Patel, MD

1. What is UAE?
Uterine artery embolization.

2. What is UFE?
Uterine fibroid embolization.

3. Explain the difference between UAE and UFE.
Technically there is no difference between UAE and UFE. Theoretically people refer to UFE as a procedure to embolize uterine fibroids and UAE as embolization of the uterine artery for any cause of bleeding from the uterine artery, whether it is for fibroids or another cause.

4. Define uterine leiomyoma.
Leiomyoma (fibroid) is a benign tumor of the uterine smooth muscle. Leiomyomas are the most common benign tumors of the female genital tract.

5. What is the prevalence of fibroids?
Fibroids affect 20–40% (millions) of the female population.

6. What percentage of patients with fibroids are symptomatic?
25% of patients with fibroids are symptomatic.

7. In what age group are fibroids most prevalent?
Fibroids are most frequent between 30 and 40 years of age. They typically resolve after menopause.

8. How many hysterectomies are performed annually for fibroids?
In the United States 600,000 hysterectomies are performed annually. Approximately 33% of the procedures performed are for fibroids.

9. How are fibroids diagnosed?
- Clinical history and physical exam
- Pelvic ultrasound
- Magnetic resonance imaging (MRI)
- Laparoscopy or hysteroscopy

10. Where are fibroids located?
- Submucosal
- Intramural
- Subserosal

11. How are the symptoms related to the location of fibroids?
Submucosal: heavy and prolonged menstrual bleeding, increased miscarriage rate; fibroids may be pedunculated and/or prolapsed into cervix.
Intramural: most common type; may present with heavy menstrual bleeding as well as pelvic pain, back pain, and pressure.

Subserosal: typically do not cause vaginal bleeding; however, they do cause pelvic pain, back pain, and pressure on adjacent bowel and bladder.

12. Summarize the current treatment plan for fibroids.
1. No symptoms: follow with pelvic exam and ultrasound.
2. Mild symptoms: over-the-counter (OTC) medications and/or oral contraceptive pills (OCPs).
3. Moderate symptoms: Lupron (gonadotropin-releasing hormone [GnRH] agonist). Recurrence is common when the drug is stopped.
4. Severe symptoms: surgery or uterine artery embolization. Surgical options include:
   - Myomectomy: associated with higher morbidity, significant blood loss, and may not treat the culprit fibroid
   - Hysterectomy: curative but irreversible

13. Who reported the first cases of UFE?
Ravina et al. from France in 1995 noticed that, during preoperative embolization of the uterine artery for fibroids to decrease surgical blood loss, patients became symptom-free.

14. Who reported the first UFE experience in the United States?
Goodwin et al. in 1997 reported the results of 11 patients.

15. Explain the concept of uterine fibroid embolization.
Transcatheter blockage of both uterine arteries deprives fibroids of their blood supply, leading to caseous necrosis followed by hyaline sclerosis and shrinkage of the fibroids.

16. What happens to the uterus when both uterine arteries are embolized?
The uterus is spared by its ability to weather the vascular assault. No definite mechanism is known.

17. List three alternatives to UFE.
Hysterectomy, myomectomy, and hormonal therapy (progestational compounds and GnRH agonist).

18. Summarize the advantages and disadvantages of hysterectomy.
Advantages
1. Completely cures the disease.
2. Eliminates any possibility of future neoplasm.
3. Facilitates postmenopausal hormonal replacement therapy.

Disadvantages
1. Invasive procedure.
2. Higher risk and longer recovery.

19. Summarize the advantages and disadvantages of myomectomy.
Advantages
1. Uterus-sparing.

Disadvantages
1. Increased blood loss.
2. Higher risk and longer recovery.
3. May not treat the culprit fibroid.
4. Recurrent symptoms often develop, with 20–25% of patients eventually requiring another surgical procedure (usually hysterectomy).

20. Summarize the advantages and disadvantages of hormonal therapy.
Advantages
1. Noninvasive.
2. Short-term relief for symptomatic women not wanting surgery.
3. Treatment of perimenopausal women.
4. Adjuvant therapy to myomectomy to decrease tumor vascularity before surgery.

Disadvantages
1. Rapid regrowth of fibroids after discontinuation of medication.
2. Risk of developing osteoporosis and menopausal symptoms when taken on a long-term basis.

20. In evaluating a patient for UFE, what important questions need to be asked?
- Does the patient have uterine fibroids?
- Are the patient's symptoms directly related to the presence of uterine fibroids?
- Does the patient need invasive treatment for fibroids?
- Does the patient desire future childbearing?
- Does the patient have gynecologic or nongynecologic medical conditions that may predispose her to complications of either embolization or surgery?
- Does the patient have anatomic factors that predispose her to treatment failure or indicate an adjunctive procedure to ensure the success of UFE?

21. Which imaging modalities can confirm the presence of uterine fibroids?
Imaging confirmation is required by ultrasound and/or MRI. Generally ultrasound is adequate. MRI is used in the presence of:
- Global uterine enlargement without a clearly discernible uterine mass (e.g., diffuse fibroid disease, adenomyosis, malignancy)
- Concern for malignancy requiring better visualization of uterine tissue layers to detect local invasiveness.

22. How do you determine whether the patient's symptoms are directly related to the presence of uterine fibroids?
The common presenting complaints are menorrhagia and pelvic pain. Consider carefully the differential diagnosis of each.

Menorrhagia: fibroids, adenomyosis, endometrial diseases, endometrial polyps, endometrial hyperplasia, endometrial carcinoma. In many cases endometrial biopsy is required to determine the cause.

Pelvic pain and mass effect: fibroids, ovarian masses, abdominal masses, infection, endometriosis, adenomyosis. Each of these masses can produce symptoms by:
- Compression of the lumbosacral nerve plexus resulting in back pain
- Compression of the bladder with resulting urinary symptoms
- Compression of the rectum with resulting constipation

23. What factors often determine the need for invasive treatment?
Presence and degree of symptoms. Most patients with fibroids are asymptomatic or have minimal symptoms; therefore, invasive treatment is not indicated. In symptomatic patients, the decision depends on the degree to which the symptoms physically or psychologically incapacitate the patient.

24. How is the treatment decision different in perimenopausal symptomatic women?
Mild-to-moderate symptoms
1. Watchful waiting. Patients should be counseled that fibroids usually regress during and after menopause due to diminishing hormonal stimulation.
2. Hormonal therapy. Some physicians recommend hysterectomy to post- or perimenopausal women who need hormonal therapy for the following reasons:

- It is an important component of prophylaxis against osteoporosis and coronary artery disease.
- In women with endometrial hyperplasia, fear of promoting neoplasia provides further justification for hysterectomy if fibroids are also present.

Severe symptoms
1. Minimally invasive therapy such as embolization.
2. Hysterectomy.

25. Discuss the invasive treatment of choice for patients who desire future childbearing.

Currently, myomectomy is considered the invasive treatment of choice in this patient group, until further data are available. UFE should be reserved for women who refuse surgery or hysterectomy. Pregnancy has been reported in all available studies of UFE. The risk of infertility, however, persists for two major reasons.

    1. Premature menopause, which has been reported predominantly in women over 45 years of age. This phenomenon is not completely understood as yet but may be due to nontarget embolization of ovary or the direct effect of UFE on the uterus.

    2. Complications of embolization leading to hysterectomy (less than 0.5% of cases)

26. What medical conditions may predispose patients to complications of either surgery or embolization?

Surgery
- Coronary artery disease
- Chronic obstructive pulmonary disease
- Prior pelvic surgery with associated adhesions

UFE
- History of pelvic irradiation or microvascular disease (may confer higher risk for ischemic necrosis)
- Pelvic infection (chronic salpingitis or endometriosis theoretically confer higher risk for postembolization infection)
- Assessment of serum levels of beta human chorionic gonadotropin (hCG) in sexually active premenopausal women (to exclude current pregnancy)

27. List anatomic factors that predispose to treatment failure or indicate the need for an adjunctive procedure to ensure the success of UFE.
- Aberrant uterine artery
- Untreated ovarian artery supply to fibroids
- Coexistant adenomyosis
- Patient taking GnRH agonist
- Extremely large fibroid

In recent reports using MRI to study the response toUFE, submucosal fibroids, small fibroids, hypervascularity, and low T1 signal have correlated with greater fibroid volume reduction. High T1 signal has been correlated with lesser volume reduction.

28. What are the indications for endometrial biopsy in working up a patient for UFE?

Endometrial biopsy is indicated when ultrasound and MRI are incapable of making a definitive diagnosis of endometrial thickening. Unfortunately, the presence of a benign cause of menorrhagia does not exclude the possible coexistence of endometrial carcinoma. For this reason endometrial biopsy is also recommended in the following groups:
- All postmenopausal women with vaginal bleeding
- All women with irregular vaginal bleeding
- All women over 40 years of age with regular menorrhagia

29. What are the contraindication to UFE?

Pregnancy, active pelvic inflammatory disease, prior pelvic radiation, and connective tissue disease are contraindications to UFE. In addition, patients with weight loss, fatigue, other systemic symptoms, or rapid growth of a single fibroid should be treated with hysterectomy due to a higher likelihood of malignancy.

30. What are the benefits of using MRI as the modality of choice for pre- and post-UFE evaluation?

Pre-UFE evaluation
- Most accurate in localization of fibroids, whether submucosal, intramural, or subserosal.
- Has better interobserver reproducibility.
- Allows accurate and consistent measurement of fibroid size and tissue perfusion. Uterine and fibroid volumes can also be estimated.
- Can diagnose other pathologies that clinically mimic fibroid, such as adenomyosis (junctional zone thicker than 12 mm) and endometriosis.
- Contrast-enhanced MRA can help in planning for UFE and may reduce procedural load contrast and x-ray exposure; in addition, it may demonstrate aberrant uterine artery anatomy and/or the presence of ovarian artery supply to fibroids.

Post-UFE evaluation
- Assessing success of UFE and follow-up of response to UFE.

31. What are the MRI findings of fibroids after embolization?

As fibroids infarct, either spontaneously or after UFE, they degenerate with variable appearance on T2-weighted and contrast-enhanced images. The differences are due to the various types of degeneration that can occur (see table).

TYPE OF DEGENERATION	T2 SIGNAL	CONTRAST ENHANCEMENT
Hyaline degeneration	Low signal	
Myxoid degeneration	High signal	Minimal enhancement
Cystic degeneration	High signal	May show some areas that do not enhance
Red (hemorrhagic) degeneration	High T1 signal with or without low signal intensity rim on T2	
Calcific degeneration	Low signal	

32. Define menorrhagia and menometrorrhagia.

Menorrhagia: excessively prolonged or profuse menses.

Menometrorrhagia: irregular or excessive bleeding during menstration and between menstral periods.

33. What is the most common symptom of fibroids?

Abnormal uterine bleeding, characterized by menorrhagia. Worsening of menstrual cramps may accompany growth of fibroids. Menometrorrhagia may also occur, typically with pedunculated submucosal or intracavitary fibroid.

34. What are other common symptoms of fibroids?

1. **Pelvic pain**
   - *Acute:* spontaneous degeneration of fibroid, torsion of a pedunculated subserosal fibroid, prolapse of a pedunculated submucosal fibroid.
   - *Chronic* pelvic pain may also be due to fibroids. However, if it is an isolated symptom, other diagnostic considerations include pelvic inflammatory disease, endometriosis, adenomyosis, pelvic congestion syndrome, other organ involvement (e.g., genitourinary, gastrointestinal, musculoskeletal).
2. **Increased abdominal and pelvic girth** due to an enlarging uterus or fibroid
3. **Pressure symptoms**
   - *Urinary bladder pressure:* increased frequency of urination, stress incontinence, urinary retention, hydronephrosis.

- *Rectal pressure:* constipation.
- *Nerve compression:* back, flank, or leg pain.

4. **Infertility or repeated miscarriage** may also result from the presence of fibroids. They are most often associated with submucosal or intracavitary fibroids.

35. Describe the blood supply to the ovaries.

The ovaries are supplied by the two ovarian arteries. Both arise directly from the aorta a few centimeters below the origin of their respective renal arteries. However, an arterial anastomosis has been noted between the uterine artery and the ovarian circulation. This anastomosis is visible angiographically in 5–10% of cases.

36. Can the ovarian arteries supply fibroids?

Yes. Normally the ovarian arteries are 1 mm in diameter and are usually not visible in nonselective angiography. When the vessel supplies a fibroid uterus, it may be visible angiographically and as large as 4 mm in diameter.

37. Explain the importance of recognizing the arterial anastomosis between the uterine and ovarian arteries in the setting of UFE.

Nontarget embolization may occur, resulting in ischemic damage to ovaries. Ischemic damage may lead to the following:
- Transient amenorrhea
- Permanent amenorrhea (2% of UFEs)
- Premature menopause (usually seen in women 45 years and older undergoing UFE)

38. Can the radiation dose from UFE induce ovarian failure?

Induction of ovarian failure usually requires a radiation dose of 375–400 cGy. Estimates of radiation dose during UFE are approximately a tenth of that amount. Therefore, UFE is unlikely to cause ovarian failure.

39. What is the normal uterine artery diameter?

On the average the uterine artery diameter is 3 mm.

40. Why does UFE require bilateral uterine artery embolization?

The intrauterine branches of both uterine arteries freely anastomose within the body of the uterus, with excellent cross-filling between the two circulations. For this reason UFE must be successful on both sides to be effective (Fig. 1).

41. Which artery has a common origin or a short trunk with the uterine artery?

The inferior vesicle artery, which can usually be identified as a straight artery.

42. Describe the normal course of uterine artery.

From proximal to distal, the uterine artery is divided into descending, transverse, and ascending segments (Fig. 2). The **descending** segment originates from the hypogastric artery at a sharp angle of 45–90° and descends along the pelvic sidewall to the broad ligament. At the level of the broad ligament, the uterine artery turns medially and courses to the midline as the **transverse** segment. As the artery approaches the uterus, it turns and ascends along the uterus as the **ascending** segment.

43. Which segment of the uterine artery does not have branches?

Descending segment.

44. What branches arise from the uterine artery?

The cervicovaginal branches usually arise from the transverse segment but may also arise from the proximal portion of ascending segment (Fig. 3). From the ascending segment arise numerous centripetally oriented perforating vessels, the terminal branches to fallopian tube, and the terminal branches to ovarian arteries.

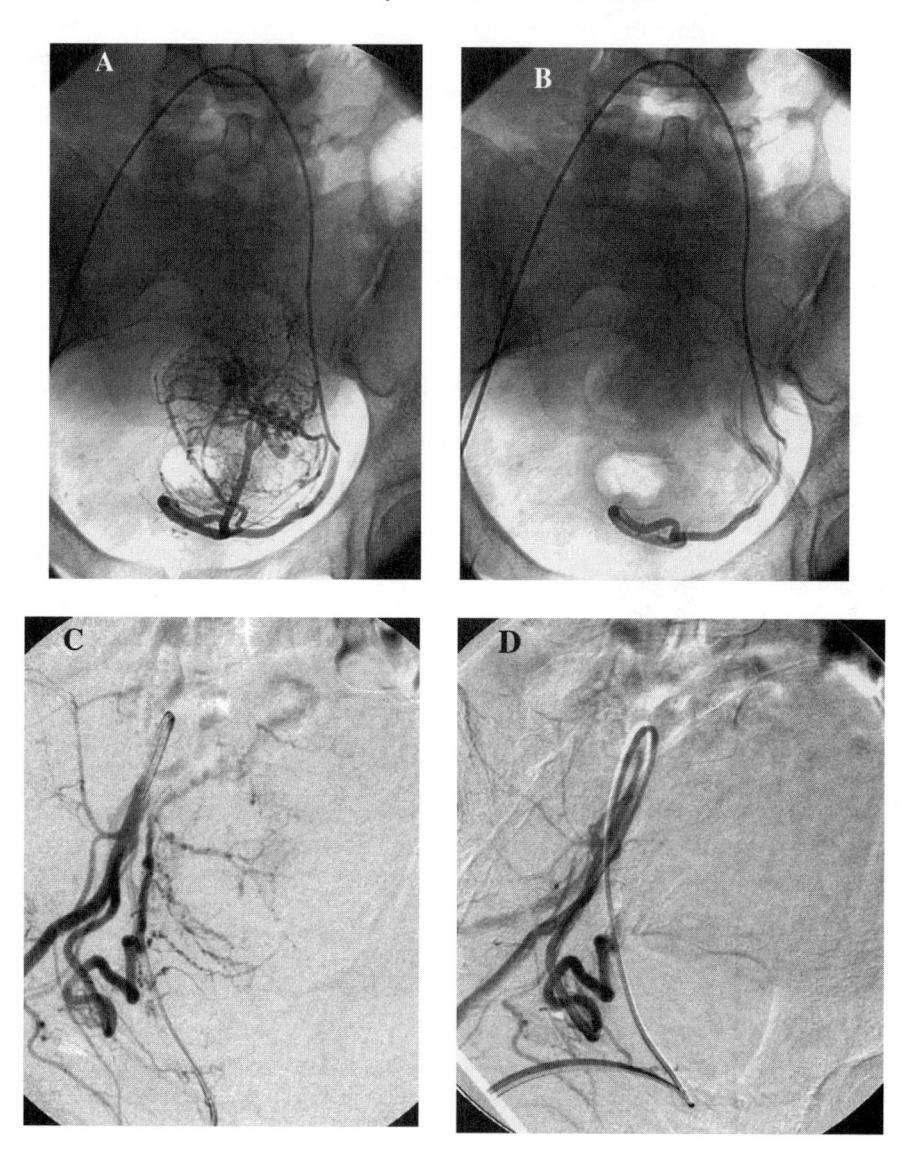

FIGURE 1. A, Selective injection into the left uterine artery demonstrated a large blush within the fibroid. **B,** After embolization there was no significant flow to the fibroid. **C,** A similar procedure was done the right uterine artery. There was less vascularity on the second side after embolization. **D,** The right side was then embolized. PVA particles (300–500 micron) were used for embolization.

45. In what percentage of cases is the ovary supplied exclusively by the uterine artery?

In 4% of women the ovarian artery is absent and the ovary is supplied exclusively by the uterine artery.

46. What percentage of women have communication between the uterine artery and the ovaries?

Approximately 46% of women have communication between the uterine artery and ovarian arteries. During angiography, however, only approximately 5–10% of these communications are visible. Occasionally a parenchymal blush of the ovaries can be seen on angiography.

FIGURE 2. Pelvic angiogram demonstrating the anatomy of the uterine artery. The uterine artery originates as an anterior division of the hypogastric artery (A). The descending portion (B) of the uterine artery runs along the pelvis side wall, travels horizontally (C) along the broad ligament, and then ascends (D) along the uterine sidewall.

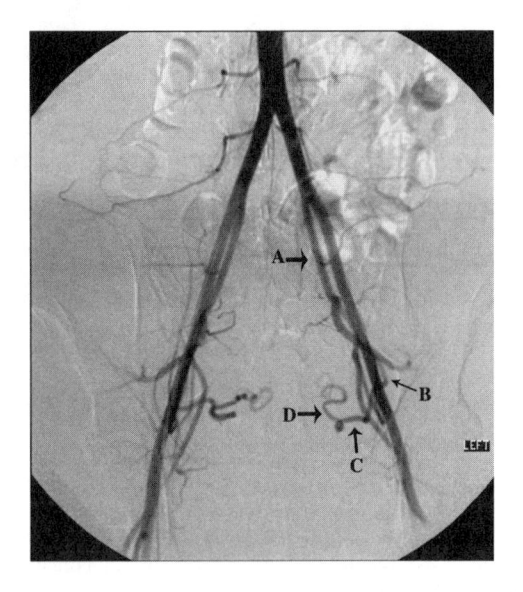

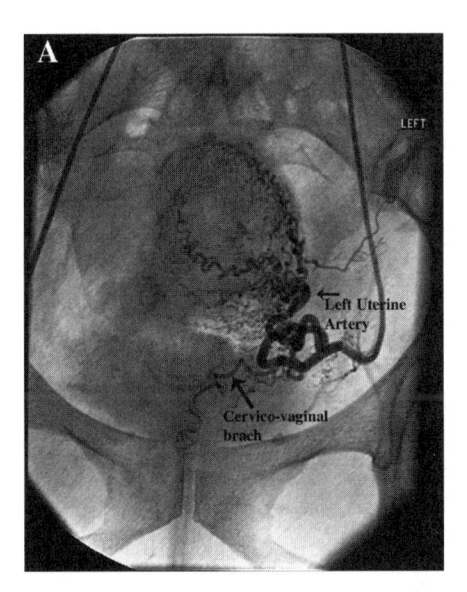

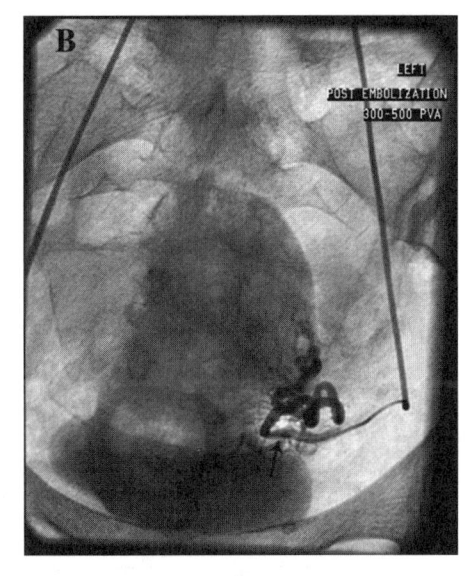

FIGURE 3. Left uterine angiogram for uterine fibroid embolization shows multiple tortuous and corkscrew-type branches supplying the fibroid. **A,** The arrow indicates the cervicovaginal branch arising from the transverse portion of the uterine artery. Would you embolize the uterine artery with the catheter in this position? **B,** A coaxial 3-French microcatheter is placed distal to the cervicovaginal branch to avoid nontarget embolization of the cervicovaginal branch. Some authors have described embolization even proximal to the cervicovaginal branch when it is not possible to pass the catheter distal to the branch. This technique usually requires bigger particles (> 500 microns) because the average size of the cervicovaginal branch is 300 microns. It also avoids nontarget embolization of the cervicovaginal branch.

47. Once the uterine-ovarian anastmosis is identified, what can be done to minimize non-target embolization of ovarian branches?
Pelage et al. found that channels of the uterine-ovarian anastomosis measure about 500 mm in diameter. They advocate the use of larger PVA particle size for UFE (such as 700–900 µm) to avoid sending particles across the anastomosis into the ovary.

48. What percentage of women have complete or partial absence of a uterine artery?
In 1–2% of women the uterine artery is completely or partially absent; this finding is a normal variant. In only about 0.4% of cases are both uterine arteries absent; in such cases, the entire vascular supply to the uterus originates from the ovarian arteries.

49. Are fibroids more vascular than the uterus?
No. Fibroids are generally hypovascular relative to the normal uterus, which accounts for their lower signal intensity on T1-weighted MRI images.

50. What is the classic anatomic origin of the uterine artery?
The uterine artery is typically the first branch of the anterior division of the internal iliac artery, arising anteromedially.

51. Give the normal diameter of the uterine artery.
The diameter of the uterine artery can greatly vary, from as small as 1–2 mm to as large as 5–6 mm. Typically, however, the diameters is about 3 mm.

52. Which part of the uterine artery is most prone to vasospasm?
Spasm usually occurs proximally in the vessel near its origin because of the straightening effect of the catheter on the sharp angle often encountered at the vessel's origin.

53. What can be done to minimize and treat spasm?
To minimize spasm
- Minimize guidewire manipulation
- Use microcatheters
- Use iso-osmolar, nonionic contrast

To treat spasm
- Wait for spasm to resolve on its own
- Inject vasodilators such as nitroglycerin
- Occasionally, slow injection of saline or contrast can break the spasm

54. Describe the mechanism of action of GnRH agonist in the treatment of fibroids.
GnRH agonist leads to decreased levels of luteinizing hormone (LH) and follicle-stimulating hormone (FSH), which in turn decrease estrogen. The decrease in estrogen leads to hyaline degeneration of fibroids and reduction of fibroid size after 3 months of therapy.

55. What vascular changes have been demonstrated in patients who take GnRH agonist?
Doppler ultrasound has shown a decrease in uterine and fibroid arterial blood flow and increased arterial resistance index, decreased arterial size, and increased atherosclerotic changes.

56. What happens to fibroids when GnRH agonists are discontinued?
Within 3 months of discontinuing GnRH therapy, the uterus and fibroids return to approximately 88% of pretreatment size.

57. Why do some authors suggest the discontinuance of GnRH agonist for at least 3 months before UFE?
The vascular changes due to GnRH agonist lead to a decrease in uterine blood flow; hence the effect of embolization may be diminished because of decreased particle delivery to distal uterine vasculature.

58. What is the ideal position of the catheter tip during embolization?

The ideal position of the catheter tip is at the medial aspect of the horizontal segment of the uterine artery, past the cervicovaginal branch if it can be identified. Occasionally the ideal position cannot be reached due to tortuosity and risk of spasm. Safe embolization is still possible, but greater care must be taken to avoid reflux or nontarget embolization.

59. What embolic agents are available for UFE?

- Polyvinyl alcohol (PVA)
- Tris-acryl collagen-coated microspheres (embospheres)
- Gelfoam
- Contour SE (Fig. 4)

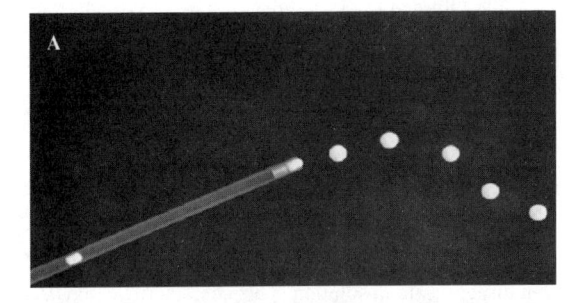

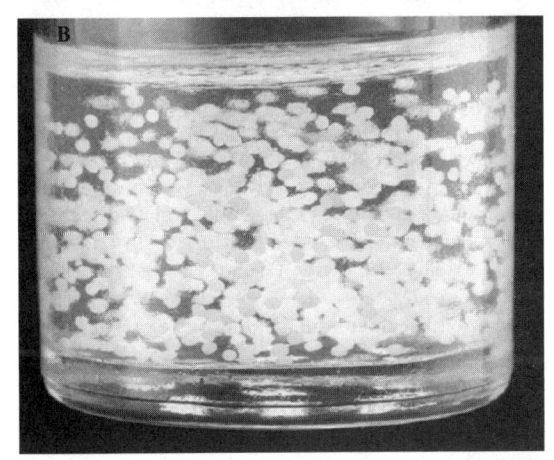

FIGURE 4. A, Contour SE microspheres passing through and exiting a microcatheter. **B,** Contour SE microspheres suspended in saline/contrast. **C,** Contour SE microspheres (700–900 μm) after exiting a FasTracker-325 microcatheter.

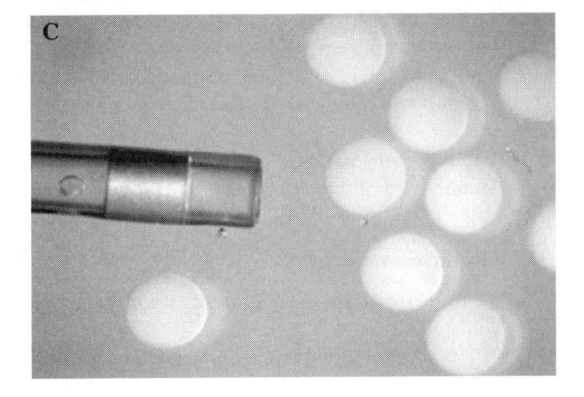

60. Describe the mechanism of action of PVA.

The intravascular injection of PVA initiates local inflammation and thrombosis that result in target vessel occlusion. There have been some reports of recanalization several months after embolization. Recanalization tends to occur within the interstices of the lumen that contain thrombus and not the latticework of PVA particles, which is not biodegradable.

61. Describe the mechanism of action of embospheres.

Embospheres are hydrophilic and nonabsorbable. Intravascular administration causes a thrombotic reaction that is similar in nature to that induced by PVA.

62. How does gelfoam work?

Gelfoam are temporary agents. They initiate an acute arteritis of the arterial wall that ultimately induces thrombosis. Resorption of gelfoam typically occurs by 6 weeks after embolization with minimal tissue reaction.

63. Discuss the theoretical advantages of embospheres vs. PVA.

1. PVA particles are somewhat jagged and tend to clump together during embolization, which makes their effective size larger than it would otherwise be. The increase in effective size leads to more proximal embolization and potentially allows collateral vessels to bypass the embolic occlusion. This problem can be somewhat overcome by greater dilution.

2. PVA particles result from milling a sheet of PVA plastic and then passing the particles through successively smaller sieves. Smaller particles may initially cling together in the dry state but disaggregate in solution. This characteristic may lead to a more distal embolization and possibly unintended organ infarction and/or nontarget delivery.

3. Embospheres are gelatin-like, hydrophilic spheres. They are softer and more deformable than PVA and easier to administer. These characteristics also lead to reduced clumping and aggregation after administration. In addition, manufacturing ensures uniformity within given size range.

64. Discuss the role of gelfoam in UFE.

The experience with UAE for a variety of indications other then fibroids reveals that pregnancies have occurred. In this setting gelfoam has been the most commonly used agent because of its potential to preserve fertility due to its temporary effect. Some authors use gelfoam for patients wishing to preserve fertility who are not candidates for or do not wish to undergo myomectomy. Of interest, there have been several published reports of pregnancies after UFE using PVA. Hence recommendation for choice of agent remains speculative.

65. What is the embolization endpoint?

Embolize until fibroid hypervascularity is eliminated, leaving flow in the main uterine artery sluggish but patent.

66. What is the risk related to radiation dose during UFE?

Worldwide experience shows no increase in pelvic tumors or congenital birth defects. The radiation dose from UFE is 10–30 times less then radiotherapy for Hodgkin's disease of the pelvis. Studies in patients with Hodgkin's disease have not shown an increase in infertility or genetic defects.

67. Why is a Foley catheter useful during uterine fibroid embolization?

Contrast administered during embolization is cleared by the kidneys into the bladder. Since the bladder overlies the uterus, it is technically difficult to visualize the uterus once the bladder is filled with contrast. Therefore, a Foley catheter keeps the bladder empty.

68. What medications are commonly used for UFE?

Although medication regimens differ substantially from hospital to hospital, most regimens include preprocedural, intraprocedural, postprocedural, and home medications.

Uterine Artery Embolization for Fibroids

69. List commonly used preprocedural medications.
- EMLA cream over the access site in the preprocedure holding area minimizes the initial pain from local anesthetic such as lidocaine.
- Metoclopramide (Reglan), 10 mg orally in the preprocedure holding area, has an antiemetic effect against postembolization nausea.
- Cefazoline (Ancef), 1gm IV; if the patient is allergic to penicillin, use vancomycin, 1gm IV.

70. List commonly used intraprocedural medications.
- Anxiolytic and sedative: midazolam (Versed)
- Narcotic: fentanyl (Sublimaze)
- Nonsteroidal anti-inflammatory drug (to reduce inflammation in response to infarction from organ embolization): ketorolac (Toradol), 2 IV doses of 30 mg each (doses are administered after each uterine artery is embolized)
- Antiemetic: ondansetron (Zofran), 2–4 mg IV if needed

71. What medications are commonly used after UFE?
- Analgesics: patient-controlled analgesia (PCA) pump, most commonly with morphine, hydromorphone (Dilaudid), or fentanyl. In addition to the PCA pump the patient is given the option of at least one supplemental oral analgesic: Percocet (oxycodone combined with acetaminophen) or Percodan (oxycodone combined with aspirin). Both acetaminophen and aspirin are antipyretics, which are helpful for the low-grade fever of postembolization syndrome.
- Antipyretics: if not included in the combination with analgesics.
- Anti-inflammatory agents: ketorolac (Toradol), 10 mg orally every 6 hours (not to exceed 5 days due to potential adverse effect of platelet inhibition and gastrointestinal bleeding from peptic ulcers).
- Antiemetic: it is sometimes difficult to distinguish nausea due to narcotic analgesia from pure postembolization nausea. If the former is suspected, the narcotic analgesic should be switched. If postembolization nausea is suspected, an antiemetic can be used. Most common ones include ondansetron (Zofran), 4 mg IV or IM, and prochlorperazine (Compazine), 10 mg IV or IM (not to exceed 40 mg/day).

72. What medications are commonly prescribed for home use?
- Analgesic, anti-inflammatory, and antipyretic: oxycodone with acetaminophen (Percocet) in 5-mg/325-mg dose, 1 to 2 tablets every 3 hours, interlaced with ketorolac (Toradol), 10-mg tablets every 6 hours (not to exceed 40 mg/day). The schedule is set for 24–48 hours. As more severe pain recedes, the time between doses can be prolonged, the number of oxycodone tablets reduced per dose, or the Percocet discontinued.
- Antiemetic: prochlorperazine (Compazine), 10 mg orally every 6 hours as needed or, if not tolerated by mouth, 25-mg suppository
- Stool softener: should be prescribed due the constipation effect of analgesics.

73. Define postembolization syndrome.
Postembolization syndrome is a symptom complex that may follow UFE. It variably consists of pain, nausea, vomiting, fever, malaise, and leukocytosis. Differentiation of postembolization syndrome from true infection is usually possible on clinical grounds.

74. Explain the importance of fever in relation to UFE.
Approximately 15–30% of patients develop fever and high white blood cell (WBC) count, typically the second day after UFE. These findings may be related to the release of tissue-breakdown products from degenerating uterine fibroids. Most patients respond to acetaminophen and hydration. Rarely, postembolization syndrome may be quite severe with fever as high as 104° F and WBC count exceeding 20,000 cells/mm^3. Such patients also frequently have malaise and fatigue. If the patient has a vaginal discharge or if fever, pain, and malaise are progressive, broad-

spectrum antibiotics should be prescribed, blood cultures drawn, and the patient followed closely.

75. What is the time course for pain following UFE?
Abdominal and pelvic cramping occurs shortly after embolization and increases over about 2 hours. The intensity typically stays at a moderately high level for 3–4 hours, then gradually decreases to a less intense level, which lasts for 4–5 hours.

76. Does pain predict the outcome of UFE?
No. Uterine or dominant fibroid volume has not been shown to correlate with the degree of postprocedural pain, nor does the severity of pain predict outcome.

77. Do fibroid composition and vascularity play a role in size reduction after UFE?
Yes. Cellular, viable fibroids, which are hypervascular and enhance after contrast administration, have shown greater volume reduction compared with nonviable, degenerating fibroids, which do not enhance with contrast administration.

78. How is fibroid volume measured?
Length × width × height × 0.52. Large volume reductions result from relatively smaller changes in diameter.

79. What is the average length of time for symptomatic improvement after UFE?
Most patients report symptomatic improvement at 3 months after UFE.

80. What are the clinical signs of uterine necrosis, fibroid infection, or fibroid expulsion?
In general, there should be few or no symptoms after 7 days after UFE. Any patient with persistent fever, progressive or unremitting abdominal pain, or purulent discharge should be evaluated promptly and treated aggressively.

81. Which type of fibroids is at the greatest risk for expulsion?
Submucosal fibroids are thought to be at greatest risk for expulsion, and in some patients expulsion may cause cervical impaction and uterine obstruction.

82. What is the rate of permanent amenorrhea after UFE?
The average rate ranges from 1% to 2%, with a definite trend toward a higher incidence in women over the age of 45 years.

83. Which malignancy can mimic symptoms of fibroids or coexist with fibroids?
Leiomyosarcoma can mimic fibroid disease. Endometrial carcinoma and cervical cancer can also coexist with fibroid disease and be a cause of menorrhagia.

84. What is the incidence of malignant tumors in premenopausal women whose uterus was removed due to fibroids?
The incidence of malignancy found at pathologic evaluation of uteri removed for fibroids is about 3 in 1,000.

85. At what age is endometrial cancer common?
85% of cases arise after menopause. The peak incidence occurs between the ages of 55 and 65. Less than 10% are found under the age of 40.

86. What screening guidelines can be used to identify most, if not all, patients with cervical or endometrial neoplasms?
Pap smear and endometrial evaluation (possibly including biopsy, hysteroscopy, or dilatation

and curettage) should be part of the routine pre-UFE workup for all patients over 40 and for any patient with an abnormal bleeding pattern.

87. How can you exclude leiomyosarcoma?
No imaging study can reliably separate leiomyoma from sarcoma.

88. Is the rate of fibroid growth a useful predictor of leiomyosarcoma?
No.

89. Are laparoscopy and biopsy justified as routine pre-UFE steps to rule out leiomyosarcoma?
The diagnostic yield for laparoscopy and biopsy is too low to justify such an invasive procedure as a routine pre-UFE step.

90. What are the two possible outcomes if a sarcoma is inadvertently embolized?
1. If complete infarction results, the embolization may be an effective primary treatment and the presence of sarcoma may never be discovered.
2. If (as is more likely) the sarcoma is not completely infarcted, the neoplasm continues to grow and the clinical failure warrants further follow-up. Therefore, if a woman who has had a technically successful UFE shows a lack of response to embolization and continues to have both fibroid growth and menorrhagia, the possibility of an unsuspected malignancy must be considered. The consensus has been that the 3- to 6-month delay in diagnosis does not affect the prognosis.

91. Is gas within the uterus a normal finding on imaging studies performed in the first week after UFE?
Yes. This finding is not an indication for therapeutic intervention unless there are associated signs and symptoms of sepsis.

92. How long after embolization may gas persist within the uterine cavity before it is considered abnormal?
This timeframe has yet to be defined. However, regression or an increase in the amount of parenchymal gas on serial scans may help differentiate whether or not a serious problem is present.

93. What is the rate of infection after UFE requiring hysterectomy?
In several studies, 0.7% of patients had infection or severe ischemia requiring hysterectomy.

94. What are the causes of failure with UFE?
- Incomplete embolization
- Luminal recanalization
- Extremely large uterine fibroids
- Presence of uterine leiomyosarcoma
- Presence of coexisting disorder (adenomyosis)
- Persistence of collateral blood supply (ovarian artery in 5% of cases)

95. What is the technical success rate of UFE?
98%.

96. What is the clinical success rate with UFE?
- 90% require no further treatment.
- 90% show a decrease in mass effect.
- 85% show a significant decrease in bleeding.

97. What is the average volume reduction with UFE?
- Uterus: 35–40%
- Fibroids: 40–50%

98. Describe the role of UAE in patients with adenomyosis.
Recent studies show that embolization successfully addresses symptoms, although the failure rate is higher than with embolization of fibroids. The definite treatment of adenomyosis is hysterectomy.

99. Summarize concerns related to embolization of pedunculated fibroids.
Ischemic changes can disrupt the stalk, thereby releasing the fibroid into the peritoneal cavity (in the case of subserosal fibroid) or endometrial cavity (in the case of submucosal fibroid), leading to fibroid expulsion or cervical impaction.

100. What recommendation has been made in regard to embolization of pedunculated fibroids?
Recommendations have varied, but stalk width greater then one-third to one-half the diameter of the fibroid is considered acceptable to most authors.

BIBLIOGRAPHY

1. Lipman JC, Smith SJ, Spies JB, et al: Uterine fibroid embolization: Follow-up. Tech Vasc Intervent Radiol 5:44–51, 2002.
2. Matson M, Nichilson A, Belli A: Anastomosis of the ovarian and uterine arteries: A potential pitfall and cause of failure of uterine embolization. Cardiovasc Intervent Radiol 23:393–396, 2000.
3. Siskin GP, Bonn J, Worthington-Kirsch RL, et al: Uterine fibroid embolization: Pain management. Tech Vasc Intervent Radiol 5:35–43, 2002.
4. Spies JB, Roth AR, Gonsalves SM, et al: Ovarian function after uterine artery embolization for leiomyomata: Assessment with use of serum follicle stimulating hormone assay. J Vasc Intervent Radiol 12:437–442, 2001.
5. Spies JB, Roth AR, Jha RC, et al: Leiomyomata treated with uterine artery embolization: Factors associated with successful symptom and imaging outcome. Radiology 222:45–52, 2002.
6. Sterling KM, Vogelzang RL, Chrisman HB, et al: Uterine fibroid embolization: Management of complications. Tech Vasc Intervent Radiol 5:56–66, 2002.
7. Vedantham S, Sterling KM, Goodwin SC, et al: Uterine fibroid embolization: Preprocedure assessment. Tech Vasc Intervent Radiol 5:2–16, 2002.
8. Worthington-Kirsch RL, Andrews RT, Siskin G, et al: Uterine fibroid embolization: Technical aspects: Tech Vasc Intervent Radiol 5:17–34, 2002.

17. ENDOVASCULAR MANAGEMENT OF TRAUMA

David E. Lee, MD

1. What group of patients may be candidates for interventional management of trauma?

Patients suffering from blunt, penetrating, or iatrogenic trauma may be eligible for interventional therapy. Stable and unstable patients may be treated. Continued resuscitation efforts may be utilized in the angiography suite while the procedure is being performed.

2. How do you perform angiography to diagnose arterial injuries in patients with traumatic injuries?

All potential sites of bleeding must be investigated with angiography with a directed exam performed at suspected sites of injury. If rupture of a large vessel (e.g., arota) is suspected, nonselective angiography may be performed to exclude massive hemorrhage. More commonly, selective/superselective catheterization of smaller vessels is performed to identify arterial sources of bleeding more accurately and to facilitate a focused approach to treatment.

3. What interventional therapeutic options are available to treat traumatic arterial injuries?

Embolization is the mainstay of treatment for arterial traumatic injuries. The use of transcatheter embolization is preferable when the patient cannot tolerate a surgical procedure or if transcatheter therapy can limit the amount of tissue or organ parenchyma loss. More recently, the development of stent grafts has allowed vessel repair instead of occlusion for injured arterial vessels.

4. What types of embolization agents are available for use in traumatic injuries?

- **Coils.** Stainless steel coils provide rapid occlusion, are delivered in a controlled manner and come in numerous different sizes to accommodate different size vessels.
- **Gelfoam.** This agent is used when the injuries are distal or multiple and in the presence of many collateral pathways. Gelfoam may be delivered as either a slurry or as a single pledget. It is a preferred agent because of its temporary effect, which lasts approximately 1–2 weeks.
- **Guglielmi detachable coils (GDCs).** These detachable coils have been used to pack pseudoaneurysms.
- **Thrombin.** Used on an investigational basis, this substance can cause thrombosis when injected via a microcatheter
- **N-butyl cyanoacyrlate.** Commonly referred to as "glue," this substance has been used on an investigational basis to embolize bleeding sites.

5. Where are interventional techniques most commonly used in trauma patients?

Interventional techniques are most commonly used for pelvic trauma, abdominal solid organ injury (e.g., liver, spleen, kidney; Figs. 1 and 2), and facial trauma.

6. Why is percutaneous management of pelvic arterial injuries advantageous?

Arteriography (Fig. 3) can quickly and accurately identify sites of hemorrhage. After diagnostic angiography, embolization can then be quickly performed. The advantage of a percutaneous technique is that the peritoneal lining remains intact and can provide a tamponade effect.

7. When is pelvic arteriography indicated?

Arteriography is indicated in either blunt or penetrating pelvic injuries with a high suspicion of arterial hemorrhage.

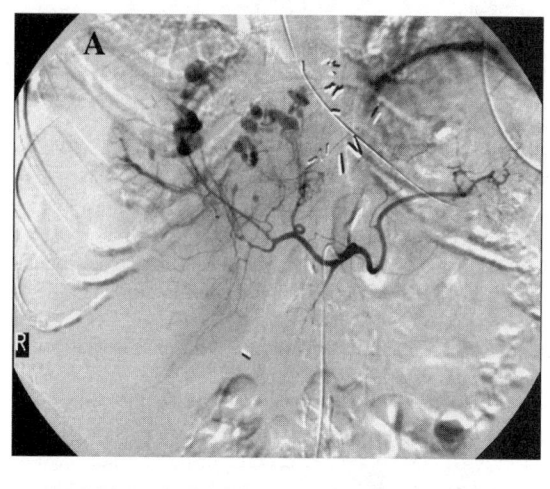

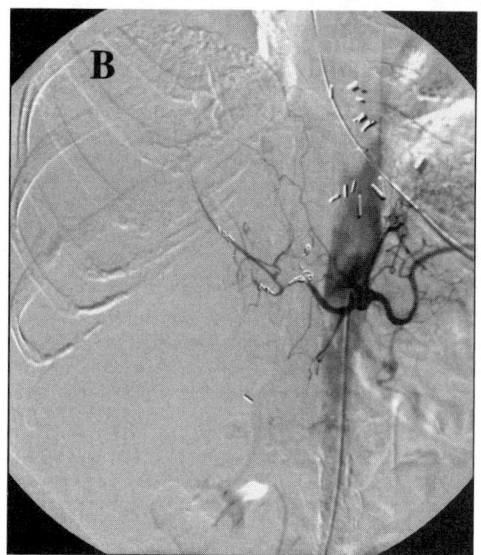

FIGURE 1. A patient underwent surgery for injuries sustained in a motor vehicle accident. After surgery he remained hypotensive and was brought to the angiography suite. **A,** The initial angiogram of the celiac artery showed massive pooling of contrast consistent with bleeding. **B,** After embolization, no further contrast extravasation was identified.

8. How is a percutaneous intervention of the pelvis performed?

A pelvic arteriogram is performed initially, followed by selective catheterization of the internal iliac arteries. If sites of bleeding are identified, they may be embolized. If no site of bleeding is localized in an unstable patients, nonselective embolization of the internal iliac arteries may be performed. Repeat angiography is performed to ensure that the site of bleeding has been effectively embolized.

9. Which arteries are most commonly injured in pelvic trauma?

The superior gluteal, internal pudendal, obturator, and lateral sacral vessels.

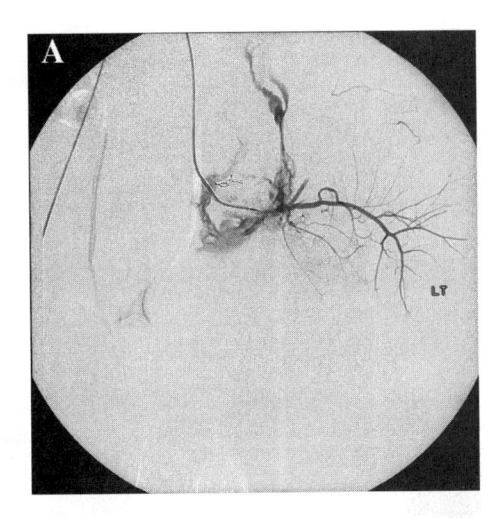

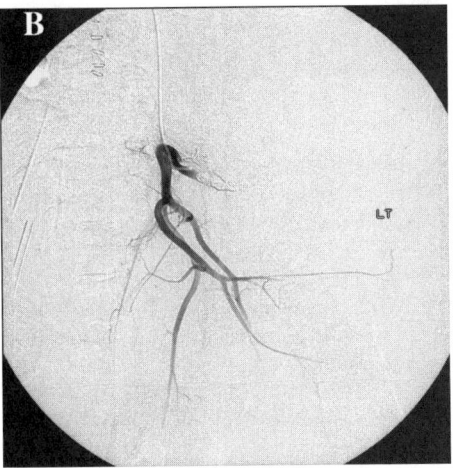

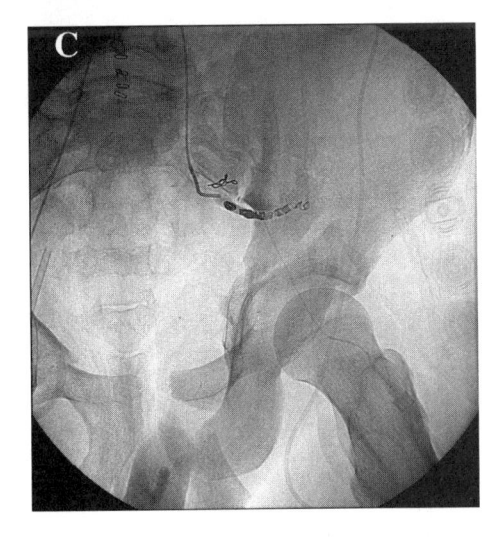

FIGURE 2. A 28-year-old patient involved in a motor vehicle accident sustained pelvic trauma, and vital signs were unstable. The patient was referred for pelvic angiography and possible embolization. **A,** Selective left hypogastric artery angiogram demonstrated active extravasations of contrast. **B** and **C,** Successful embolization was achieved from distal to proximal using multiple coils. Overall 7–11% of pelvic fractures require embolization. Only 2% of lateral compression fractures are associated with demonstrable arterial hemorrhage compared with 20% of anteroposterior compression, vertical shear, or combined mechanism injuries. Angiography is sensitive and specific in the evaluation of major arterial injuries. One series of 280 arteriograms reported sensitivity of 98.3%, a specificity of 98.5%, a positive predictive value of 95%, and a negative predictive value of 99.5% in detecting major arterial injuires.

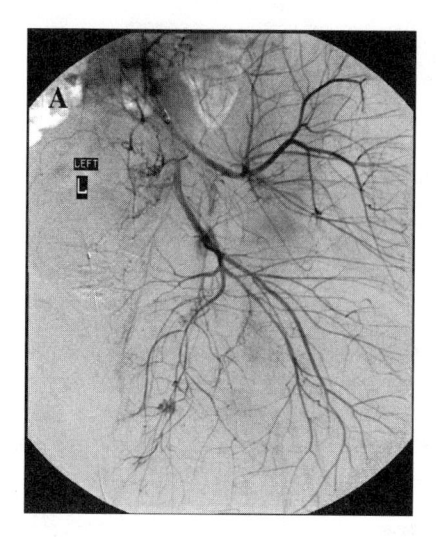

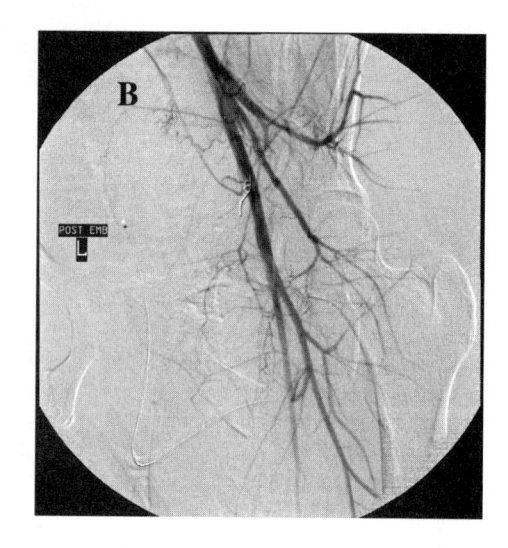

FIGURE 3. A patient involved in a motor vehicle accident sustained significant pelvic fracture. **A,** Selective angiogram of the left hypogastric artery demonstrated punctate collections of contrast. **B,** After embolization contrast extravasation resolved.

10. Is distal or proximal embolization more effective in trauma patients?

Distal embolization is clearly more effective. It may be performed with either a gelfoam slurry or microcoils for distal arterial branches. Proximal embolization is to be avoided due to the extensive collateral network in the pelvis, which renders proximal embolization ineffective.

11. What type of success can be expected with pelvic embolization?

Control of hemorrhage can be expected with arteriography and embolization in upward of 90% of patients.

12. What complications are associated with pelvic percutaneous interventions?
- Ischemia
- Infarction
- Infection
- Nontarget embolization
- Contrast-induced renal failure

13. What are the indications for percutaneous interventions in patients with abdominal trauma?

The decision to perform angiography is based on both the mechanism of injury and the patient's hemodynamic status. Unstable patients should receive an emergency laparotomy. By contrast, stable patients are evaluated with computed tomography (CT). Angiography is rarely performed unless contrast extravasation is noted on the CT scan.

14. What type of hepatic injuries may be treated by embolization?
- Extravasation
- Pseudoaneurysms
- Arteriovenous fistulas
- Arteriobiliary fistulas

15. Why is transcatheter embolization safe for hepatic injuries?

The liver is well suited to embolization because of its dual blood supply. Embolization is not likely to result in infarction unless there is also an injury to the portal vein.

16. What is the success rate for embolization of hepatic arterial injuries?

The success rate for hepatic embolization is 88% with few reported complications.

17. What is the indication for percutaneous treatment of splenic injuries?

Percutaneous treatment of splenic injuries (Fig. 4) is controversial. Injury previously requiring splenectomy will leave the patient at an increased life-long risk of sepsis. Percutaneous management of splenic injuries is organ-sparing. Investigators have embolized the splenic artery just

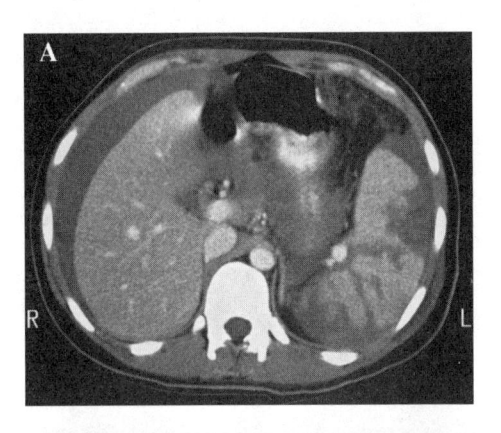

FIGURE 4. A 25-year-old man involved in a motor vehicle accident sustained blunt trauma to the abdomen. **A,** CT demonstrated splenic injury with hemoperitoneum, and an angiogram was requested for embolization. **B,** Angiogram demonstrated multiple small aneurysms. **C,** Aneurysms were successfully embolized. The spleen is the most frequently injured solid parenchymal organ within the abdomen. Most injuries are due to blunt trauma. Splenic injury is associated with rib fractures in 40% of cases. Twenty-five percent of patients with left renal injury also have splenic injury.

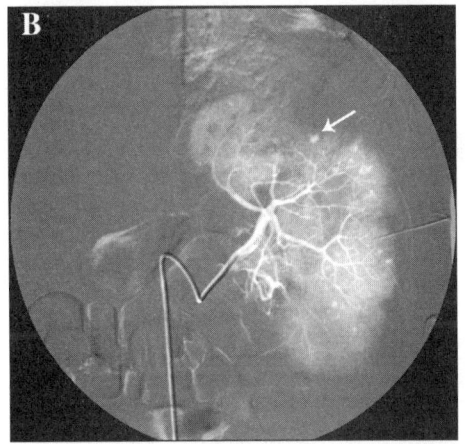

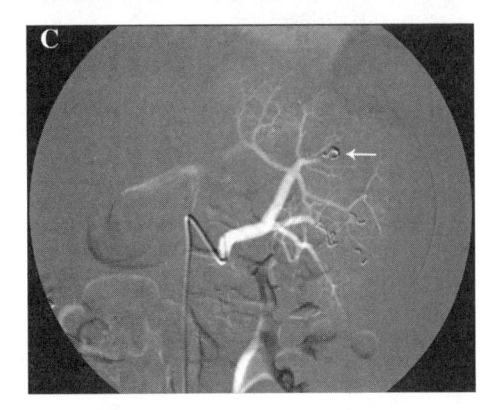

distal to the dorsal pancreatic artery with reported success rates of 87–94%. Embolization distal to the dorsal pancreatic artery allows pancreatic and gastric collaterals to supply the spleen.

18. **List the indications for percutaneous treatment of renal injuries.**
    - Extravasation
    - Pseudoaneurysm

19. **Is proximal or distal embolization preferred in the kidney?**
    Distal or superselective embolization is preferred since the kidney is an end-organ and therefore more prone to infarction. Microcatheters are often used for this indication.

20. **What embolic agents are utilized for renal embolization?**
    Embolic materials most commonly include microcoils and gelfoam.

21. **What is the success rate of renal embolization?**
    Success rates for renal embolization range from 85% to 100%.

22. **What complication of treatment is unique to renal embolization?**
    Hypertension.

23. **What clinical signs are suspicious for extremity arterial injury?**
    - Diminished pulses
    - Bruit
    - Expanding hematoma
    - Significant bleeding
    - Neurologic deficit

24. **How can extremity injuries be treated percutaenously?**
    Management is limited to embolization (Fig. 5), as determined by the nature and location of the injury. Arterviovenous fistulas and pseudoaneurysms must be embolized both proximal and distal to the lesion to prevent retrograde filling of collateral vessels.

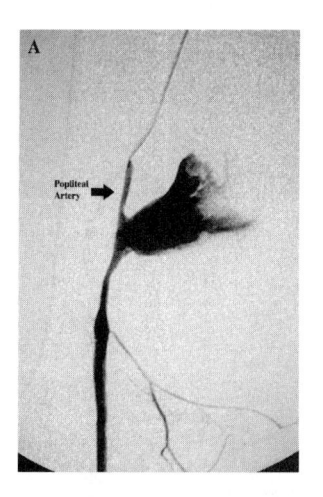

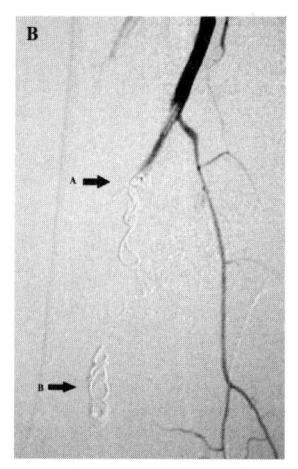

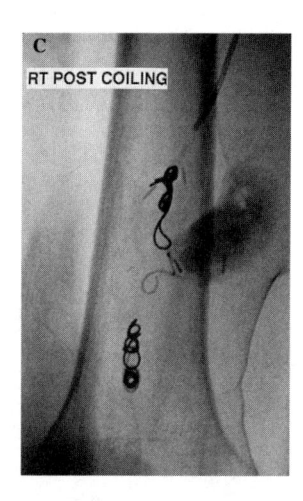

FIGURE 5. A 26-year-old man was shot in the back of the knee by his girlfriend as he was walking away from her after a fight. Examination in the emergency department revealed a tender mass in the popliteal fossa with absent distal pulses. **A,** Angiogram demonstrated traumatic injury to the popliteal artery with active extravasation. **B** and **C,** Embolization from distal to proximal with multiple coils successfully resolved the extravasation.

25. What is the success rate for embolization of extremity injuries?
Success rates range from 85% to 100%.

26. What type of head and neck injuries are best suited for embolization?
Embolization is very useful for zone III injuries, which may be difficult to access with operative management. Branches of the external carotid artery are amenable to embolization due to the rich collateral network. However, it is important to ensure that there are no extra- to intracranial anastomoses.

BIBLIOGRAPHY

1. Carlin BI, Resnick MI: Indications and techniques for urologic evaluation of the trauma patient with suspected urologic injury. Semin Urol 13:9, 1995.
2. Corr P, Hacking G: Embolization in traumatic intrarenal vascular injuries. Clin Radiol 43:262, 1991.
3. Eastham JA, Wilson TG, Larsen D, et al: Angiographic embolization of renal stab wounds. J Urol 148:268, 1992.
4. Hagiwara A, Yukioka T, Shoichi O, et al: Nonsurgical management of patients with blunt splenic injury: Efficacy of transcatheter arterial embolization. Am J Roentgenol 167:159, 1996.
5. Pachter HL, Hosfstetter SR: The current status of nonoperative management of adult blunt hepatic injuries. Am J Surg 169:442, 1995.
6. Schwartz RA, Teitelbaum GP, Katz MD, et al: Effectiveness of transcatheter embolization in the control of hepatic vascular injuries. J Vasc Intervent Radiol 359, 1993.
7. Sclafani AP, Sclafani SJA: Angiography and transcatheter arterial embolization of vascular injuries of the face and neck. Laryngoscope 106:168–173. 1996.
8. Sclafani SJA, Shaftan GW, McAuley J, et al: Interventional radiology in the management of hepatic trauma. J Trauma 24:256, 1984.
9. Sclafani SJA, Weisberg A, Scalea TM, et al: Blunt splenic injuries: Nonsurgical treatment with CT: Arteriography and transcatheter arterial embolization of splenic artery. Radiology 181:189,1991.
10. Teitelbaum GP, Reed RA, Larsen D, et al: Microcatheter embolization of non-neurologic traumatic vascular lesions. SCVIR 4:149, 1993.

18. TREATMENT OF TUMORS WITH INTERVENTIONAL RADIOLOGY PROCEDURES

Talia Sasson, MD, and Marlon Maragh, MD

1. What is heptocellular carcinoma?
Heptocellular carcinoma (HCC) is a primary tumor of the liver that in 99% of cases is associated with hepatitis B infection and hepatitis C cirrhosis. Median survival without treatment is approximately 6 months (compared with 26 months in surgically resected patients).

2. What is the curative treatment for HCC?
Surgical intervention (resection, liver transplant) is the only curative treatment for HCC. Resection is limited to 10–20% of patients.

3. How is chemoembolization performed?
Chemotherapy agents and gelfoam are injected directly into the hepatic artery (Fig. 1). Chemoembolization is a palliative treatment, not a cure, for liver cancer.

4. Describe the technique of transcatheter arterial chemoembolization.
The most common method is intra-arterial (hepatic artery) injection of emulsion of chemotherapy and oil, followed by embolization of the vessels feeding the tumor with gelfoam.

5. Which three chemotherapy drugs are used?
Usually mitomycin C, cispatin, and doxorubicin.

6. What is the advantage of transcatheter arterial chemoembolization?
It causes tumor necrosis while sparing normal liver tissue.

7. Since the hepatic artery and portal vein supply blood to the liver, why is only the hepatic artery accessed?
A tumor receives the majority of its blood supply from the hepatic artery.

8. How does the chemotherapy dose for tumor compare between chemoembolization and intravenous administration?
The tumor dose is 20 to 200 times greater in chemoembolization.

9. Why embolize?
Since no blood washes through the tumor, the chemotherapy drugs stay within the site for a longer period (up to 1 month), intensifying tumor necrosis secondary to ischemia.

10. What are the indications for transcatheter arterial chemoembolization in patients with HCC?
- Unresectable tumors
- Adjuvant therapy before liver transplant or before resection
- Tumor recurrence after surgery

11. What are the contraindications for transcatheter arterial chemoembolization?
- Biliary obstruction, which may cause biliary necrosis leading to biloma or abcesses
- Hepatic enchephlopathy or elevated total bilirubin, both of which make the patient more susceptible to fulminant liver failure

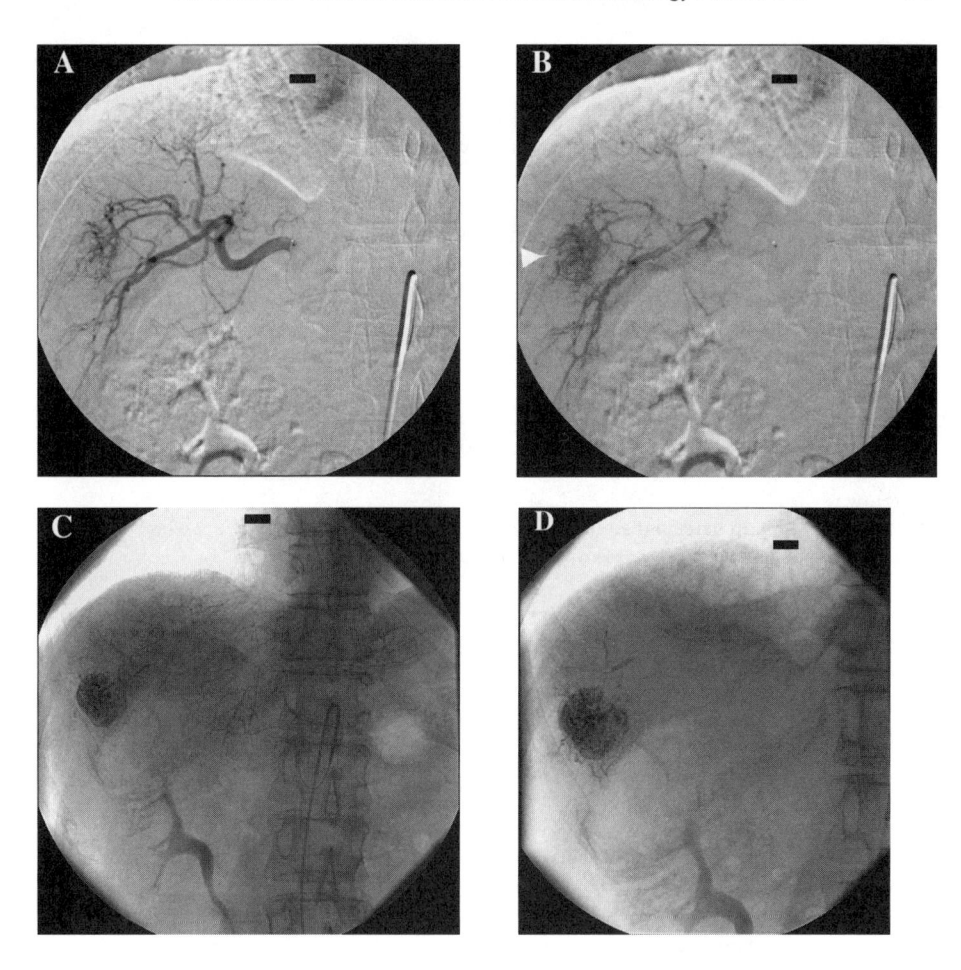

FIGURE 1. A 47-year-old man with a history of hepatitis C presented for chemoembolization of a hepatocellular carcinoma involving the right lobe of the liver. **A** and **B,** Selective angiography identified the hypervascular mass *(arrowhead)*. **C** and **D,** the mass was successfully treated with chemoembolization.

- Portal vein thrombosis, which increases the risk of hepatic failure. After chemoembolization, patients are more dependent on portal blood flow.

12. **List the complications of transcatheter arterial chemoembolization.**
    Hepatic failure, liver abscess, and gastrointestinal bleeding.

13. **Which patients are at high risk for acute hepatic failure after chemoembolization?**
    Patients with 50% of the liver replaced by tumor and patients with severe hepatic insufficiency as measured by liver function tests.

14. **What is the incidence of serious events?**
    5–7%.

15. What factors contribute to the prognosis of patients treated with transcatheter arterial chemoembolization?
Tumor size less then 5 cm is associated with a favorable outcome as well as a solitary lesion and tumor hypervascularity. Patients with poor liver function are at high risk for fulminant hepatic failure.

16. Which antibiotics are given prophylactically?
Intravenous cefazolin (Ancef), 1 gm every 8 hours, and metronidazole (Flagyl), 500 mg every 12 hours.

17. What embolization materials may be used?
- Polyvinyl alcohol (PVA) 300–500 microns
- Biospheres, 300–500 or 500–700 microns
- Gelfoam (gelatin sponge powder),
- Ethiodol (iodinated, oily x-ray contrast medium)

18. Why perform an arteriogram of the celiac and superior mesenteric arteries?
To evaluate hepatic artery anatomy and to visualize the portal vein.

19. What other vessels must be avoided?
Gastroduodenal, right gastric, and supraduodenal arteries. Embolization of these vessels may cause ischemia of the stomach or small bowel.

20. Is it possible to chemoembolize the right hepatic artery proximal to the cystic artery?
Yes. However, the risk of chemical cholicystitis secondary to gallbladder embolization is increased.

21. If disease is seen throughout the liver, what is the procedure?
Chemoembolization is performed on one lobe at a time.

22. When is the other diseased lobe treated?
Approximately 4 weeks after the initial therapy.

23. What is the 30-day mortality rate?
1–4%.

24. What should you do after the procedure?
Obtain a radiograph to evaluate the distribution of embolization medication.

25. Define postembolization syndrome.
Some patients have a post embolization syndrome, including fever, abdominal pain, nausea, and vomiting.

26. How can you treat these symptoms?
- IV hydration, antiemetics
- Patient-controlled analgesia (PCA) pump
- Antipyretics (avoid acetaminophen)

27. What situation requires a repeat embolization?
Tumor regrowth.

Treatment of Tumors with Interventional Radiology Procedures

28. Does transcatheter arterial chemoembolization affect survival rates of patients with HCC?

Controversy surrounds this method of treatment for HCC. Various nonrandomized studies strongly suggest that transcatheter arterial chemoembolization prolongs the lives of patients with HCC, whereas a number of randomized studies suggested that this treatment is not effective for HCC.

29. Discuss the role of transcatheter arterial chemoembolization in liver metastases.

Due to poor results of systemic chemotherapy in patients with liver metastases from colorectal carcinoma, ocular melanoma, neuroendocrine tumor, and gastrointestinal sarcomas, experimental treatment of liver metastases with transcatheter arterial chemoembolization has been done. Initial studies evaluating transcatheter arterial chemoembolization of colorectal metastases to the liver show promising early response.

30. Discuss the role of transcatheter arterial chemoembolization in liver metastases from carcinoid.

Transcatheter arterial chemoembolization for patients with liver metastases and carcinoid syndrome results in relief of symptoms in 90–100% of cases. Hormone levels were reduced in 90% of patients, and tumor reduction was observed in 60–80%. Studies that compared transcatheter arterial chemoembolization with hepatic artery embolization showed that the response rates in both treatments were comparable.

31. When should transcatheter arterial chemoembolization be considered for a patient with liver metastases?

Transcatheter arterial chemoembolization should be considered only for patients with metastatic disease that is confined to the liver and for patients with minimal extrahepatic metastases in which the liver disease is considered the primary source of morbidity.

32. What types of percutaneous ablation therapy are used for hepatic tumors?
- Direct injection into the tumor of chemical agents such as ethanol, hypertonic saline, and acetic acid
- Thermal techniques such as radiofrequency microwaves or cryotherapy

33. Which imaging modalities are used for percutaneous ablation therapy?

Percutaneous ablation therapy can be done with ultrasound, computed tomography (CT; Fig. 2), or magnetic resonance imaging (MRI) guidance.

34. Explain the purpose of thermal ablation therapy.

The purpose is to destroy the entire tumor without damaging adjacent vital structures.

FIGURE 2. Computed tomography of the liver in a patient with metastatic disease (from colon cancer) confined to the liver. The R_f ablation needle is seen in the right lobe liver lesion.

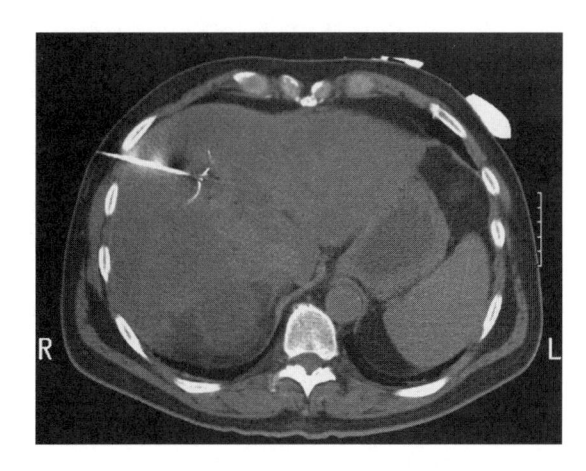

35. What are the ablative margins?
Ablative margins refer to the 0.5–1 cm of normal tissue surrounding the tumor that is also treated to ensure that all malignant cells are destroyed.

36. Define coagulation necrosis.
Irreversible thermal damage to cells that accrue immediately when the cells are exposed to temperatures between 60°C and 100°C.

37. What happens at temperatures greater then 105°
Tissues may boil, causing vaporization, or undergo carbonization. This decreases energy transmission and results in suboptimal ablation.

38. What diameter of coagulation can a single radiofrequency electrode produce?
1.6 cm. Because of poor heat conduction by the tissue, energy falls off rapidly from the electrodes. There is a limit to the energy used because increasing the tissue temperature too high results in suboptimal ablation.

39. What strategies may be used to increase the diameter of coagulation produced by radiofrequency electrodes?
- Improve heat conduction
- Increase the energy
- Decrease tumor tolerance to heat

40. What strategies enable us to use more energy?
Use of several electrodes in the same lesion or use of a radiofrequency umbrella electrode. The umbrella electrodes have several hooks that act as speared electrodes and increase the ablation diameter by 3–5 cm (Fig. 3).

41. What strategies can decrease heat lost?
Reduced blood flow during radiofrequency treatment decreases heat loss. Blood flow can be reduced with an occlusion balloon or arterial embolization.

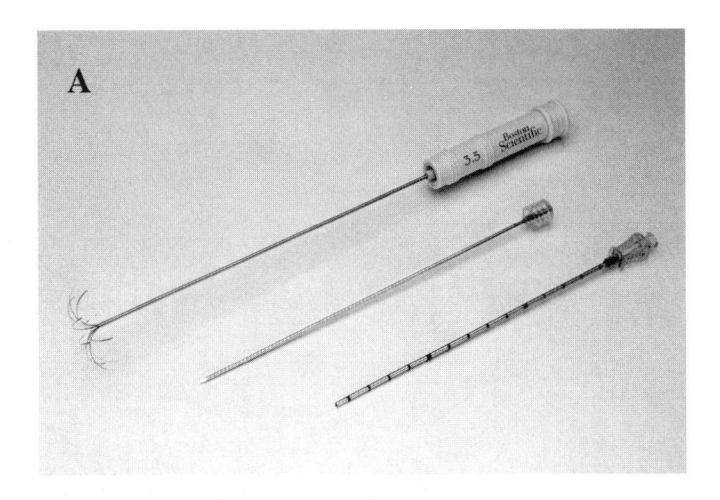

FIGURE 3. The radio frequency ablation (RFA) needle. **A,** The set consists of the RFA needle with coxial guide needle. **B,** Magnification view demonstrating the needle with umbrella appearance. **C** and **D,** The needle in the lesion. (Courtesy of Boston Scientific.)

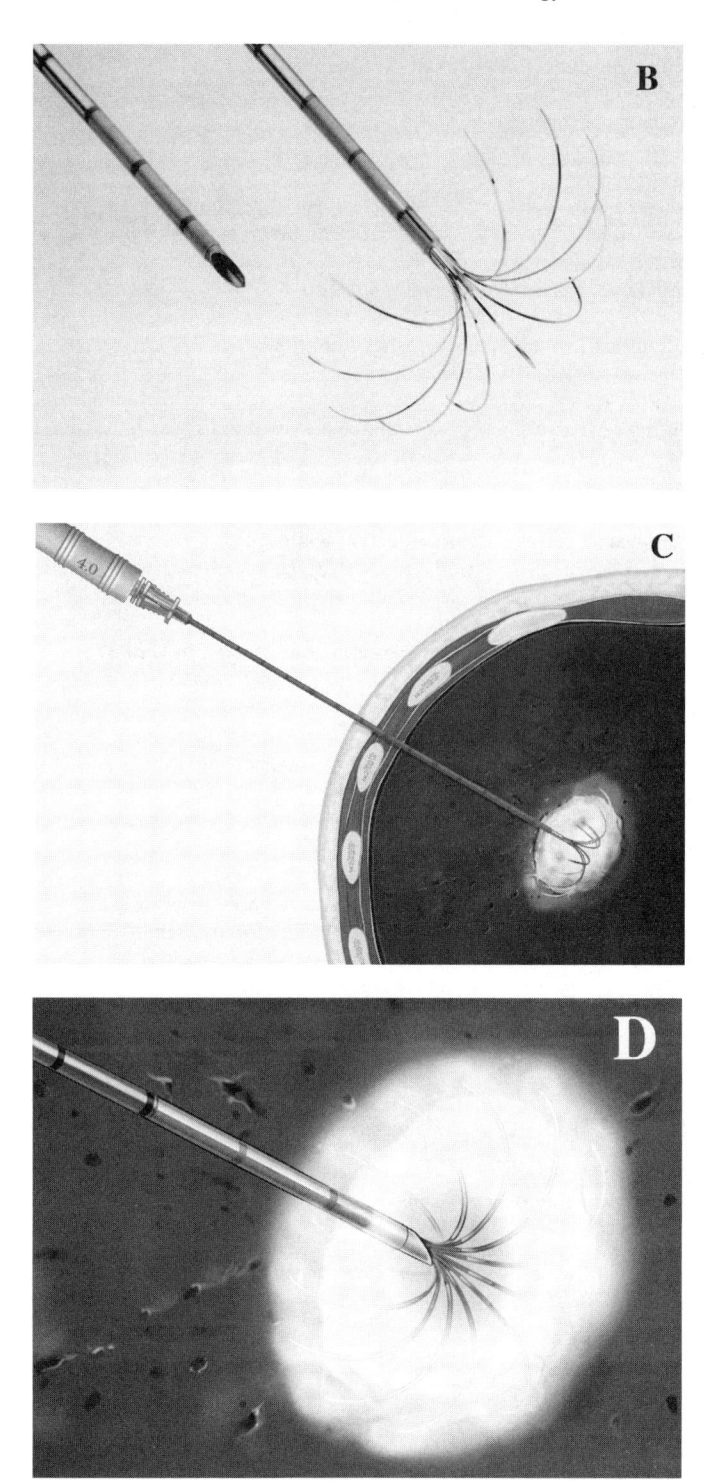

FIGURE 3. (continued)

42. List the roles of imaging during radiofrequency therapy.
- Targeting of the lesion
- Evaluation of treatment
- Follow-up

43. How is tumor necrosis assessed after radiofrequency ablation?
Contrast-enhanced CT demonstrates the necrotic tumor as hypodense. MRI demonstrates a hypointense area in T1-weighted images and an iso- or hyperintense area in T2-weighted images. These areas should not enhance with gadolinium.

44. List the complications of radiofrequency ablation in the liver.
Hemorrhage, abscess, and bile peritonitis.

45. Which patients are candidates for radiofrequency therapy for liver tumor?
- Patients with small lesions (< 5 cm)
- Patients with fewer than 4 lesions

46. What is the percutaneous ethanol injection technique?
Percutaneous placement of a needle into the center of a tumor with injection of absolute ethanol.

47. What imaging modality is used for percutaneous ethanol injection?
Ultrasound or CT.

48. How much ethanol is injected?
$V = \frac{4}{3} \pi (r+0.5)^3$, where V = volume and r = radius.

49. What is the advantage of percutaneous ethanol injection over radiofrequency ablation?
Smaller needle.

50. Which patients are candidate for percutaneous ethanol injection?
The selection criteria are similar to those for radiofrequency therapy.

51. What are the results of percutaneous ethanol injection?
High rate of technical success (90%), with a 0–17% rate of local recurrence.

BIBLIOGRAPHY

1. Bast RC, Kufe DW, Pollock RE, et al (eds): Cancer Medicine, 5th ed. Hamilton, Canada, B.C. Decker, 2000.
2. Bolondi L, Piscaglia F, Camaggi V, et al: Review article: Liver transplantation for HCC. Treatment options on the waiting list. Aliment Pharmacol Ther 17(Suppl 2):145–150, 2003.
3. Donckier V, Van Laethem JL, Ickx B, et al: Local ablative treatments for liver metastases: The current situation. Acta Chir Belg 103(5):452–457, 2003.
4. Gupta S, Yao JC, Ahrar K, et al: Hepatic artery embolization and chemoembolization for treatment of patients with metastatic carcinoid tumors: The M.D. Anderson experience. Cancer J 9(4):261–267, 2003.
5. Schwartz JM, Ham JM: Treatment of hepatocellular carcinoma. Curr Treat Opt Gastroenterol 6:465–472, 2003.
6. Shen BY, Li HW, Regimbeau JM, Belghiti J: Recurrence after resection of hepatocellular carcinoma. Hepatobil Pancreat Dis Int 1:401–405, 2002.
7. Stuart K: Chemoembolization in the management of liver tumors. Oncologist 8:425–437, 2003.
8. Sumie S, Yamashita F, Ando E, et al: Interventional radiology for advanced hepatocellular carcinoma: Comparison of hepatic artery infusion chemotherapy and transcatheter arterial lipiodol chemoembolization. Am J Roentgenol 181:1327–1334, 2003.

19. VASCULAR CLOSURE DEVICES

Labib Syed, MD

1. **What are closure devices?**
Closure devices are a new technology to aid in the closure of arterial puncture sites following diagnostic and interventional endovascular procedures.

2. **Explain the basic purpose of closure devices.**
To ensure an accelerated hemostasis at the groin puncture site after removal of the indwelling sheath.

3. **Describe the standard of care for treating the groin puncture site after an arteriotomy for a diagnostic or interventional endovascular procedure.**
External compression, most commonly applied manually for a minimum of 10 minutes. The time increases if the patient is coagulopathic. The patient must also remain supine and under constant nursing supervision for 6 hours.

4. **Give the complication rate of simple manual compression at the groin puncture site.**
5%.

5. **What is the most common complication? What are the more serious complications?**
The most common complication is the development of a small hematoma. More serious complications include development of: arterial pseudoaneurysms, arteriovenous fistulas, and infections.

6. **What types of arterial closure devices are available?**
Suture-mediated closure devices (SMCDs) and non-suture-mediated closure devices (NSMCDs).

7. **What was the first SMCD?**
The Perclose systems (Abbott Laboratories, Abbott Park, IL), which include the Closer and the Prostar XL (Fig. 1).

8. **Explain the premise of the Perclose systems.**
The basis of the Perclose systems is the delivery of needles and suture into the vessel to permit hemostasis.

9. **What is the basic difference between the Closer and Prostar XL?**
Closer is used for 5- to 6-French sheaths, whereas Prostar XL may be used with 8- and 10-French sheaths. The Prostar XL has an added advantage in that it may be used in patients who are anticoagulated.

10. **What are the mean times to hemostasis (minutes) and ambulation (hours) with use of Perclose systems?**
- Hemostasis: 4.4 + 3.7 min
- Ambulation: 1.8 + 3.2 hours

11. **Name the second group of SMCDs.**
Sutura (Fig. 2).

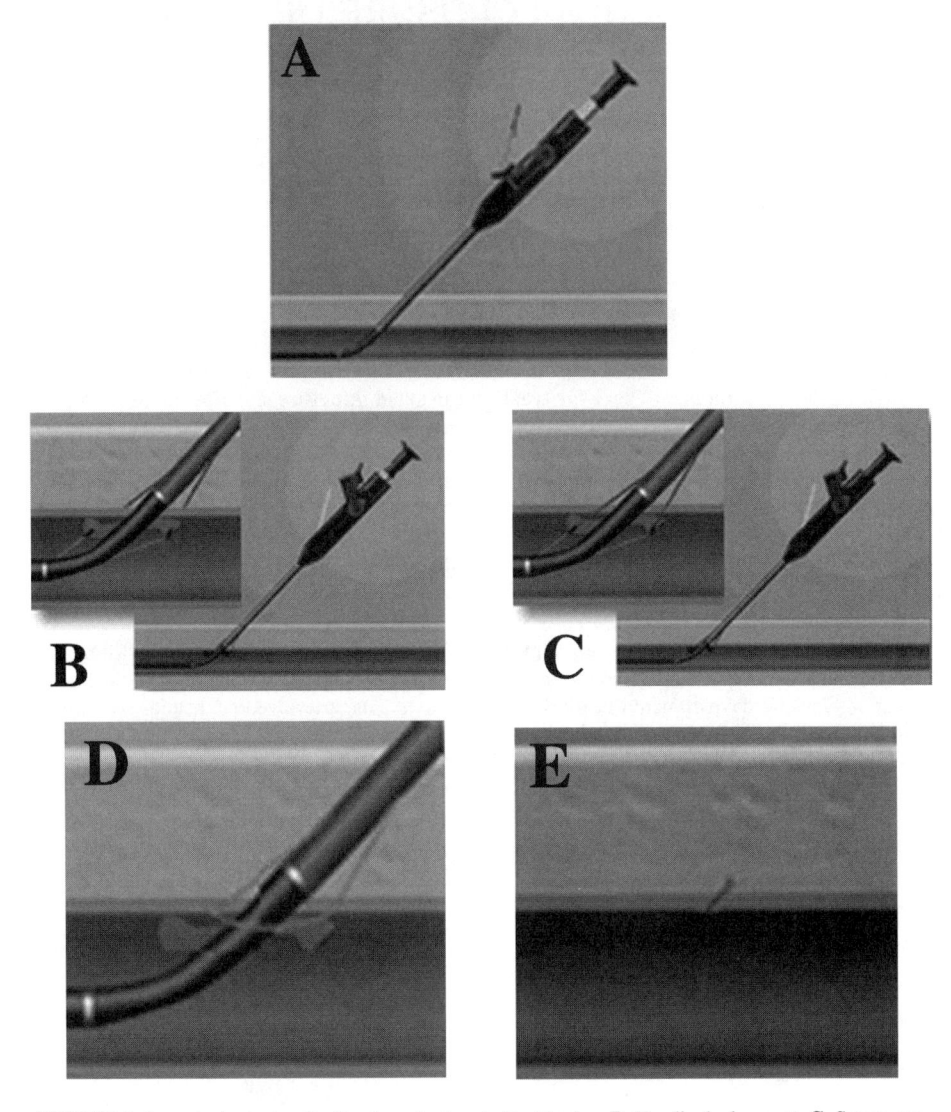

FIGURE 1. Steps in deploying the Perclose device. **A,** Positioning. **B,** Needle deployment. **C,** Suture capture. **D,** Needle removal. **E,** Hemostasis. (Courtesy of Abbott Laboratories.)

12. **What are the major differences between Perclose and Sutura?**
    Perclose may be used for sheaths up to 12 French in size, whereas Sutura may be deployed in sheaths up to 24 French in size.

13. **Explain the underlying mechanism of NSMCDs.**
    NSMCDs create a form of mechanical barrier to "plug" the arteriotomy puncture site, much as the body creates a platelet plug to maintain hemostasis.

14. **What are the most common types of NSMCDs?**
    AngioSeal (St. Jude Medical, St. Paul, MN) and VasoSeal (Datascope, Mahwah, NJ; Fig. 3).

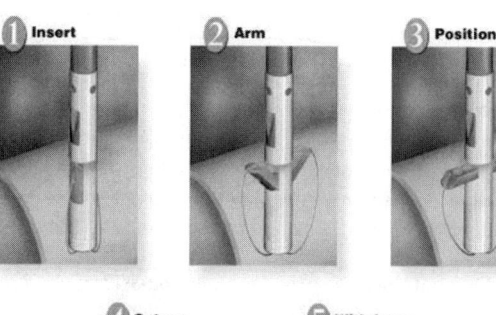

FIGURE 2. Steps involved in deploying the Sutura device. (Courtesy of Sutura, Inc.)

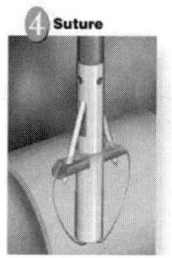

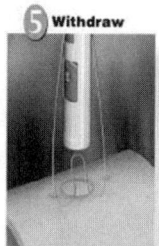

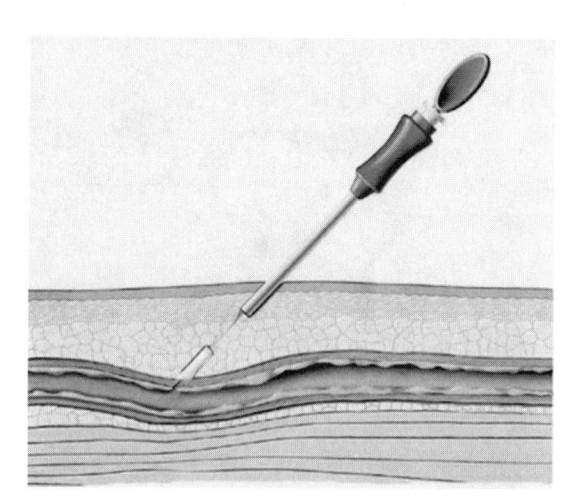

FIGURE 3. Vasoseal closure device. (Courtesy of Datascope, Inc.)

15. How does AngioSeal function?
An anchor plate placed within the vessel provides tension on a collagen plug holding it in place on the outside of the vessel wall, thus ensuring hemostasis. The anchor plate and collagen plug are left within the body to biodegrade.

16. What is the time period for the biodegradation of the anchor plate and collagen plug?
Within 30 days complete biodegradation should have occurred.

17. What is the most common complication of AngioSeal?
Migration of the indwelling anchor plug down the vessel, resulting in embolization at the popliteal trifurcation.

18. What is the major difference between AngioSeal and VasoSeal?
The VasoSeal uses a similar collagen seal but without a biodegradable prosthesis.

19. Name the third type of NSMCD.
The Duett device (Vascular Solutions, Minneapolis, MN; Fig. 4).

20. How does the Duett function?
A3-French catheter is advanced through an indwelling arterial sheath, and a balloon located at the end of the catheter is inflated and positioned inside the artery at the puncture site to temporarily stop bleeding. A liquid procoagulant is then delivered to the outside of the puncture site to stimulate the body's natural clotting process. The catheter and sheath are then removed.

21. Of what does the procoagulant consist?
Collagen and thrombin.

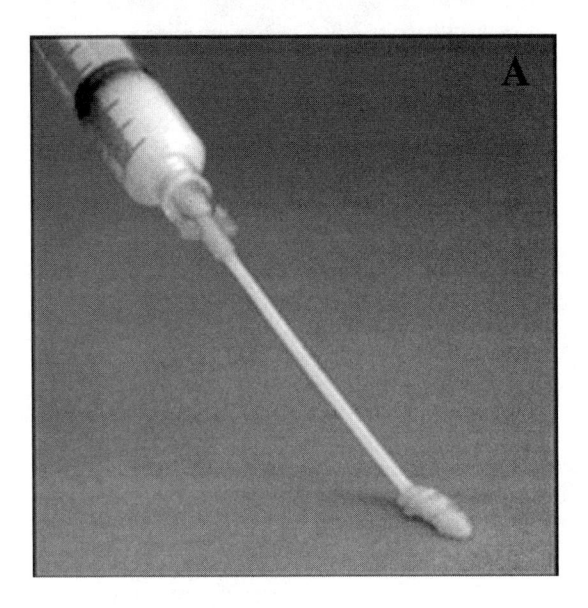

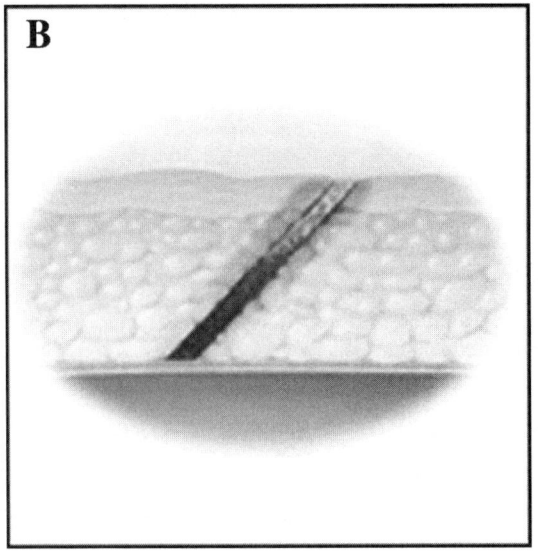

FIGURE 4. A and **B,** The Duett device. (Courtesy of Vascular Solutions.)

22. List the contraindications to use of the Duett device.
- Sensitivity to materials made from cattle
- Coagulopathies
- Blockages in or previous surgeries on a leg
- Leg pain when walking
- High blood pressure
- Pregnancy

BIBLIOGRAPHY

1. Cleveland G, Hill S, Williams S: Arterial puncture closure using a collagen plug. II: VasoSeal. Tech Vasc Intervent Radiol 6(2):82–84, 2003.
2. Dickey KW: Arterial hemostasis using the Duett sealing device. Tech Vasc Interv Radiol 6(2):85–91, 2003.
3. Hoffer EK, Bloch RD: Percutaneous arterial closure devices. J Vasc Intervent Radiol 14:865–85, 2003.
4. Mackrell PJ, Kalbaugh CA, Langan EM III, et al: Can the Perclose suture-mediated closure system be used safely in patients undergoing diagnostic and therapeutic angiography to treat chronic lower extremity ischemia? J Vasc Surg 38(6):1305–1308, 2003.
5. Rilling WS, Dicker M: Arterial puncture closure using a collagen plug. I: Angio-Seal. Tech Vasc Intervent Radiol 6(2):76–81, 2003.
6. Starnes BW, O'Donnell SD, Gillespie DL, et al: Percutaneous arterial closure in peripheral vascular disease: A prospective randomized evaluation of the Perclose device. J Vasc Surg 38:263–271, 2003.
7. Taylor LM Jr, Mueller-Velten G, Koslow A, et al, for the Beriplast B Investigators: Prospective randomized multicenter trial of fibrin sealant versus thrombin-soaked gelatin sponge for suture- or needle-hole bleeding from polytetrafluoroethylene femoral artery grafts. J Vasc Surg 38:766–771, 2003.
8. Wagner SC, Gonsalves CF, Eschelman DJ, et al: Complications of a percutaneous suture-mediated closure device versus manual compression for arteriotomy closure: A case-controlled study. J Vasc Intervent Radiol 14:735–741, 2003.

20. VENOUS ACCESS

Waqar A. Shah, MS, MD

1. What information should you know about the patient before attempting venous access?
The history should include indications for the procedure, anticoagulation status, and laboratory values, including hematocrit, platelet count, international normalized ratio (INR), prothrombin time (PT), and partial thromboplastin time (PTT).

2. What laboratory values are acceptable for venous puncture?
Acceptable values vary, depending on the interventional radiologist performing the procedure. However, a platelet count over 50, INR under 1.5, PT below 25 seconds, and PTT below 40 seconds are acceptable to most interventionalists.

3. List the indications for obtaining vascular access.
- Delivery of medications (e.g., antibiotics, chemotherapeutic drugs)
- Delivery of total parenteral nutrition (TPN)
- Withdrawal of blood samples
- Hemodialysis

4. List the devices used for venous access.
- Midline catheters
- Peripherally inserted central catheters (PICCs)
- Implantable ports
- Acute and chronic dialysis catheters
- Acute and chronic central venous catheters

5. List factors that influence the choice of device for venous access.
- Frequency of therapy. Daily access favors an external device. Weekly or monthly use favors an implantable device.
- Length of therapy. A few weeks to several months of usage warrant nontunneled chest wall catheters, PICCs, and tunneled chest wall catheters. Months to years of use warrant tunneled central lines and subcutaneous ports.
- Type of therapy
- Patient level of activity and comfort. PICCs are small and prone to mechanical failure. Larger tunneled catheters are more durable but also can break at the hub. Ports are the most durable.
- Ability to care for the device. Ports require the least maintenance.
- Personal preference

6. What materials are used to construct venous catheters?
Polyurethane and silicone rubber are the most abundant materials.

7. How are the two materials different?
Silicone rubber is a biocompatible blend of silica and polymethylsiloxane with a high coefficient of friction. It is also kink-resistant. However, silicone rubber catheters are thick-walled.

Polyurethane is a newer material that is stronger than silicone. It allows a larger lumen with the same outer diameter, yielding strong, thin-walled catheters. It is a high-molecular-weight macroglycol linked to urethane. The result is high flow rates.

8. How are the catheter tips designed? Explain the advantages and/or disadvantages of each design.

End-hole catheters have an open-ended tip that allows easier placement and sizing due to the ability to trim the catheter to size.

Valved-tip catheters have specially designed slits at the tip that allow blood to be aspirated and solutions infused. They do not allow blood to enter the catheter when it is not in use. As a result, routine heparinization is not required to prevent catheter thrombosis. The tip cannot be trimmed to size.

Staggered-tip dual-lumen catheters are specifically designed for therapies requiring simultaneous rapid aspiration and infusion with limited admixture (e.g., hemodialysis and pheresis; Fig. 1).

9. When should a chest wall catheter be tunneled?

Whenever the catheter is intended to stay in place for more than 4 weeks.

10. What is the purpose of the cuff on a tunneled catheter?

The cuff incites the growth of fibrous tissue, which stabilizes the catheter and allows it to stay in position for longer periods. Some catheters offer a second antimicrobial cuff that is positioned at the skin exit site, serving as an antimicrobial barrier. Studies have not shown the the antimicrobial cuff reduces infection.

11. When should ultrasound be used in attempts to gain venous access?

Whenever possible. Ultrasound guidance has been proved to be a tremendous aid in minimizing complications of gaining venous access.

12. What kind of ultrasound probe should be used to gain venous access?

A high-frequency, 7.5-MHz linear transducer.

13. How is ultrasound used to gain venous access?

The ultrasound probe is kept sterile under a cover with coupling gel. The puncture should be performed with the transducer in a transverse orientation perpendicular to the vessel being punctured. Lidocaine should be used for local anesthetic in the region below the probe and where the

FIGURE 1. Arrow indicates the staggered-tip, dual-lumen Vaxcel hemodialysis catheter. Also note the ideal position of the catheter, with the staggered tip facing the atrial lumen. If the tip is positioned facing the arterial wall, the result may be malfunctioning of the catheter because its tip may adhere to the atrial wall on suction.

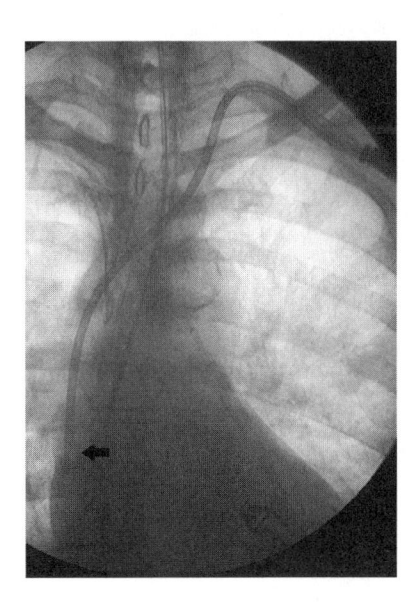

skin will be entered. Venous structures can be discerned by gentle compression. If the vessel does not compress under ultrasound, it is either an occluded vein or an artery

14. What if arterial blood is drawn into the syringe during attempts at venous access?
1. Withdraw the needle immediately.
2. Apply manual pressure for at least 5 minutes.
3. Monitor the patient's hemodynamic status.
4. Watch breath sounds in order to recognize a hemothorax.

15. How will I know if I have given the patient a pneumothorax?
Sometimes you will not know until you obtain the postprocedure chest x-ray. However, in the vast majority of cases, you obtain a rush of air in the syringe as you advance or withdraw while aspirating. Careful monitoring of the patient also gives you the answer.

16. What do I do if I have given the patient a pneumothorax?
If it is a tension pneumothorax, decompress with a 16-gauge angiographic catheter in the second intercostal space in the midclavicular line. If it is less than 10%, administer 100% oxygen and follow with serial x-rays. If it is greater than 10%, a chest tube is indicated.

17. Does it matter if the patient has an inferior vena cava (IVC) filter if I am trying to gain subclavian or internal jugular vein access?
Yes. You should be aware of the patient's history and try to avoid any possible complications. On the chance that the guidewire goes past the heart and into the IVC, the IVC filter may be encountered.

18. What can be done if I forget to cover the needle after the vein is accessed and fear that the patient may have gotten enough air to cause an air embolism?
Attempt to withdraw air by suctioning from the catheter. If the patient goes into cardiac arrest, follow the protocol for advanced cardiac life support (ACLS). If the patient is stable, position the patient in left lateral decubitus position with Trendelenberg. This position traps air in the right ventricle. A chest x-ray in this position can show the air if it is present. Note that air dissolves with time.

19. How much air in the venous system will cause an air embolism?
Usually greater than 20 ml.

20. What happens if I see a dysrhythmia on the cardiac monitor as I place the line?
Atrial or ventricular dysrhythmias are associated with wires and catheters in the right atrium and/or right ventricle and usually resolve when the catheter is pulled back into the superior vena cava (SVC). If dysrhythmia persists, medical management may be necessary.

21. What is the normal position of the internal jugular vein with respect to the carotid artery?
See Fig. 2.

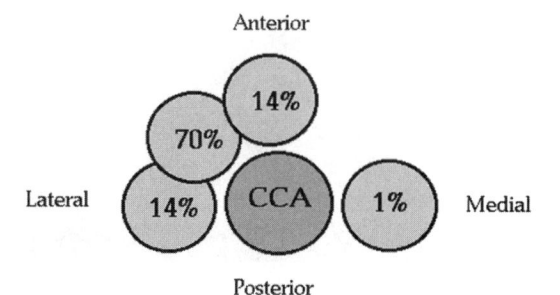

FIGURE 2. Position of the internal jugular vein in relation to the common carotid artery.

22. **List the contraindications to internal jugular venous access.**
    - Untreated sepsis
    - Venous thrombosis (Fig. 3)
    - Previous ipsilateral neck surgery (Fig. 4)

23. **What is the proper position for gaining internal jugular venous access?**
    The patient should be supine, in Trendelenberg position, and the head should be turned to the contralateral side at least 45° to provide adequate exposure to the neck.

24. **How is the internal jugular vein accessed using the central approach?**
    1. Using sterile technique, identify the anatomy of the neck, including the external jugular vein, sternocleidomastoid muscles, and carotid artery.
    2. Prepare and drape the apex of the triangle formed by the heads of the sternocleidomastoid muscles.
    3. Using a 25-gauge needle and 1% lidocaine, anesthetize the skin and subcutaneous tissue at the apex of the triangle.
    4. It is particularly important to withdraw before injecting into the neck because the vessel may be very superficial in this region.
    5. Identify the carotid artery and retract it medially with your free hand. At this time, ultrasound guidance is extremely useful.

25. **What happens if the carotid artery is punctured?**
    Withdraw the needle immediately and apply pressure. Surgical intervention may be necessary if the bleeding is not controlled. Use of a micropuncture kit greatly reduces the chance of complications.

26. **Explain the micropuncture technique.**
    The micropuncture technique involves using a micropuncture needle and 0.018-inch wire,

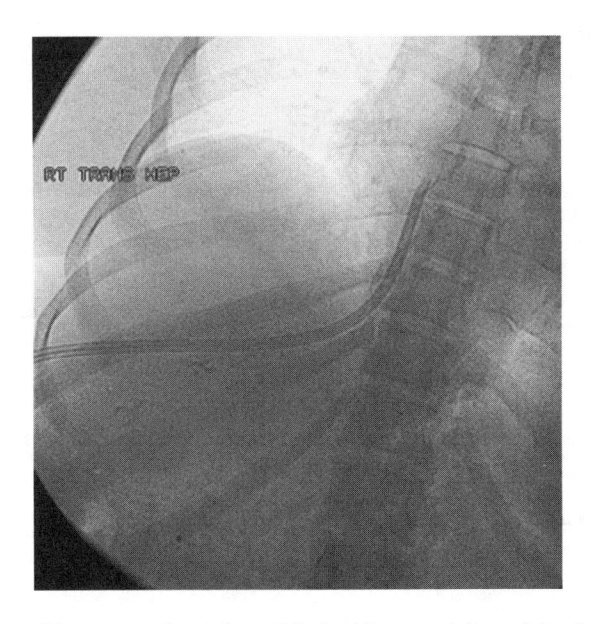

FIGURE 3. A 41-year-old woman on chronic hemodialysis with no remaining peripheral access because of previous multiple lines leading to thrombosis and occlusion. A translumbar catheter was also placed and failed to function properly. Hence, a transhepatic venous catheter was placed for hemodialysis.

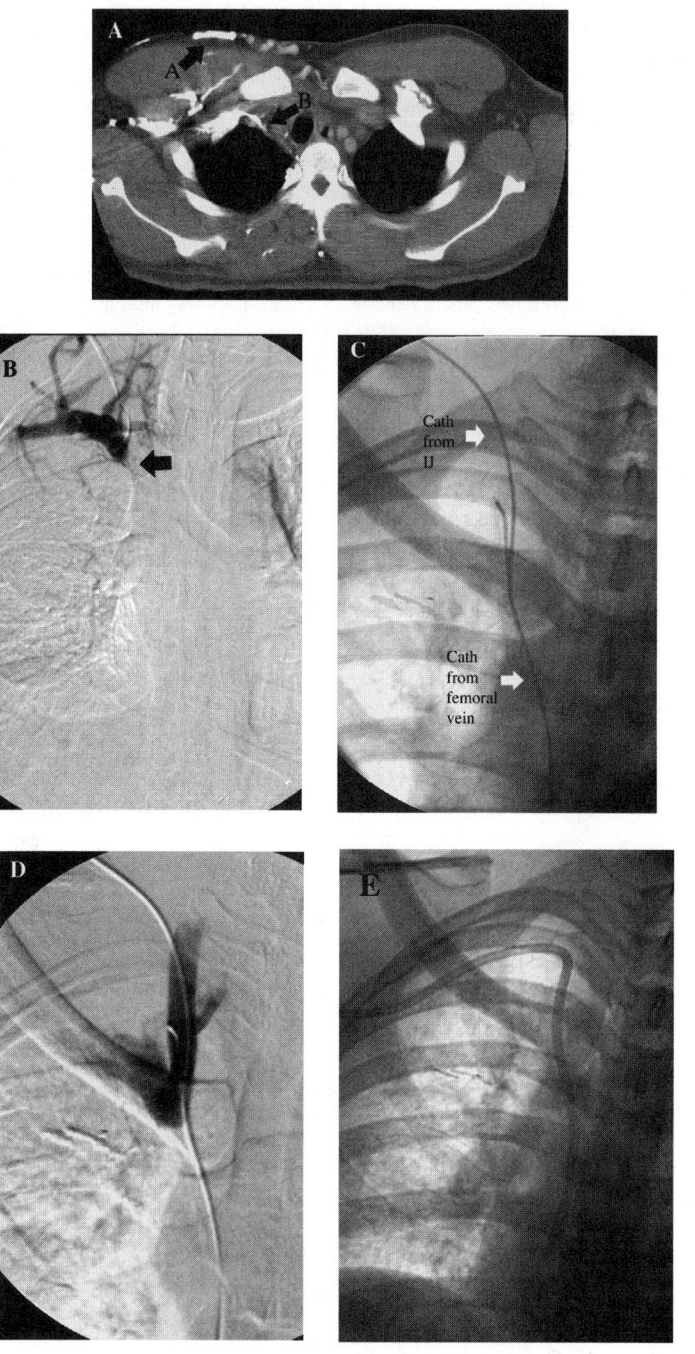

FIGURE 4. Dialysis patient with a history of left neck dissection for lymphoma presents for a central line placement. Because of previous left neck surgery, access was obtained on the right and demonstrated occlusion of the right subclavian brachiocephalic junction (**A** and **B**). Because of the left neck surgery the plan was to recanalize the occluded right internal jugular vein. The occlusion was recanalized from above and below (**C**) and confirmed to be in the lumen by contrast injection (**D**). Angioplasty of the occlusion was performed, and a dialysis catheter was placed (**E**).

exchanging for an 8-French sheath, and upgrading to the 0.035-inch wire instead of gaining direct access with the 18-gauge needle.

27. What is Horner's syndrome? Explain the cause.
Horner's syndrome consists of two signs: a constricted pupil and slight drooping of the eyelid. These signs are caused by damage to the sympathetic nervous system as it supplies the eye on the affected side of the head. The patient may exhibit signs of Horner's syndrome temporarily if the carotid sheath is punctured. Signs usually resolve without intervention.

28. How is the femoral vein accessed?
1. In a sterile fashion, shave, prepare, and drape the left or right groin.
2. Identify the relevant anatomy, including the inguinal ligament.
3. Palpate the femoral artery. The femoral vein runs approximately 1 or 2 cm medial to the femoral artery.
4. Anesthetize the skin and subcutaneous area just medial to the palpated pulse with a 25-gauge needle. Ultrasound guidance can be extremely helpful at this time.
5. Using an 18-gauge needle, puncture the skin and advance cranially at a 45° angle to the skin while aspirating.

29. What should be done if the femoral artery is punctured and/or a hematoma develops?
1. Withdraw the needle.
2. Hold pressure for at least 5–10 minutes before checking for hemostasis.
3. If after 5 minutes, the artery is still bleeding, hold pressure for another 10 minutes.
4. Continue doubling the time of holding pressure between checking until the bleeding stops.

30. What is a peripherally inserted central catheter (PICC)?
PICCs are venous lines that are inserted through a peripheral vein of the upper extremity (antecubital, basilic, cephalic veins). The tips are placed in a central location (superior vena cava, right atrium). PICCs are available in 2- to 7-French sizes with single or dual lumens.

31. Give the major indications for a PICC.
Daily access for a few weeks or up to 6 months.

32. What can be delivered through a PICC?
Fluids, blood and blood products, total parenteral nutrition, antibiotics, chemotherapeutic agents, AIDS and Lyme disease protocols, and combination therapies.

33. List the potential complications of PICC use.
Insertion-related trauma and/or bleeding, occlusion, catheter fracture, and infection.

34. What is best position for the patient during placement of the PICC?
Sitting or reclining with the arm externally rotated and abducted to approximately 45° to the axis of the body. The elbow should be extended.

35. How is the PICC placed?
1. With sterile technique, place a tourniquet on the arm proximally and identify a vein in the forearm that is continuous with the basilic or cephalic vein. Ultrasound guidance may be used.
2. Prepare and drape the area of interest.
3. Obtain a rough measurement from the insertion site to the superior vena cava.
4. Using a 25-gauge needle and 1% lidocaine, anesthetize the skin on both sides of the vein of interest.
5. Cannulate the vein with the 14-gauge introducer catheter as if starting an IV.
6. Remove the needle and advance the plastic portion of the introducer.
7. Insert the silastic catheter through the plastic introducer.

36. List risk factors for thrombosis of central venous lines.
Cancer (Fig. 5), diabetes, oral contraceptives, pregnancy, and smoking.

37. Give the major indication for use of implantable ports.
Intermittent access for 1 month to years.

38. What can be delivered through an implantable port?
High-volume or viscous solutions, blood and blood products, total parenteral nutrition, antibiotics, chemotherapeutic agents, AIDS and Lyme disease protocols, and combination therapies.

39. List the advantages of implantable ports (Fig. 6).
- Reduced risk of infection
- Fewer reminders of disease/cosmetically more appealing
- Reduced need for care

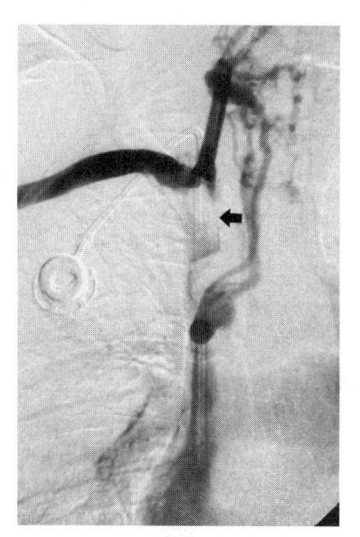

FIGURE 5. A 37-year-old woman with ovarian cancer had Port-a-Cath for chemotherapy with access in the right internal jugular vein. She presented with swelling of the neck and right upper extremity. Venogram of the right upper extremity demonstrated thrombosis of the right brachiocephalic vein extending into the superior vena cava.

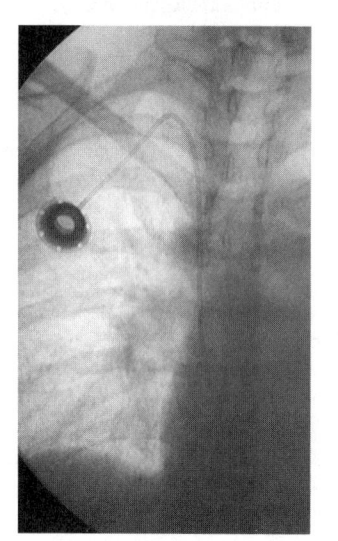

FIGURE 6. Single-lumen Port-a-Cath placed via right internal jugular vein, with the port in the anterior chest wall on top of the second anterior rib for support during access.

- Reduced risk of accidental damage or removal
- Lifestyle advantages

40. What are the potential complications of implantable ports?

Trauma and bleeding at the venous entry site, infection, catheter occlusion, catheter separation and/or fracture, and trauma related to pocket creation, tunneling and/or suturing.

41. List the advantages of dialysis catheters.
- Easiest access to create
- Immediate use
- No needle puncture required

42. What are disadvantages of dialysis catheters?
- Highest complication rate
- Lower flow rates
- Lowest patency rates
- Increased risk of infection
- Cosmetically unattractive

43. List the insertion complications of chronic dialysis catheters.

Air embolism, bleeding, vessel perforation (Fig. 7), hemothorax/pneumothorax (Fig. 8), hematoma, introduction of infection, cardiac arrhythmias, and tamponade.

44. What are the ongoing complications of chronic dialysis catheters?

Catheter or vessel thrombosis (Fig. 9), infection, vessel or tissue injury, and catheter damage.

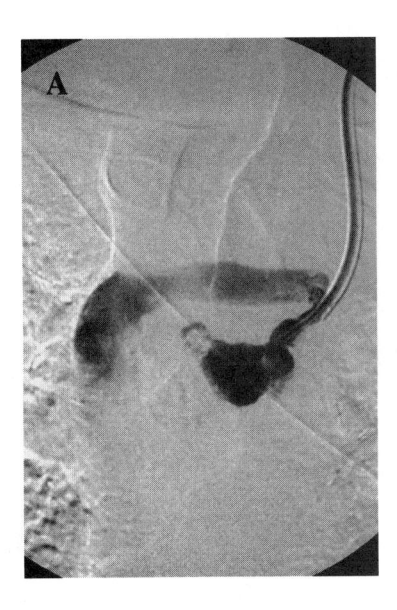

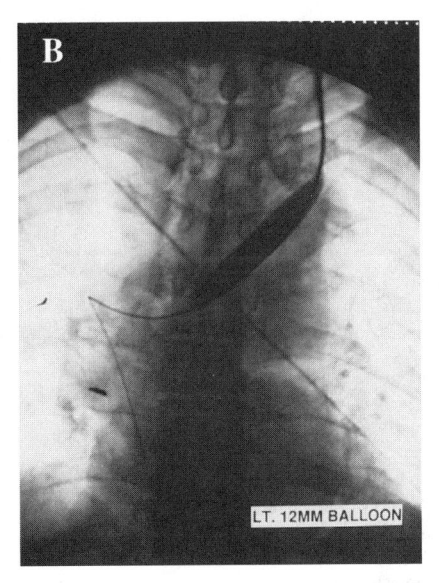

FIGURE 7. A 65-year-old man with chronic end-stage renal disease, with multiple previous lines for hemodialysis, presented for tunnel hemodialysis catheter placement. Due to the absence of adequate veins in the right neck, the left internal jugular vein was used. Because of difficulty in advancing the catheter past the curve in the left brachiocephalic vine, contast was injected and demonstrated active extravasations (**A**) consistent with rupture. A 12-mm x 4 cm angioplasty balloon was immediately placed (**B**) and resulted in successful tamponade of the bleeding. A right femoral vein catheter was then placed, and the patient was admitted for observation. He was then discharged home in stable condition.

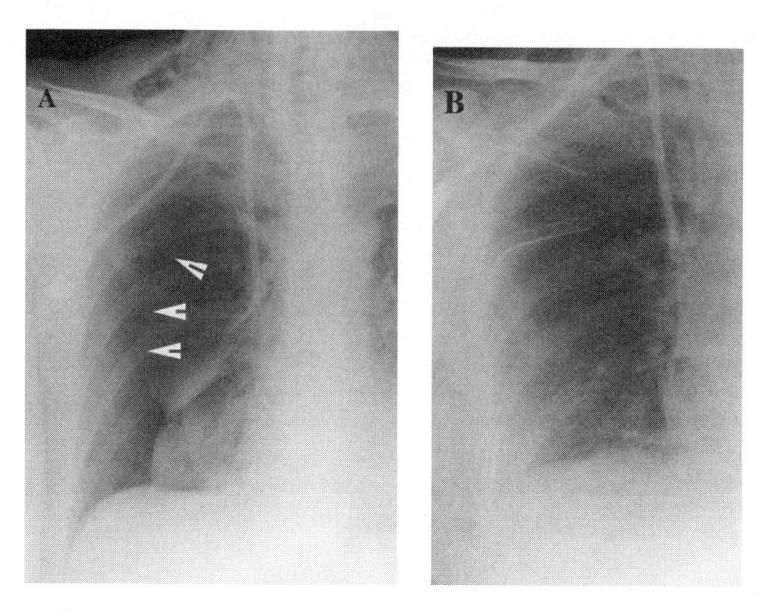

FIGURE 8. A, Arrows indicate pneumothorax on a chest x-ray obtained after placement of a tunnel catheter. **B,** The pneumothorax was successfully treated by placing a chest tube.

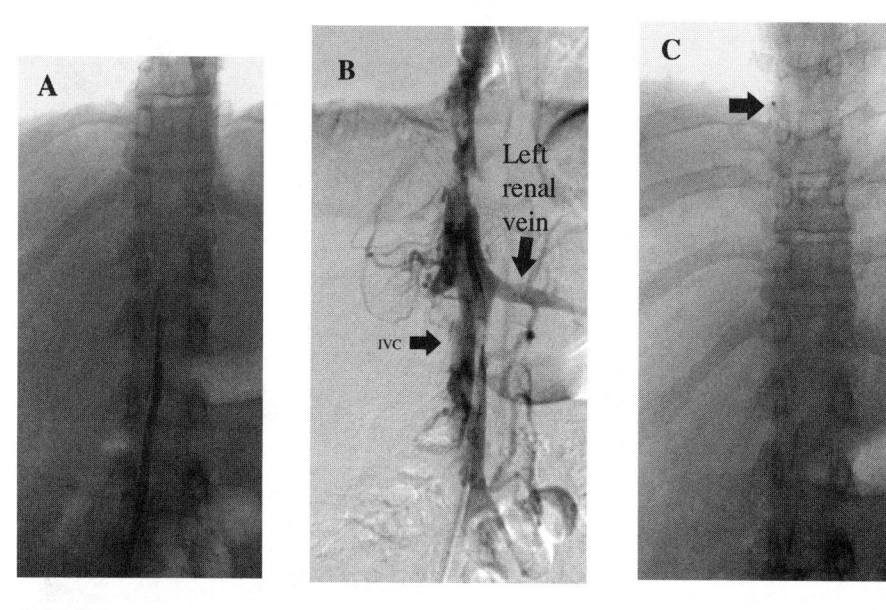

FIGURE 9. A 42-year-old woman on chronic hemodialysis has chronically occluded upper extremity veins; hence, the right common femoral vein access catheter was placed. The patient presented with a poorly functioning catheter. Contrast injected through the catheter demonstrated thrombosis of the inferior vena cava (IVC) secondary to the catheter (**A** and **B**). TPA was initiated for thrombolysis. Markers indicate the distal end (**C**) and the proximal end (**D**) of the infusion catheter. The patient was brought back on the next day, and a cavagram was performed (**E** and **F**). The cavagram demonstrated minimal residual thrombus with distal stenosis. The stenosis was treated with angioplasty (**G**) with a moderate response (**H**). It was decided not to place a stent and to keep the patient on anticoagulation.

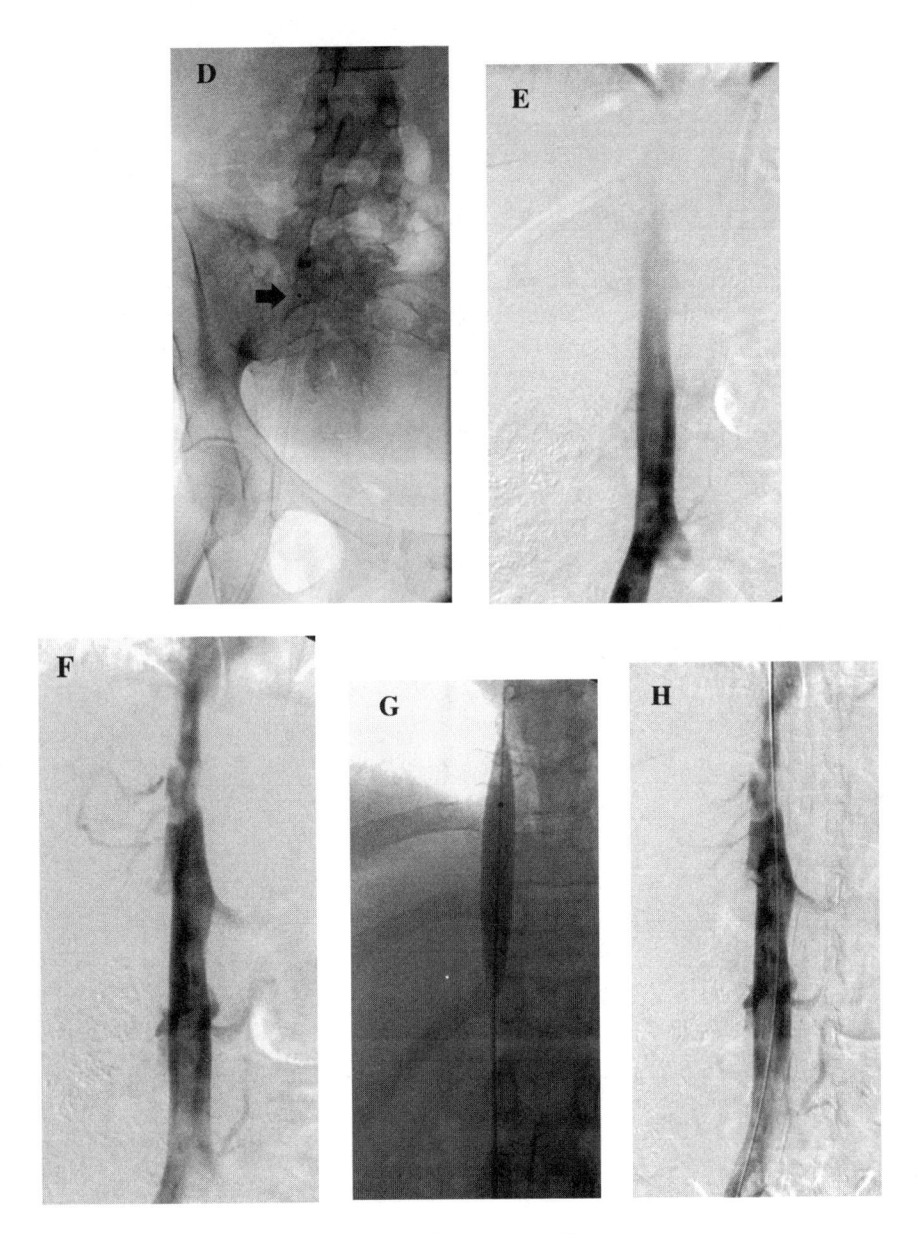

FIGURE 9. (continued)

45. What care should be provided for the exit site of the catheter?
Aqueous-based providone iodine with an occlusive dressing. No alcohol-based antiseptics should be used.

46. Identify the gold standard for hemodialysis access.
Creation of an arteriovenous fistula—surgical anastomosis of an artery and vein.

168   Venous Access

47. What causes venous catheter thrombosis?

Any foreign body causes activation of the coagulation pathway. Red blood cells, platelets, white blood cells, fibrogen, and fibrin adhere to the surface of the catheter. Often a fibrin sheath can form around the catheter at any site along the catheter from its site of venous entry to its tip. Fibrin sheaths have more of an effect on hemodialysis and apheresis catheters than others because of the high flow required (Fig. 10).

48. When is a dialysis catheter considered to malfunction?

The National Kidney Foundation's Dialysis Outcome Quality Initiative criteria for catheter thrombosis state that if the flow volume of the dialysis catheter is less than 300 ml/min in the arterial port it is malfunctioning. No specific flow volume has been established for low-flow central catheters. However, the inability to draw or flush is an indication of malfunction.

49. What can give false positives regarding catheter occlusion?

Catheter kink (Fig. 11), a malpositioned tip (Fig. 12), or constricting suture.

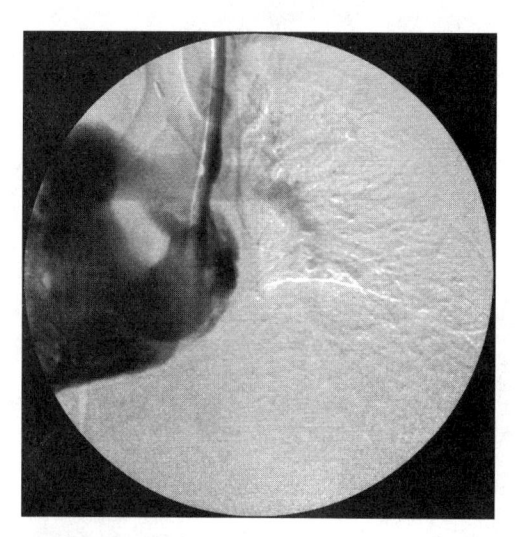

FIGURE 10. Note the contrast traveling upward along the catheter. The proximal movement of the contrast is characteristic of a fibrin sheath.

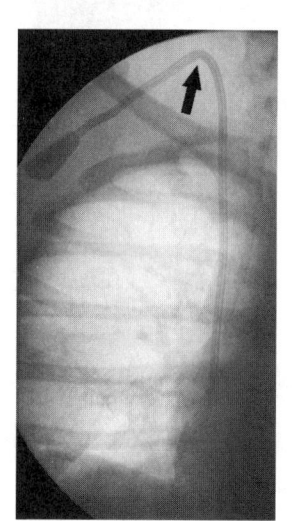

FIGURE 11. Right internal jugular vein access with poorly functioning port due to a kink in the catheter at the access site *(arrow)*.

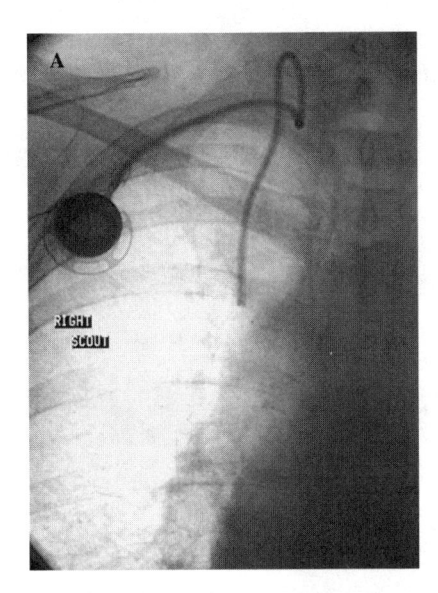

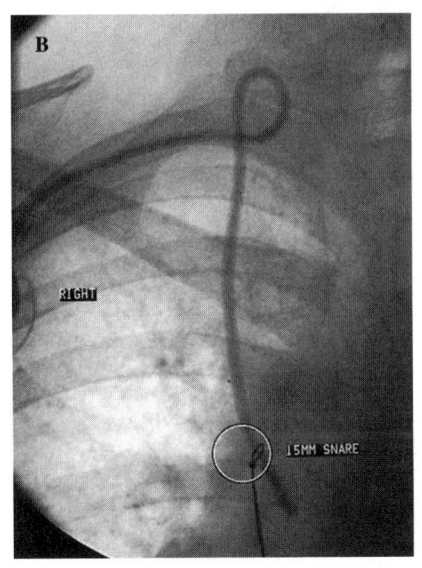

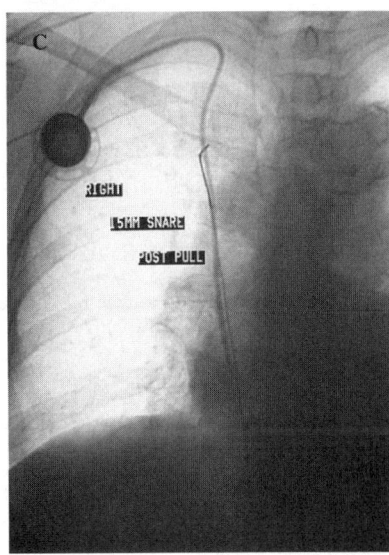

FIGURE 12. A patient with breast cancer and nonfunctioning Port-a-Cath presented for evaluation with contrast injection. On fluoroscopy the port was noted to be malpositioned with a loop at the access site (**A**). A snare was placed from the common femoral vein approach, and the catheter tip was snared (**B**) and repositioned (**C**).

50. How can flow be restored to a malfunctioning catheter?

Pharmacologic therapy with 5,000 U of urokinase is the initial choice. The therapy can repeated with longer infusion times and up to 60,000U of urokinase over 4 hours. Recombinant tissue plasminogen activator (rt-PA) can also be used with an infusion of 2.5 mg (low dose) in 50 ml of normal saline over 3 hours (Fig. 13).

When pharmacologic therapy fails, **mechanical means** can be used. Fibrin sheath stripping involves accessing the femoral vein and placing a wire snare around the indwelling catheter and

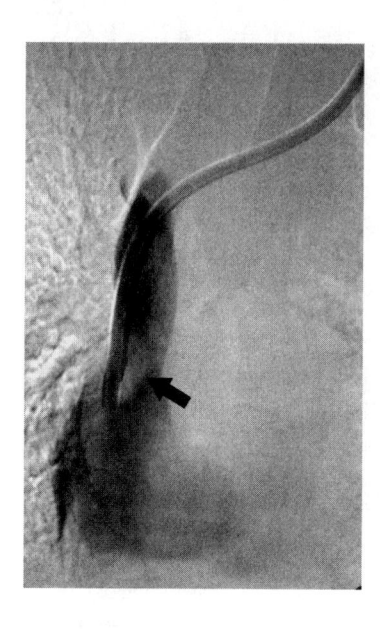

FIGURE 13. A 50-year-old man on chronic hemodialysis presented with catheter malfunction. Contrast injection through the catheter under fluoroscopy guidance demonstrated nonopacification at the catheter tip due to a clot *(arrow)*.

subsequently pulling the fibrin sheath off of the catheter. Two stiff glide wires can be used to exchange the catheter over a wire while preserving access. A balloon occlusion catheter can be used to disrupt the fibrin sheath from within.

BIBLIOGRAPHY

1. Chen H, Sonnenday C: Manual of Common Bedside Surgical Procedures, 2nd ed. Philadelphia, Lippincott Williams & Wilkins, 2000.
2. Chrisman HB, Omary RA, Nemcek AA, et al: Peripherally inserted central catheters: Guidance with use of US versus venography in 2,650 patients. J Vasc Intervent Radiol 10:473–475, 1999.
3. Davis SN, Vermeulen L, Banton J: Activity and dosage of alteplase dilution for clearing occlusions of venous-access devices. Am J Health Syst Pharm 57:1039–1045, 2000.
4. Farrell J, Gellens M: Ultrasound-guided cannulation versus the landmark-guided technique for acute haemodialysis access. Nephrol Dial Transplant 12:1234–1237, 1997.
5. Gordon AC, Saliken JC, Johns D, et al: US-guided puncture of the internal jugular vein: complications and anatomic considerations. J Vasc Intervent Radiol 9:333–338, 1998.
6. Haskal ZJ, Leen VH, Thomas-Hawkins C, et al: Transvenous removal of fibrin sheaths from tunneled hemodialysis catheters. J Vasc Intervent Radiol 7:513–517, 1996.
7. Semba C, Katzen B: Venous access. Tech Vasc Intervent Radiol 1(3), 1998.
8. Semba C, Razavi M: Central venous and dialysis related access: Current and emerging interventions. Tech Vasc Intervent Radiol 5(2), 2002.

21. ARTERIOVENOUS HEMODIALYSIS ACCESS

John Fitzgerald, MD

1. **List the options for hemodialysis access.**
   - Native arteriovenous fistulas
   - Arteriovenous bridge grafts
   - Cuffed central venous catheters

2. **When should hemodialysis access planning be initiated?**
   Surgical referral should be made when the creatinine clearance is < 25 ml/min, serum creatinine exceeds 4 mg/dl, or within 1 year of anticipated need for dialysis.

3. **Discuss the role radiologic studies in preoperative planning.**
   Venography is indicated if the physical exam or history supports the possibility of venous stenosis. Indications include the following:
   - History of subclavian central line placement
   - Multiple prior phlebotomies or peripheral intravenous line placements
   - History of transvenous pacemaker or automatic implantable cardioverter defibrillator (AICD)
   - Edema in the extremity of planned access
   - History of arm, neck or thoracic trauma
   - Collateral veins in extremity of planned access or differential upper extremity size

   Magnetic resonance venography (MRV) and Doppler ultrasound are alternative studies in cases of contrast sensitivity.

   Arteriography is rarely required but may be needed if physical exam demonstrates decreased peripheral pulses.

4. **What is considered the ideal hemodialysis access?**
   A radial-cephalic wrist (Brescia-Cimino) fistula placed in the nondominant extremity approximately 4 months before the need for dialysis.

5. **List the options for arteriovenous placement in order of desirability.**
   - Brescia-Cimino wrist fistula
   - Brachiocephalic elbow fistula
   - Transposed brachial-basilic native fistula *or* an arteriovenous polytetrafluoroethylene (PTFE) graft fistula

6. **What are long-term patency rates for the various arteriovenous options?**
   Cumulative 3-year patency rates for all options are roughly equivalent:
   - Brescia-Cimino: 64–72% (at 3 years), 37–72% (at 5 years)
   - Brachiocephalic: 50–70% (at 3 years), 34–53% (at 5 years)
   - Transposed brachial-basilic: 43–64% (at 3 years)
   - PTFE graft fistula: 40–59% (at 3 years)

   These numbers, however, include native fistulas that fail to achieve primary patency after maturation. Native fistulas that achieve primary patency have 3-year patency rates in excess of 80%. The brachiocephalic native fistula is not as well studied, but uncontrolled studies indicate similar results.

7. **Define native fistula maturation.**
   Successful maturation implies sufficient dilation of the draining vein for dialysis needle cannulation and increased flow in the draining vein (access flow) to permit dialysis. Access flow

needs to be approximately 100 ml/min higher than the dialysis blood pump flow rate, which in the United States is typically 400 ml/min.

8. How long does maturation take? What percentage of native fistulas fail to achieve primary patency?

Maturation time varies but typically occurs within 2–4 months. Failure of maturation depends on age, gender, race. and type of native fistula. On aggregate, 20–30% of fistulas fail to achieve primary patency.

9. Explain the most important predictor of primary patency.

Vessel size is important to achieving primary patency. Ideally, the diameter of the artery should be at least 2 mm, and the vein should be at least 2.5 mm. Beyond these minimum limits, however, a bigger diameter does not imply better outcomes.

10. What interventions can reduce the failure rate?

Preoperative vascular mapping with ultrasound increases the likelihood that a native fistula will be placed vs. a graft fistula. Three of four studies that used such vascular mapping noted native fistula placement in the mid-60th percentile; in the fourth study 34% of patients received a native fistula. The studies were not conclusive that vascular mapping improves primary patency rates.

It is believed that extremity exercise during maturation and/or ligation of side channels off the draining vein may improve maturation success, but no studies support these theories.

11. List the possible complications once primary patency is achieved in a native fistula.
- Venous stenosis
- Infection
- Steal phenomenon

12. How often and at what location may stenosis develop in a native fistula?

Approximately 40% of the stenoses are central (typically in the subclavian vein; Fig. 1) and normally are the sequelae of prior cannulations for central access. The vast majority of the remainder occur within several centimeters of the anastomosis of the vein to the artery and are secondary to neointimal hyperplasia.

13. Is infection a common cause of native fistula failure?

Native fistula failure requiring surgical revision because of infection is rare (< 1%). Native fistula revision or ligation is indicated only with evidence of septic emboli. Less than 10% of native fistulas develop infections.

14. Summarize the standard treatment for infection of a native fistula.

Six weeks of antibiotic therapy targeted at the cultured or suspected organism.

15. Define the steal phenomenon.

Steal phenomenon is distal limb ischemia due to the shunting of a disproportionate amount of arterial blood back to the heart. Steal becomes more common as the site of the anastomosis is moved more proximally.

16. What are the clinical manifestations of the steal phenomenon?

Manifestations are those defining ischemia: decreased extremity temperature and pulse, pallor, tingling, or pain.

17. What intervention is required to address clinically significant steal phenomenon?

Emergent fistula ligation is required if acute nerve ischemia is suspected on clinical presentation. Angiography to exclude proximal arterial stenosis is warranted, with angioplasty and stent

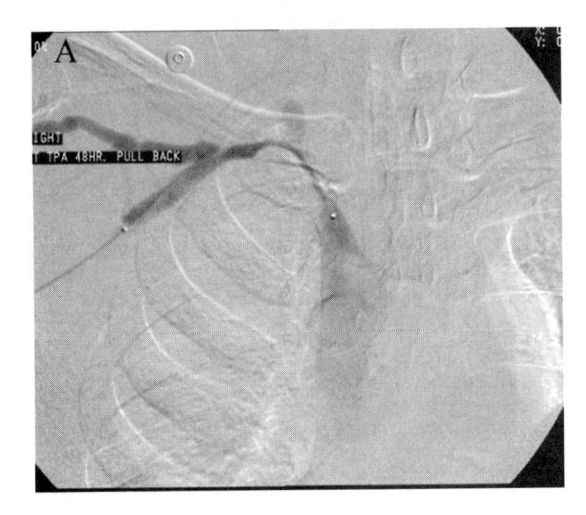

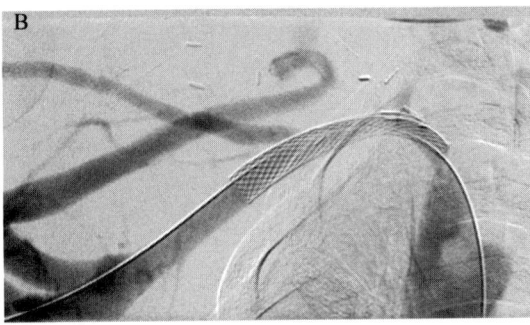

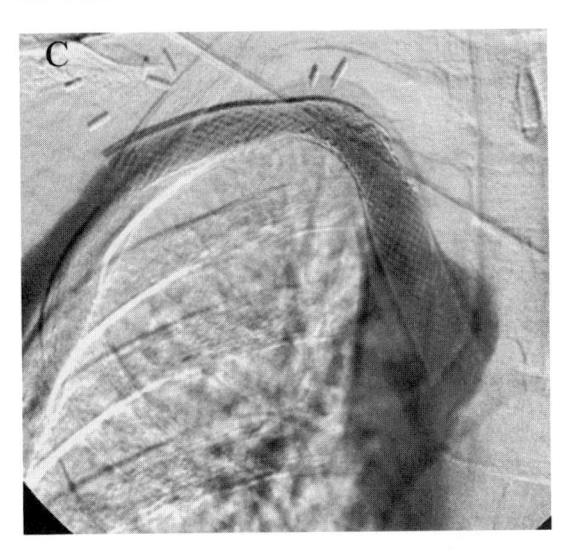

FIGURE 1. Dialysis patient with subclavian occlusion. Tissue plasminogen activator was infused overnight (**A**). Residual stenosis was treated initially with angioplasty; then a stent was placed (**B**). The patient returned 2 weeks later with increasing arm swelling. The stent was extended (**C**) with resolution of the symptoms.

placement as required to improve arterial inflow. Surgical interventions consisting of an arterial jump graft or banding of the venous outflow tract may be performed.

18. How is PTFE graft maturation defined?

The process is not true maturation as much as resolution of postoperative edema and adhesion of the graft to the subcutaneous tunnel. Ideally, 14 days should be permitted before attempting cannulation of the graft for dialysis.

Dialysis before resolution of the edema makes palpation and identification of the graft difficult. Hematoma development before the graft adheres to the subcutaneous tunnel can cause compression of the graft with possible thrombosis. Swelling and edema that do not resolve by 2 weeks are indications for venography to occlude occult central venous stenosis.

19. List the complications associated with PTFE graft fistulas.
- Venous stenosis (Fig. 2)
- Infection
- Pseudoaneurysm formation (Fig. 3)
- Steal phenomenon

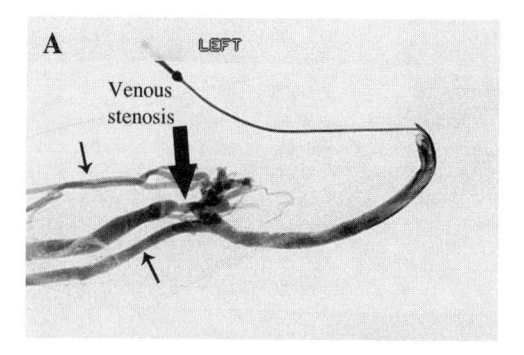

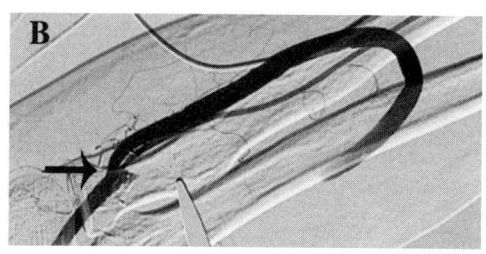

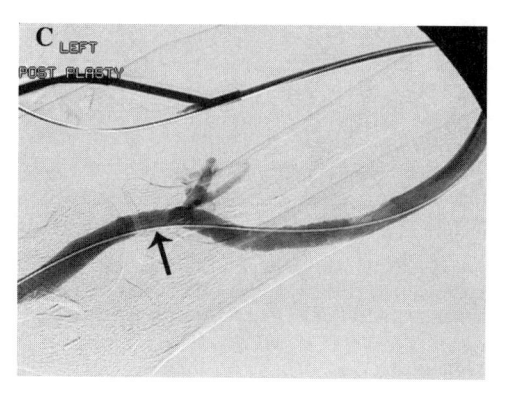

FIGURE 2. A patient with forearm loop graft for hemodialysis presents with poor flow rates during dialysis. **A,** Fistulogram demonstrates venous outflow stenosis *(big arrow)* with multiple collaterals *(small arrows)*. **B,** Arterial anastomosis is normal. Angioplasty of the venous outflow stenosis was performed. **C,** Follow-up fistulogram reveals no significant residual stensosis, and multiple collaterals are no longer seen.

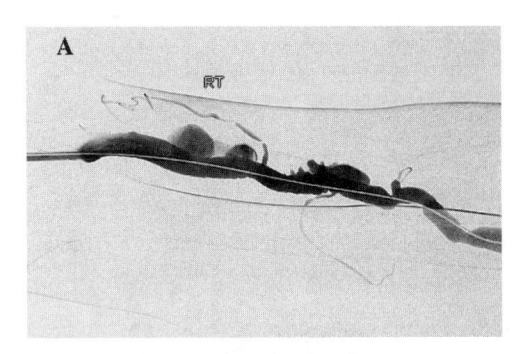

FIGURE 3. A, Pseudoaneurysm of an arteriovenous fistula. **B,** The pseudoaneurysm was covered with a stent graft. The graft remained patent 3 months after placement.

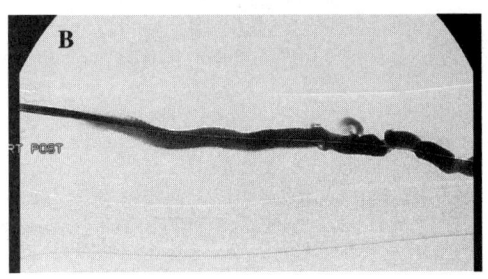

20. How often and at what location does venous stenosis develop in graft fistulas?

The majority (50–70%) of cases develop at the graft anastomosis due to neointimal hyperplasia; the remainder develop centrally.

21. With reference to native fistulas, what is the significance of graft fistula venous outflow stenosis?

- The 3-year patency rates cited in question 6) come at the expense of increased interventions.
- The incidence of procedures to maintain patency (angioplasty, thrombolysis, thrombectomy, surgical revision) is 2.4–7.1 times that of native fistulas per access year.
- The complication-free patency rate of a graft fistula is 77% at 1 year, 51% at 2 years, and 39% at 3 years.

22. How is an infected graft treated?

With surgical resection of the infected graft and antibiotics. PTFE grafts have a higher rate of infection than native fistulas (8% for native fistulas vs. 20% for graft fistulas).

23. Summarize the risks and appropriate treatment of pseudoaneurysms with graft fistulas.

The primary risk is significant hemorrhage due to rupture. Risk of rupture is increased with needle cannulation of the pseudoaneurysm, pseudoaneurysms with rapid increase in size, and pseudoaneurysms that exceed twice the diameter of the graft. Other complications include overlying skin degeneration from vascular compromise and superimposed infection of the pseudoaneurysm. The appropriate therapy is surgical revision.

24. Explain the rationale behind monitoring hemodialysis fistulas (native or graft) for signs of developing stenosis.

Better outcomes result from treatment of venous stenoses before the development of thrombosis. If no thrombosis exists, the 6-month rate of unassisted patency following percutaneous transluminal angioplasty (PTA) is between 40% and 50%. With thrombosis present, angioplasty provides a 3-month unassisted patency rate of 30–40%.

25. What tests are used to monitor hemodialysis fistula function?
- Access flow measurement
- Static or dynamic venous pressure
- Recirculation
- Physical exam and dialysis performance

26. Which test is most sensitive?
An access flow without decrement over time is the best indicator of satisfactory fistula performance for both native and graft fistulas.

27. Are the remaining tests equally useful for native vs. graft fistulas?
No—because of the flow characteristics of the fistulas.

28. Discuss the usefulness of venous pressure measurement.
Elevated venous pressure is more useful for predicting venous outflow stenosis for graft fistulas. Native fistulas have the capacity to develop venous outflow collaterals. Consequently, a stenosis in the venous outflow may not result in elevation of the venous pressure.

29. Discuss the usefulness of recirculation measurements.
Recirculation measures retrograde flow between the paired dialysis needles and occurs when the access flow is equal to or less than the dialysis blood pump flow. Graft fistulas are at risk for thrombosis when the access flow falls below 600 ml/min. Assuming a dialysis blood pump flow of 400 ml/min, recirculation becomes positive late in the game. This problem does not exist for native fistulas, in which the threshold for thrombosis is access flow of 200 ml/min. In this case, recirculation may be of value.

Similarly, the presence of a thrill throughout the length of a graft implies an access flow of at least 450 ml/min. Such a value is equivocal if the thrombogenic threshold is 600 ml/min.

30. In the setting of stenosis, when is intervention warranted?
PTA or surgical revision is warranted if the stenosis is greater than 50% of the luminal diameter and is associated with the following abnormalities:
- Previous thrombosis in the access
- Elevated venous circulation pressure
- Abnormal recirculation measurements
- Abnormal physical exam findings
- Unexplained decrease in dialysis dose measurements
- Decreasing access flow

31. Which intervention is preferable?
No study clearly demonstrates the superiority in unassisted patency for either surgical revision or PTA. Surgical revision typically involves relocation of the anastomotic site on the vein, which decreases the amount of vein available for future access fistulas. For this reason, surgical revision is held to a higher standard than PTA (50% unassisted patency at 12 months vs. 50% unassisted patency at 6 months for PTA).

PTA has the disadvantage of encouraging neointimal hyperplasia. Repetitive angioplasties may be required to maintain patency. PTA failure is defined as more than 2 interventions required within a 3-month period prompting surgical revision.

32. Discuss the differences between treatment of thrombosis in native and graft fistulas.
No significant differences exist between surgical thrombectomy/revision or percutaneous declot on graft fistulas (Fig. 4). Patency is restored in 90% of cases. Native fistulas, however, are more difficult to treat, and surgical revision to a more proximal fistula may be required. Studies of percutaneous pharmacomechanical declot procedures are limited, but results indicate efficacy.

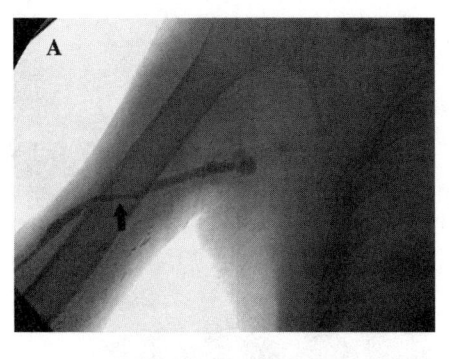

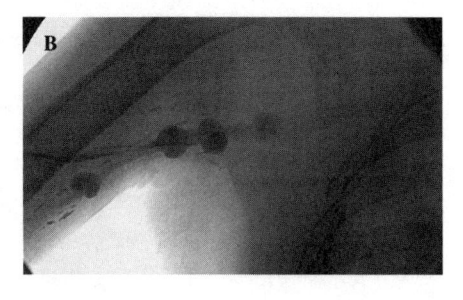

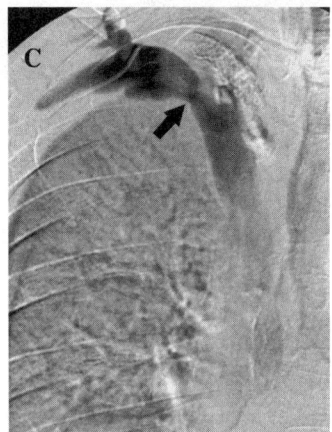

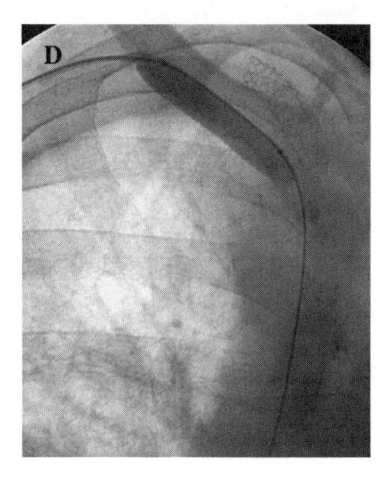

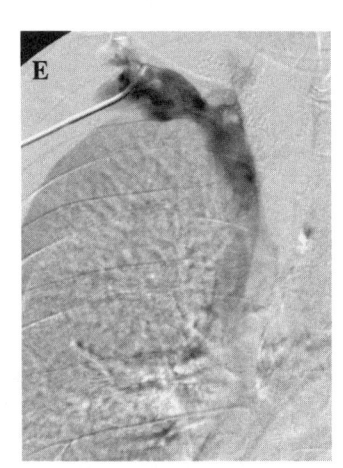

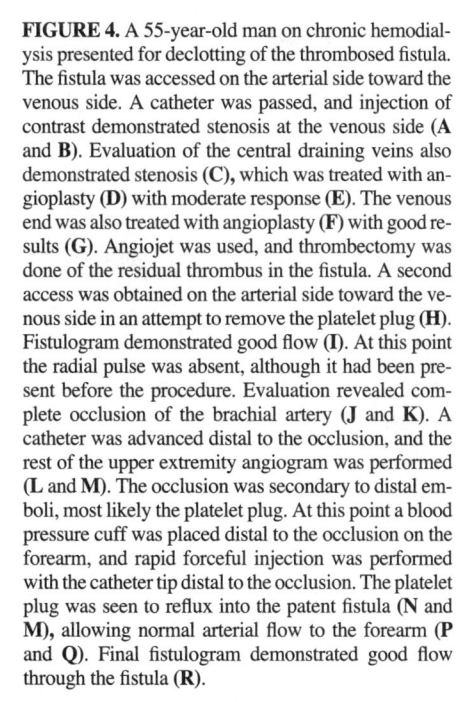

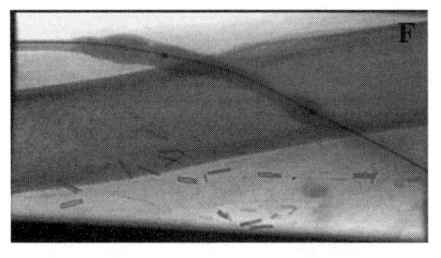

FIGURE 4. A 55-year-old man on chronic hemodialysis presented for declotting of the thrombosed fistula. The fistula was accessed on the arterial side toward the venous side. A catheter was passed, and injection of contrast demonstrated stenosis at the venous side (**A** and **B**). Evaluation of the central draining veins also demonstrated stenosis (**C**), which was treated with angioplasty (**D**) with moderate response (**E**). The venous end was also treated with angioplasty (**F**) with good results (**G**). Angiojet was used, and thrombectomy was done of the residual thrombus in the fistula. A second access was obtained on the arterial side toward the venous side in an attempt to remove the platelet plug (**H**). Fistulogram demonstrated good flow (**I**). At this point the radial pulse was absent, although it had been present before the procedure. Evaluation revealed complete occlusion of the brachial artery (**J** and **K**). A catheter was advanced distal to the occlusion, and the rest of the upper extremity angiogram was performed (**L** and **M**). The occlusion was secondary to distal emboli, most likely the platelet plug. At this point a blood pressure cuff was placed distal to the occlusion on the forearm, and rapid forceful injection was performed with the catheter tip distal to the occlusion. The platelet plug was seen to reflux into the patent fistula (**N** and **M**), allowing normal arterial flow to the forearm (**P** and **Q**). Final fistulogram demonstrated good flow through the fistula (**R**).

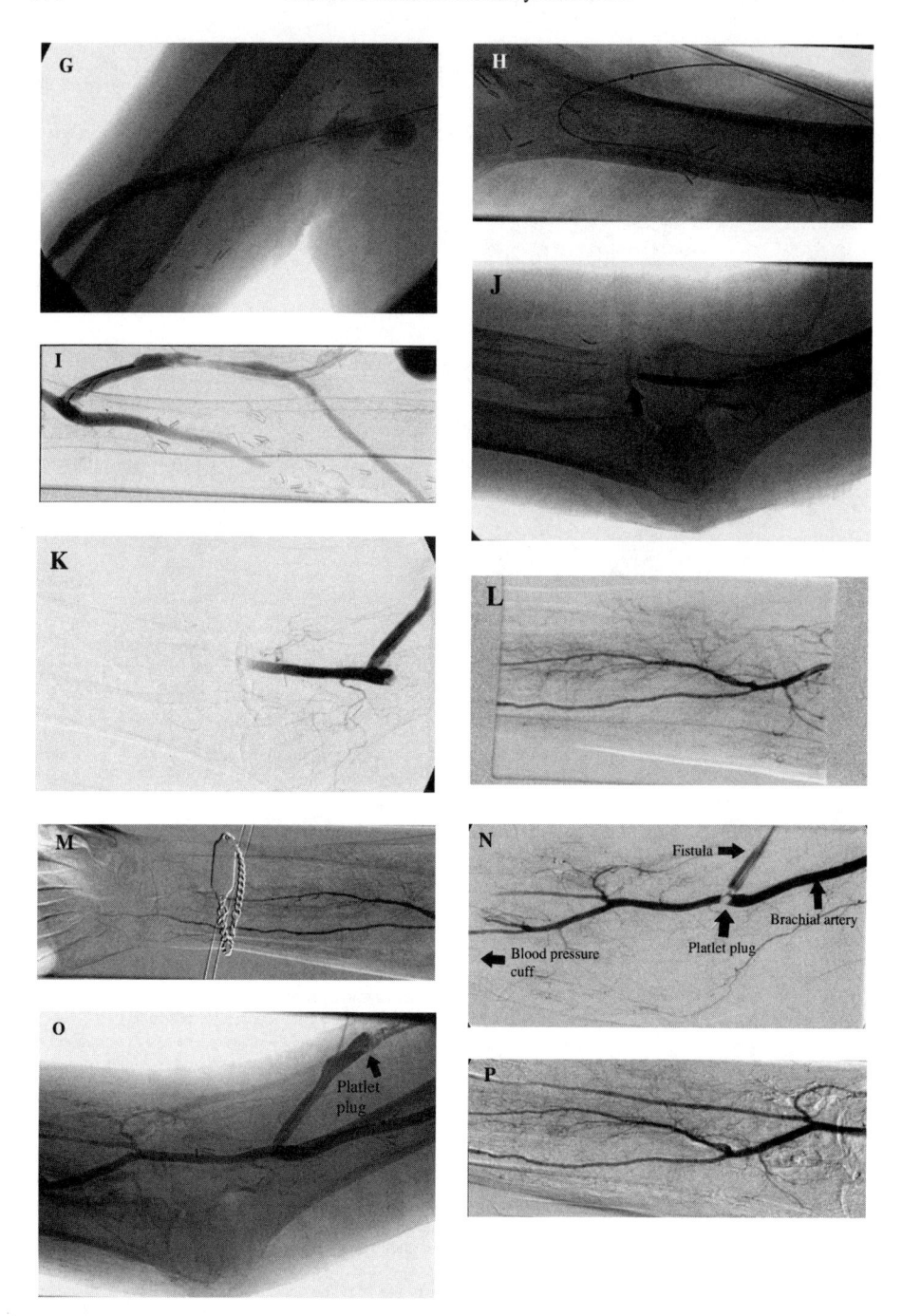

FIGURE 4. (continued)

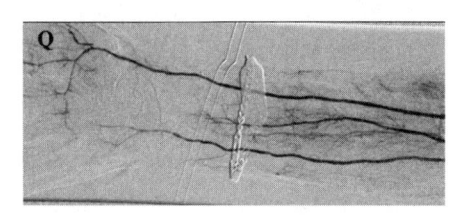

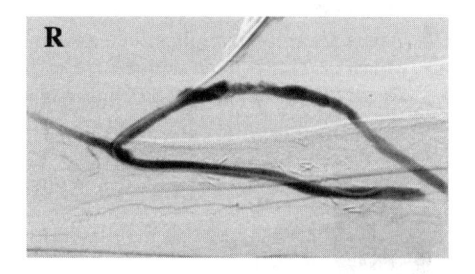

FIGURE 4. (continued)

33. What treatment options are available for central venous stenosis?

Avoid all of them. Surgical revision may require thoracotomy, and percutaneous angioplasty alone has a 6-month patency rate of 1 in 4. If the venous stenous has elastic recoil, stenting may be of value with a 12-month patency rate of 1 in 5 (Fig. 5).

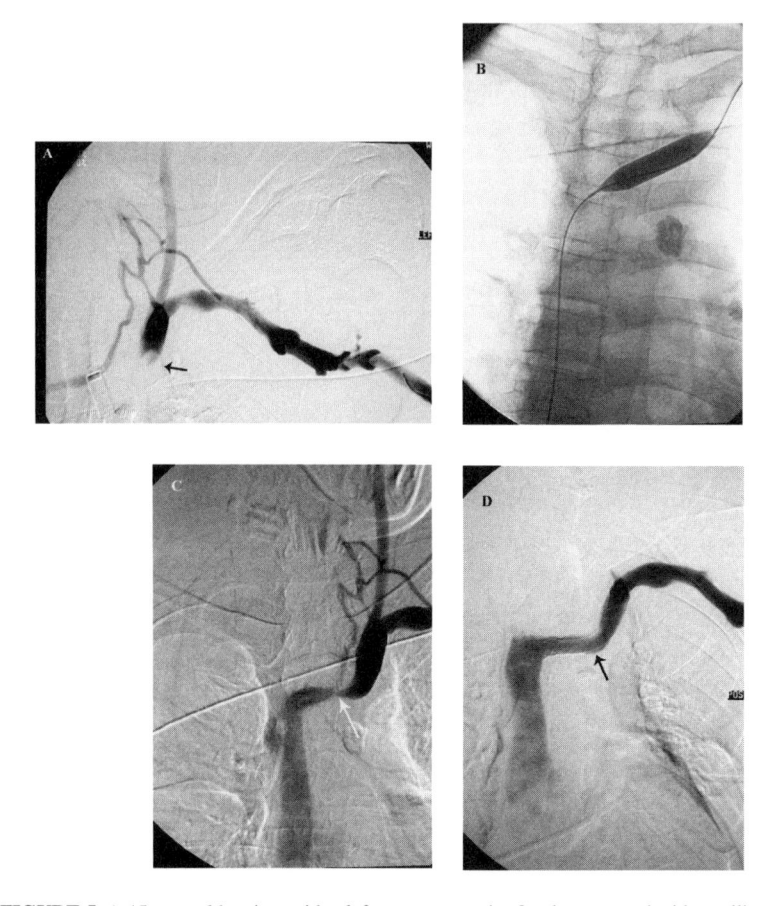

FIGURE 5. A 45-year-old patient with a left upper extremity fistula presented with swelling of the left arm. Venogram of the left upper extremity demonstrated complete occlusion of the left brachiocephalic vein (**A**). A guidewire was passed through the occlusion, and angioplasty was performed (**B**). Postangioplasty venogram (**C**) demonstrated significant residual stenosis. The decision was made to place a stent because of the patient's symptoms and limited access for a new fistula. **D,** Post-stent venogram demonstrates good results without significant residual stenosis.

34. Apart from the complications associated with central line placement, what functional drawbacks are associated with cuffed catheters?

Reduced circulation rates (300 ml/min) with either increased dialysis time or decreased dialysis dose.

BIBLIOGRAPHY

1. Allon M, Robbin M: Increasing arteriovenous fistulas in hemodialysis patients: Problems and solution. Kidney Int 62:1109–1124, 2002.
2. Feldman HI, Kobrin S, Wasserstein A: Hemodialysis vascular access morbidity. J Am Soc Nephrol 7:523–535, 1996.
3. Murphy GJ, White SA, Nicholson ML: Vascular access for haemodialysis. Br J Surg 87:1300–1315, 2000.
4. NKF-DOQI clinical practice guidelines for vascular access. Am J Kidney Dis 37(Suppl 1):S150-S191, 1997.

22. DEEP VENOUS THROMBOSIS AND CLINICAL MANAGEMENT

Vicken N. Pamoukian, MD

1. **Define deep venous thrombosis (DVT).**
   DVT is a thrombosis of the deep veins of the circulatory system.

2. **Why is the diagnosis of DVT important?**
   DVT—with its sequela, pulmonary embolism (PE)—is the leading cause of preventable in-hospital mortality in the United States.

3. **Who was Rudolf Ludwig Karl Virchow?**
   Virchow was a nineteenth-century German physician, anthropologist (he discovered the ruins of Troy), liberal politician, and author of 2000 books and papers. By the age of 25, he had already named over 100 conditions in medicine still in use today.

4. **List the elements of Virchow's triad.**
   Venous stasis, endothelial injury, and hypercoagulable state

5. **Does the body have any protective mechanism against generalized thrombosis?**
   Yes—there is a perfect homeostasis between the thrombogenic and fibrinolytic pathways. This homeostasis allows thrombosis to be followed immediately by a fibrinolytic reaction to lyse the clot.

6. **Where does a DVT usually start?**
   DVT usually begins in the deep veins of the calf around the valve sinus cusps.

7. **What happens to most DVTs?**
   Eighty percent of DVTs dissolve by the circulatory lysis action; only 20% propagate.

8. **What is the window of "clot" opportunity?**
   Between the 4th and 8th day after clot formation. The thrombus is not adherent to the vessel wall and may dislodge and embolize.

9. **What is the lifetime risk of DVT?**
   Most DVTs are occult; however, the chance that a person will develop a DVT is 1 in 20.

10. **What are the numbers in the United States?**
    Two million people are afflicted with DVT in the U.S.; 600,000 have a pulmonary embolism (PE); and the mortality is 200,000.

11. **What about in-hospital patients?**
    From 20 to 70% of hospitalized patients have venous thrombosis.

12. **How long does it take for the patient to succumb to untreated significant PE?**
    Death may ensue within 30 minutes; thus, early diagnosis is paramount.

13. **Identify Homan's sign.**
    Pain on dorsiflexion of the foot.

14. How accurate is Homan's sign in predicting DVT?
Although quoted on all rounds, it is found in only 33% of patients.

15. List the significant signs and symptoms of DVT.
Unilateral edema, vessel tenderness, Homan's sign, warmth or erythema of the leg, fever, and PE.

16. Define phlegmasia cerulea dolens.
Reddish-purple hue of the extremity due to massive acute iliofemoral venous obstruction and venous engorgement.

17. Define phlegmasia alba dolens.
Painful, white, cold extremity that follows phlegmasia alba. This condition is associated with arterial spasm of the lower extremity from massive acute iliofemoral thrombus. Absent pulses are common. Phlegmasia alba dolens is an ominous sign.

18. How often is PE the primary manifestation of DVT?
In 10% of patients, PE is the first manifestation of a DVT. In contrast, in patients with documented PE, only 45–70% have a radiologic finding of DVT.

19. List the general risk factors for DVT.
- Age > 40 years
- Immobilization > 3 days
- Pregnancy and postpartum period
- Major surgery in past 4 weeks

20. List the medical conditions that increase the risk for DVT.

Cancer	Congestive heart failure
Cerebrovascular accident	Sepsis syndrome
Myocardial infarction	

21. What trauma-related factors increase the risk for DVT?
- Multiple trauma
- Burns
- Central nervous system/spinal cord injury
- Fracture of long bones

22. List the hematologic risk factors for DVT.
- Polycythemia rubra vera
- Antithrombin III deficiency
- Protein C and S deficiency
- Factor V Leiden
- Disorder of plasminogen activation
- Inherited disorders of coagulation

23. What surgical procedures increase the risk for DVT?
- Orthopedic procedures
- Gynecologic procedures
- Urologic procedures
- Bariatric procedures
- General surgery procedures

24. Summarize the Wells Clinical Prediction Guide for DVT.

Clinical Parameter	Score
Active cancer	1
Paralysis, recent plaster immobilization	1
Bedridden > 3 days/or major surgery < 4wks	1
Localized tenderness along deep venous system	1
Entire leg swelling	1
Calf swelling > 3 cm vs. asymptomatic leg	1
Pitting edema	1
Collateral superficial veins (non-varicose)	1
Alternative diagnosis	−2

Total Score
>3 = high probability
1–2 = moderate probability
0 = low probability

25. What is in the differential diagnosis of DVT?
The differential diagnosis is long but commonly includes abscess, aneurysm, hematoma, arthritis, tendinitis, cellulites, lymphangitis, muscle or soft tissue injury, lymphedema, and Baker's cyst.

26. Why should imaging be performed?
Positive documentation and diagnosis of DVT should be made before the start of any therapy.

27. What is the gold-standard imaging modality?
The gold-standard imaging modality remains contrast venography. However, contrast venography may trigger an allergic dye allergy, takes time to perform, and may precipitate renal injury. It has been replaced by the venous duplex ultrasound study (VDUS) as the primary test of choice.

28. How accurate is VDUS?
VDUS is suboptimal for calf veins and the venous system above the inguinal ligament. However, for proximal thigh venous system, the sensitivity and specificity of VDUS approach 98%.

29. List the specific findings of DVT on VDUS.
- Incompressibility of the vein
- Lack of flow or Doppler signal
- Intraluminal echoes
- Continuous nonaugmentable flow. When the probe is on the vein, compression of the calf should augment the flow beneath the probe. In a clot-idden vein, in which there is no flow due to obstruction, the flow is not augmented.

30. Discuss the advantages and disadvantages of the VDUS.
The **advantages** of VDUS include its ability to be done at bedside, long-term cost-effectiveness, noninvasive nature, and speed of performance.

The **disadvantages** of the VDUS are that it is not as accurate in the definition of calf vein thrombosis, lacks the ability to differentiate between old and new clot (in contrast to venography), is operator-dependent, and costs a lot to buy.

31. What other tests are available for the diagnosis of DVT?
Nuclear studies with I^{125}-labeled fibrinogen are a relatively insensitive test, and it takes longer than 24 hours to obtain results; they are no longer available in the U.S.

Magnetic resonance imaging (MRI) is expensive, lacks availability, and has technical limitations. However, MRI has been shown to be almost as accurate as contrast venography. In calf vein thrombosis, it is more sensitive than any other noninvasive test. It is the diagnostic test of choice in iliac or caval thrombosis and in pregnant patients, in whom the gravid uterus alters the hemodynamic flows within the venous system, making VDUS not applicable.

Impedance plethysmography (IPG) measures the changes in blood volume of an extremity, which are directly related to venous outflow. In the setting of proximal obstruction, venous outflow is slowed and venous capacitance is increased in the extremity. The limitations of IPG are its high false-positive results in patients with congestive heart failure and high central venous pressure. IPG cannot distinguish thrombotic occlusion from extravascular compression on the vessel. IPG is accurate only in proximal thigh venous thrombi; it misses more distal or proximal thrombi.

32. What is the most important treatment for DVT?
Prevention.

33. How does one prevent DVT at each step of patient care?
- Ambulation has been shown to decrease the incidence of DVT.
- Because venous thrombosis begins at induction of anesthesia, subcutaneous heparin should be instituted before any surgical procedure.
- The use of sequential compressive device also decreases the incidence of DVT.
- In high-risk patients, starting anticoagulation or placing a filter may be of benefit.

34. Give the first line of therapy in a patient with documented DVT.
Heparin IV drip or low-molecular-weight heparin (LMWH).

35. How does heparin work?
Heparin prevents the progression of clot and has been shown to reduce significantly the incidence of fatal and nonfatal pulmonary emboli.

36. Describe the specific mechanism of action of heparin.
Heparin activates antithrombin III, the body's primary anticoagulant. Antithrombin III inactivates thrombin and inhibits the activity of activated factor X in the coagulation process. Heparin is a mixture of polysaccharides with high-molecular and low-molecular weights. The high-molecula-weight component acts on inactivating thrombin, whereas the low-molecular-weight component acts on inactivating active factor X. The hemorrhagic complications attributed to heparin are thought to arise from the high-molecular-weight fragments.

37. What is the optimal regimen for DVT?
The optimal regimen for DVT is anticoagulation with heparin or LMWH followed by anticoagulation with warfarin for 3–6 months.

38. When should heparin be started?
Heparin should be started as soon as the diagnosis is made. It should precede the start of warfarin because the initial doses of warfarin may induce a hypercoagulable state by depleting the stores of protein C and S, which confer a natural anticoagulant state.

39. Specify the doses of heparin IV, LMWH, and warfarin.
The dose of IV heparin is a bolus of 80 U/kg followed by an infusion rate of 18 U/kg to achieve a partial thromboplastin time (PTT) of 60–80 sec. The dose of LMWH in DVT treatment is 1 mg/kg subcutaneously twice daily. The warfarin dose needs adjustment until the internal normalized ratio (INR) is maintained between 2 and 3.

40. List the contraindications to anticoagulation.
- Drug hypersensitivity
- Active bleeding

- Cerebrovascular bleeding
- Heparin-induced thrombocytopenia (HIT)

41. Define HIT.

HIT is a generalized thrombotic phenomenon in a patient previously sensitized to heparin. The clot is called a "white clot" due to its white color.

42. What should be done if the patient cannot be anticoagulated?

Caval interruption is performed. Before vena cava filters were available, surgical ligation and exclusion of the cava from the circulatory system were performed. This procedure was followed by devices designed to allow partial occlusion of the vena cava.

43. What are the complications of DVT?

DVT recurs in 20% of patients with a previously documented DVT. Postphlebitic syndrome can form with venous engorgement and ulceration of the extremity through the destruction of the venous valves and increasing venous pooling in the extremity. Finally a pulmonary embolism can develop.

BIBLIOGRAPHY

1. Bick RL, Haas: Thromboprophylaxis and thrombosis in medical, surgical, trauma and obstetric/gynecologic patients. In Hematol Oncol Clin North Am 17(1), 2003.
2. Cogo A, Bernardi E, Prandoni P, et al: Acquired risk factors for deep-vein thrombosis in symptomatic outpatients. Arch Intern Med 151:164–168, 1994.
3. Dalen JE, et al: Natural history of PE. Prog Cardiovasc Dis 17:257–270, 1975.
4. de Weber K: Effort thrombosis with sepsis. Physician Sportmed 27(5), 1999.
5. Hill SL, Holtzman GI, Martin D, et al: Selective use of the duplex scan in the diagnosis of deep venous thrombosis. Surgeon 170:201–205, 1995.
6. Hirsh J, Hoak J: Management of deep vein thrombosis and pulmonary embolism: A statement for healthcare professionals. Council on Thrombosis (in constitution with the Council on Cardiovascular Radiology), American Heart Association. Circulation 93:2212–2245, 1996.
7. Lensing AWA, Hirsh J, Buller HR: Diagnosis of venous thrombosis. In Colman RW, Hirsh J, Marder VJ, et al (eds): Hemostasis and Thrombosis: Basic Principles and Clinical Practice, 3rd ed. Philadelphia, J.B. Lippincott, 1994, pp 1297–1321.
8. Menzoian JO, Doyle JE: Venous insufficiency of the leg. Hosp Pract 24:109, 1989.
9. Milne AA, Stonebridge PA, Bradbury AW, et al: Venous function and clinical outcome following deep vein thrombosis. Br J Surg 81:847–849, 1994.
10. Zamorski MA, Opdycke RA: Advances in the prevention, diagnosis, and treatment of deep venous thrombosis. Am Fam Physician 47:457–469, 1993.

23. VENOUS SYNDROMES AND MANAGEMENT
Nikhil C. Patel, MD

1. Define superior vena cava (SVC) syndrome.
SVC syndrome is defined as obstruction of the SVC resulting from compression, invasion, or thrombosis by the processes in the superior mediastinum. SVC syndrome can produce upper body venous hypertension, which may be associated with clinical consequences of varying severity. Symptom onset may be acute or gradual, and the severity of the clinical syndrome depends primarily on the degree to which collateral pathways have formed.

2. What is pseudo-SVC syndrome?
Pseudo-SVC syndrome is an uncommon clinical entity in which tumor infiltration of cervical lymph nodes, lymphatic channels, and small veins produces a clinical picture that mimics that seen with SVC obstruction.

3. List the severe clinical symptoms of SVC obstruction.
- Facial, neck, and upper extremity swelling
- Cyanosis
- Cough
- Headaches
- Hoarseness
- Dysphagia
- Dyspnea
- Laryngeal edema
- Cerebral edema leading to syncope, visual disturbances, seizure, and even coma

4. What simple action can exacerbate the symptoms of SVC syndrome?
Putting the head in a gravitational-dependent position.

5. List the causes of SVC syndrome.
Malignant SVC obstruction (80–90% of cases) may be due to bronchogenic carcinoma, epidermoid (65–80%); small-cell carcinoma (12–30%); lymphoma (12–20%); or metastatic disease. These entities can cause the obstruction by tumor invasion, extrinsic compression, radiation fibrosis, or central venous catheter-related stenosis.
Benign SVC obstruction (10–20%) may be due to a central venous catheter (Fig. 1), pacemaker-related stenosis (Fig. 2), fibrosing mediastinitis, granulomatous infection (e.g., histoplasmosis), thoracic aortic aneurysm-related compression, or anastomotic stenosis associated with heart or heart-lung transplantation.

6. Discuss the treatment options for malignant SVC obstruction.
1. **Medical therapy** is often ineffective and is currently used for patients who are not suitable for other forms of therapy. Examples of medical therapy include anticoagulation, head elevation, steroids to relieve laryngeal edema, and diuretics for peripheral edema.
2. **Thoracic surgery** (venous bypass) involves undesirable risk and significant morbidity and cannot be justified in terminal or debilitated cancer patients.
3. **Chemotherapy** can reduce tumor size, specifically in patients with lymphoma and small-cell lung cancer. But all patients do not respond, and side effects are frequent.
4. **External beam irradiation** is associated with radiation-induced side effects, and response usually takes 2–4 weeks.

Venous Syndromes and Management   187

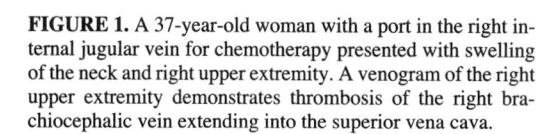

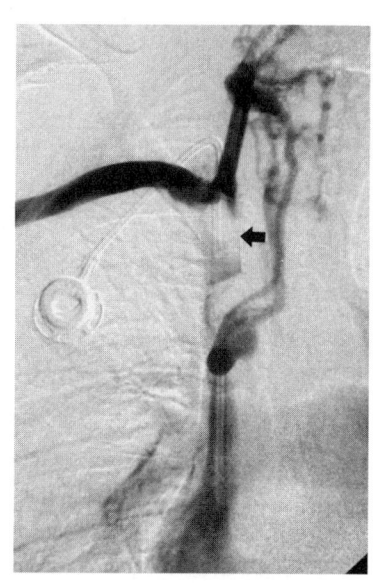

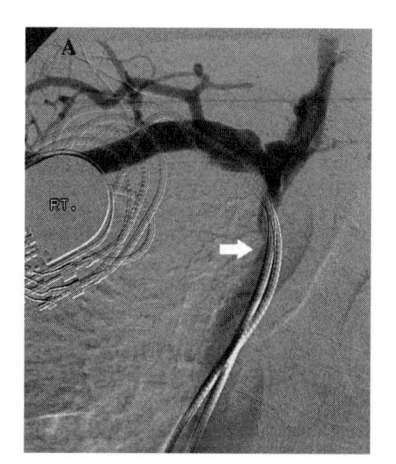

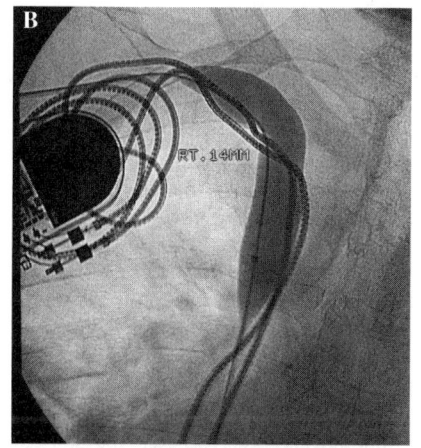

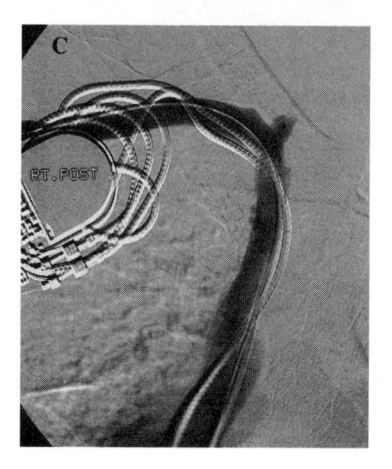

FIGURE 1. A 37-year-old woman with a port in the right internal jugular vein for chemotherapy presented with swelling of the neck and right upper extremity. A venogram of the right upper extremity demonstrates thrombosis of the right brachiocephalic vein extending into the superior vena cava.

FIGURE 2. A patient with right subclavian vein access pacemaker presents with upper extremity swelling. Venogram shows stenosis in the right proximal brachiocephalic vein (**A**). The patient is successfully treated with angioplasty (**B**) without any significant residual stenosis (**C**).

5. **Endovascular therapy** involves percutaneous transluminal angioplasty and stenting with or without thrombolysis.

7. **How successful is endovascular therapy for malignant SVC syndrome?**
   - 95–100% technical success rate (occasional failure due to inability to cross the occluded segment with guidewire)
   - Primary patency rates from 85% to 100% at 3 months
   - Secondary patency rates from 93% to 100% at 3 months

   Longer follow-up has been difficult to obtain because of the short life expectancy of patients with malignant SVC syndrome.

8. **List the treatment options for benign SVC obstruction.**
   - Surgical venous bypass using spiral saphenous vein grafts
   - Endovascular therapy

9. **How successful is surgical therapy in benign SVC obstruction?**

Primary patency rates	Secondary patency rates
1year: 61–81%	1 year: 83%
5years: 53–81%	5 years: 74%
10 years: 81%	

10. **How successful is endovascular therapy in benign SVC obstruction?**
    - Primary patency rate at 1 year: 77–91%
    - Secondary patency rate at 17-month follow-up: 85%
    - Long-term results are not yet known.

11. **List the complications of endovascular therapy for SVC syndrome.**
    Most common device-related complications
    - Stent misplacement
    - Stent migration

    Procedure-related complications
    - Thrombolysis-related hemorrhage
    - Symptomatic pulmonary embolism
    - Pulmonary edema due to increase venous flow
    - Seizures during balloon inflation in SVC
    - Periprocedural arrhythmias
    - Cellulitis and DVT related to femoral venous access

12. **What is the overall rate of complications of endovascular therapy for SVC syndrome?**
    - 7–10% in two large series
    - 1–3% mortality rate

13. **Can a single patent internal jugular vein-brachiocephalic vein-SVC axis be sufficient to prevent the head and neck symptoms of SVC syndrome?**
    Yes—as long as no flow-limiting stenosis is present.

14. **Can an upper extremity be clinically normal or minimally symptomatic in the presence of longstanding ipsilateral subclavian or brachiocephalic vein occlusion or stenosis?**
    Yes—provided that the patient has a well-developed collateral network and a patent SVC.

15. **Describe the endovascular procedural approach for SVC syndrome.**
    Bilateral upper extremity venography is usually performed either via brachial or basicilic vein access to evaluate the patency of the SVC and brachiocephalic and subclavian veins, the nature

of the occlusion (stenosis vs. occlusion), the length of the occluded segment, and the presence of acute thrombus.

16. Describe the endovascular approach in the presence of acute thrombus.
If there are no contraindications for catheter-directed thrombolysis, it can be performed as the initial means of re-establishing flow. Other options include mechanical thrombolysis using mechanical thrombectomy devices. Once the thrombus burden is resolved or improved, angioplasty and/or endovascular stenting can be performed in the presence of significant residual stenosis.

17. Can catheter-directed thrombolysis be used in chronic disease?
Yes. It can be used in the presence of thrombus to shorten the segment needing further intervention.

18. Discuss the advantages and disadvantages of self-expanding stents vs. balloon-expandable stents.
Balloon-expendable stents have better radial force, precise placement, and less foreshortening, whereas self-expanding stents have better longitudinal flexibility.

19. What can be done when the self-expanding stent is not sufficient to resist compression by the surrounding tumor?
A balloon-expandable stent can be placed internally to buttress the self-expanding stent.

20. What can be done if the occlusion is resistant to guidewire passage?
Sharp recanalization technique can be used.

21. Describe the sharp recanalization technique.
A transseptal needle may be used to literally puncture through the intraluminal material; this procedure is followed by angioplasty and/or stenting.

22. When should sharp recanalization technique be used?
It should be used only when all other measures have failed, the success of the procedure is jeopardized, and the patient's clinical symptoms due to SVC syndrome are severe enough to warrant the additional risk of extravascular puncture and injury to other thoracic structures.

23. Describe patient management in the setting of indwelling catheter with SVC syndrome.
When possible, the catheter should be removed before intervention. When removal is unacceptable, the catheter tip can be temporarily displaced into the subclavian vein using an Amplatz gooseneck snare. The catheter then is snared and returned to position after the endovascular procedure for SVC recanalization is completed (Fig. 3).

24. List treatment options for stent restenosis due to tumor ingrowth or intimal hyperplasia.
Repeat stent placement is usually performed; other options may include stent-grafts, although the viability of this approach is not yet known.

25. Define inferior vena cava (IVC) syndrome.
IVC syndrome or occlusion is a rare disorder that is most often seen in association with other underlying disease states, such as:
- Hypercoagulability disorder
- Obstruction due to tumor involvement
- Infection
- Inflammation
- Trauma

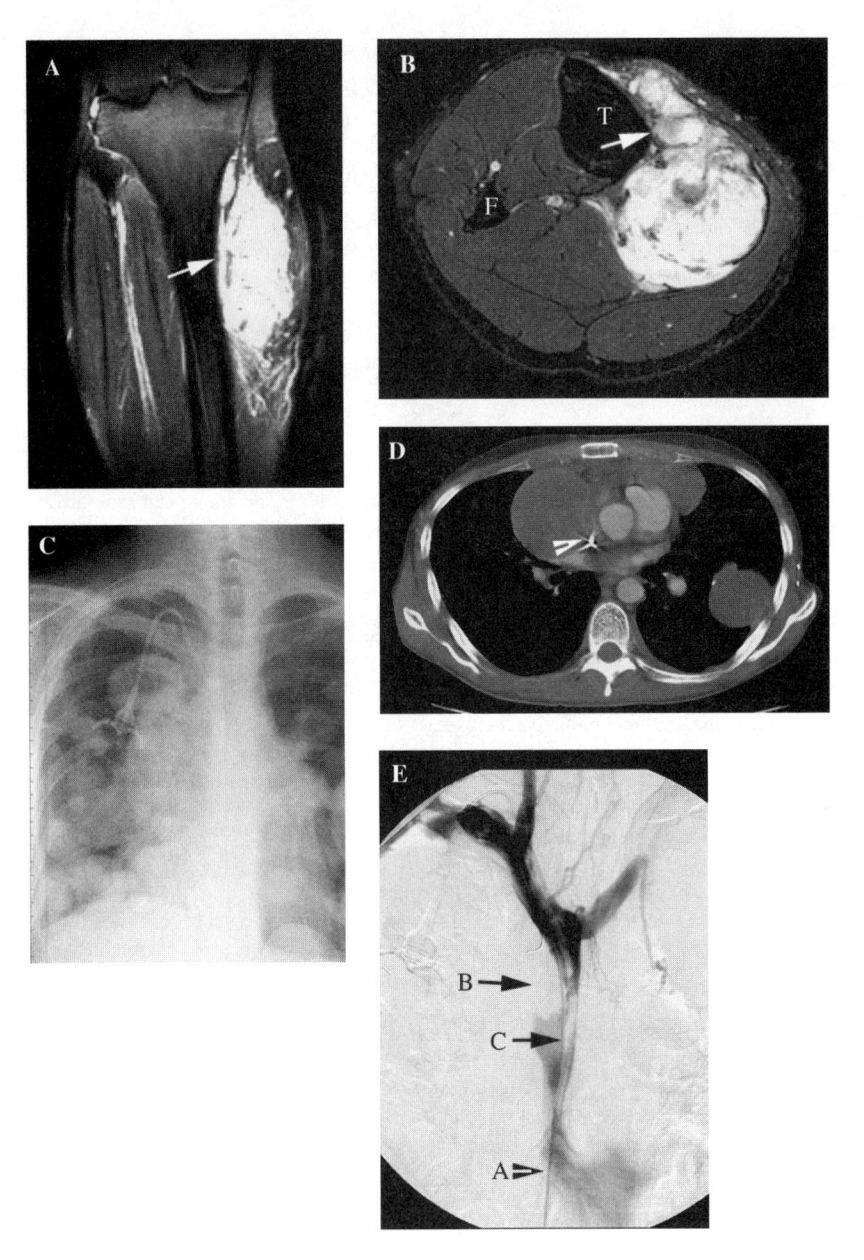

FIGURE 3. A 30-year-old man with a history of synovial cell sarcoma of the right leg and metastatic disease to the lung. A right I-J access Port-a-Cath was placed for chemotherapy. He now presents with superior vena cava (SVC) syndrome due to compression of the SVC by metastatic disease. MRI depicts the synovial cell sarcoma *(arrows)* of the right leg in coronal **(A)** and axial **(B)** planes (T = tibia, F = fibula). Chest x-ray demonstrates metastasis disease to the lung. Note the right I-J access dual-lumen Port-a-Cath in place **(C)**. CT of the chest demonstrates compression of the SVC by the extrinsic mass **(D)**. We were consulted for endovascular intervention. Cavagram **(E)** performed via access from the common femoral vein shows the catheter from below *(arrow A)*, mass compressing the SVC *(arrow B)*, and a linear filling defect representing the Port-a-Cath *(arrow C)*. The Port-a-Cath is snared and positioned out of the field for percutaneous transluminal angioplasty (PTA) and stenting of the SVC **(F)**. After PTA and placement of the wall stent, SVC cavagram demonstrates no significant residual stenosis **(G)**. The Port-a-Cath was repositioned using a snare **(H)**, and the final cavagram demonstrated excellent results **(I)**.

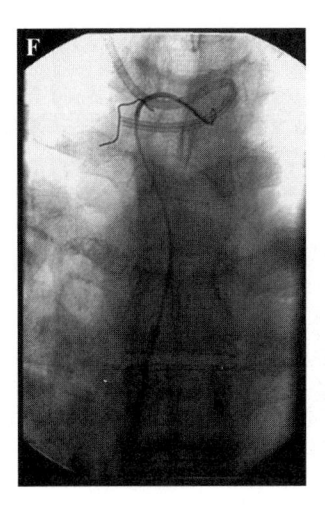

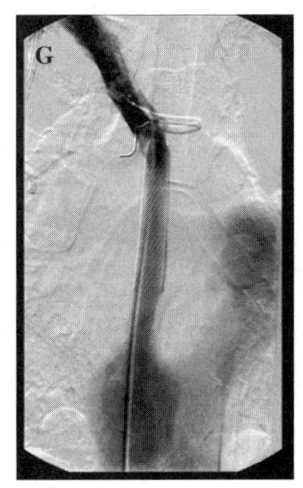

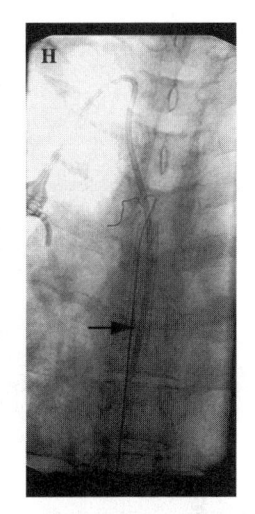

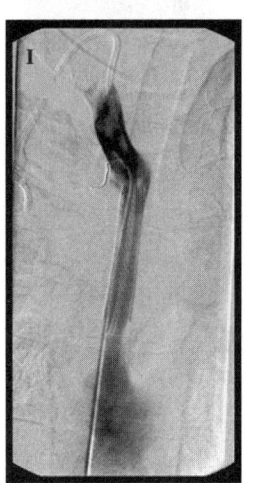

FIGURE 3. (continued)

- IVC interruption by filter or surgery
- Indwelling catheter

26. List the clinical symptoms of IVC syndrome.
- Lower extremity edema
- Lower extremity and back pain
- Weakness
- Venous stasis ulceration

27. How is IVC syndrome managed?
Management depends on the chronicity and etiology of the lesion.
- **Medical:** anticoagulation, which is largely ineffective in relieving symptoms of swelling.
- **Surgical:** venous bypass generally is associated with greater procedural morbidity and has limited success.
- **Endovascular:** more recently endovascular techniques have been applied. In acute thrombosis, catheter-directed thrombolytics is of value, whereas in longstanding occlusion percutaneous transluminal angioplasty and stent placement have been shown to be effective (Fig. 4).

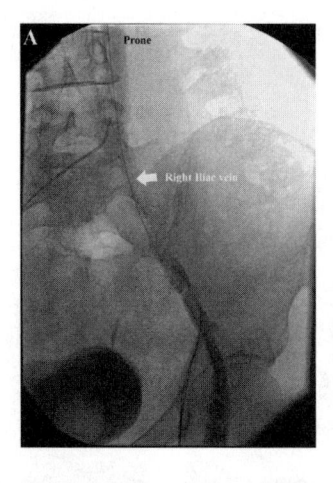

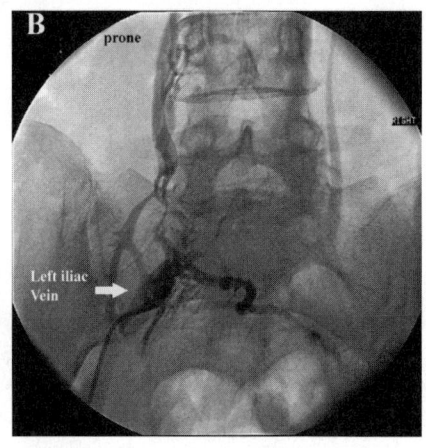

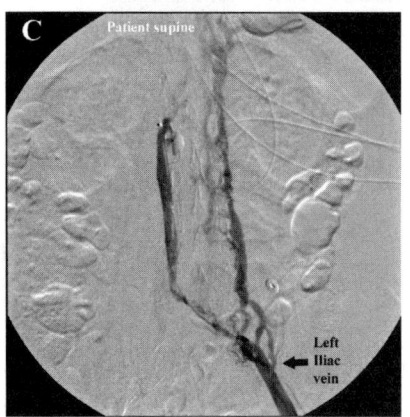

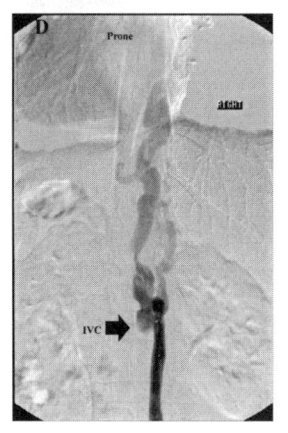

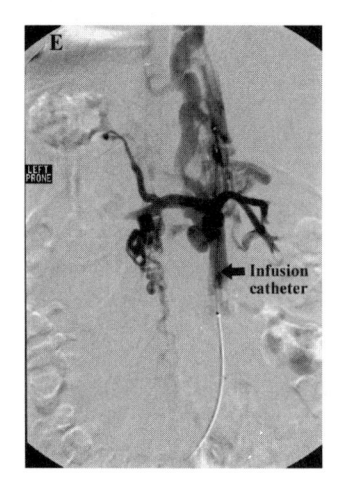

FIGURE 4. A 32-year-old woman taking oral contraceptive pills presents with bilateral lower extremity swelling. Doppler ultrasound confirmed bilateral deep venous thrombosis of the lower extremities with extension into the pelvic veins. The patient presented for bilateral lower extremity venogram and possible thrombolysis. Bilateral popliteal vein access was obtained by ultrasound guidance with the patient in the prone position. Bilateral venograms demonstrated bilateral iliac acute and chronic occlusions (**A** and **B**). Infusion of tissue plasminogen activator was started, and the patient returned on the following day for venograms (**C** and **D**) that demonstrated partial recanalization of the inferior vena cava (IVC). Infusion was continued, and follow-up demonstrated large collaterals at the distal IVC (**E**). At this point percutaneous transluminal angioplasty of the iliac veins was performed (**F**) to improve inflow without significant response (**G**); hence bilateral iliac stents were placed (**H**). The IVC was then treated by angioplasty (**I**) with good results (**J**).

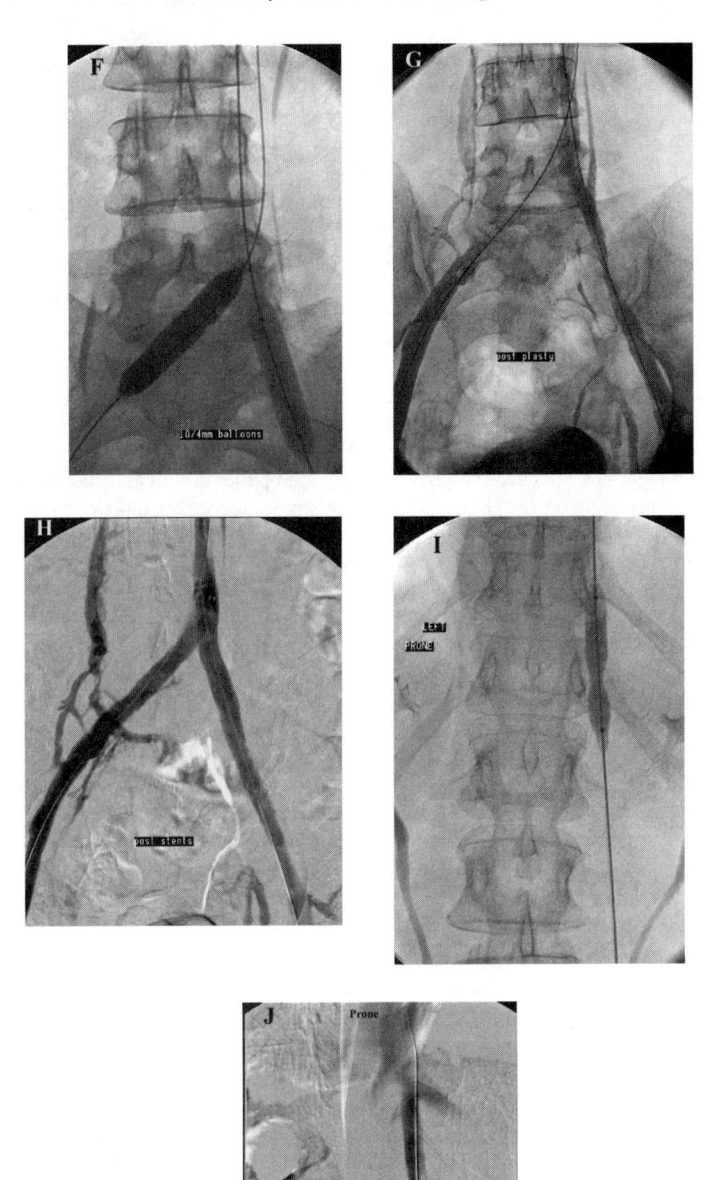

FIGURE 4. (continued)

28. Does chronic IVC occlusion exclude patients from endovascular intervention?
Chronic IVC occlusion, even up to several years, can frequently be treated successfully and effectively with good long-term clinical results.

29. What is the preferred approach for endovascular treatment in IVC occlusion?
Inferior extent of the occlusion usually determines the initial approach. Bilateral common femoral veins and popliteal veins can serve as access sites. Common femoral veins, when patent, are the preferred approach. Jugular venous access can also be used.

30. How is acute on chronic IVC occlusion treated?
An initial trial of thrombolytic therapy may be warranted if there is an indication of an acute component to the obstruction. Thrombolytic therapy may be followed by angioplasty with or without stenting of underlying stenosis or occlusion.

31. Is angioplasty alone sufficient in the treatment of IVC occlusion?
Stent placement is associated with better outcome in patients with extrinsic compression or chronic thrombosis of the IVC. Although extensive studies are lacking, previous literature suggests that angioplasty alone is insufficient in the treatment of these patients. The exception is patients with Budd-Chiari syndrome caused by membranous occlusion of IVC.

32. Describe the venography findings of May-Thurner syndrome.
Catheter-directed venography typically shows obstruction or stenosis involving the left common iliac vein near its confluence with the inferior vena cava. Presence of venous collaterals is suggestive of hemodynamically significant venous obstruction. Most of these patients present with DVT in the left lower extremity (Fig. 5).

33. Describe the percutaneous management of symptomatic May-Thurner syndrome.
The percutaneous management of May-Thurner syndrome includes obtaining percutaneous access either from the popliteal or contralateral common femoral vein with catheter-directed

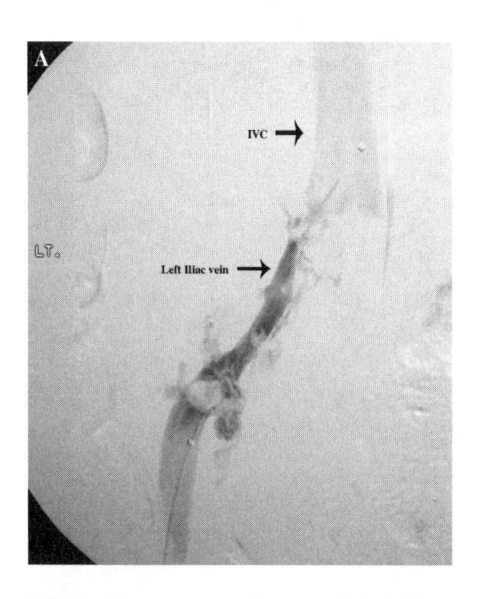

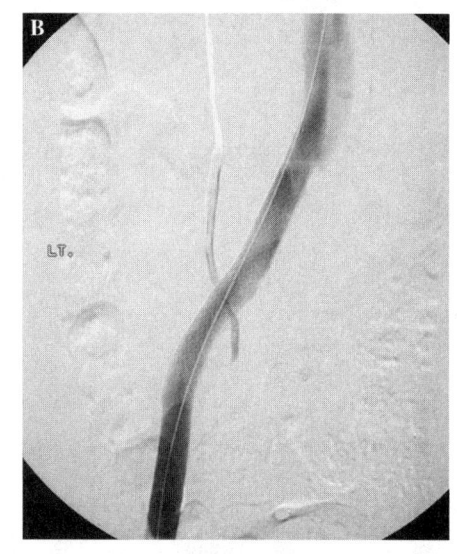

FIGURE 5. May-Thurner syndrome. **A,** Left iliac venogram demonstrates partial occlusio of the the left common iliac vein near its confluence with the inferior vena cava secondary to external compression by the right common iliac artery. A network of pelvic collaterals indicates hemodynamically significant venous obstruction. **B,** This obstruction was successfully treated with percutaneous transluminal angioplasty and stent.

thrombolysis of any thrombus, followed by stenting. The popliteal vein approach is more favored because it is antegrade to the flow of blood in the veins as well as in the direction of the opening position of the valves. The retrograde direction of the contralateral common femoral vein approach is likely to cause valve damage with passage of catheter and wires. Stents have been shown to be an effective addition to surgery and balloon dilatation. According to the National Venous Registry, a comparison of results revealed rethrombosis in 13% of patients who had stents and in 73% of those who did not.

34. Define thoracic outlet syndrome (TOS).

The subclavian artery, subclavian vein, and brachial plexus pass through a narrow boundary between the clavicle and the first rib to enter the axilla. Compression of the artery, vein, and/or the eighth cervical nerve and/or first thoracic nerve in this boundary produces a clinical scenario called thoracic outlet syndrome. This region anatomically is called the thoracic inlet (the most superior aperture of the thorax and the boundary of the roof of mediastinum). Hence some people call it thoracic inlet syndrome.

35. What is the most common form of TOS?

The most common form of TOS involves nerve compression, followed by compression of the subclavian vein and lastly compression of the subclavian artery (Fig. 6).

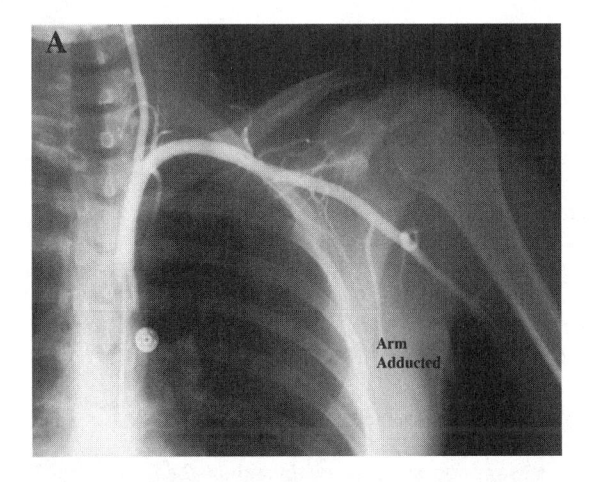

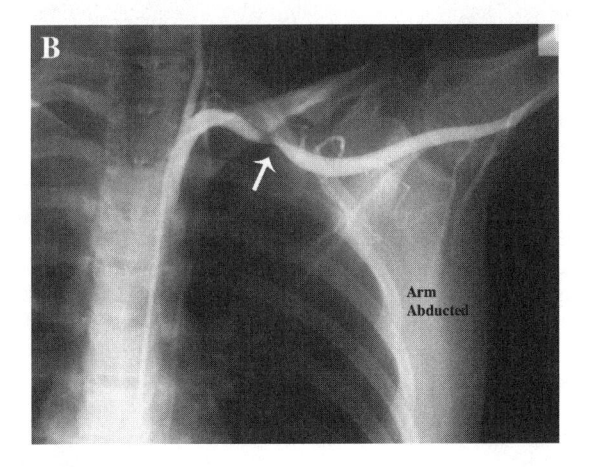

FIGURE 6. A, Angiogram of the left upper extremity in adducted position demonstrates normal subclavian artery. **B,** When the arm is abducted, moderate stenosis (arrow) is demonstrated in the subclavian artery. This scenario is consistent with thoracic outlet syndrome with arterial involvement.

36. What terms are used to describe subclavian vein compression and/or thrombosis due to TOS?

Paget-von Schrotter syndrome (named after the two physicians who described the syndrome), effort thrombosis, exertional thrombosis, effort-induced thrombosis, primary thrombus, and axillary-subclavian vein thrombosis.

37. Who is at risk for TOS?

The population at risk includes active, young, and otherwise healthy people who engage in overuse of an upper extremity. It is common in weight lifters, tennis players, pitchers, and manual laborers.

38. What percentge of DVT accounts for TOS?

Two percent of all DVTs.

39. List the signs and symptoms of TOS involving venous compression.

The signs and symptoms include nonedematous swelling, pain, discoloration, and distention of the cutaneous veins of the involved upper limb.

40. What causes TOS?

Causes can be divided into two categories: congenital and acquired.

41. List the congenital causes of TOS.

- Scalenus anticus syndrome: the most common cause, characterized by wide/abnormal insertion or hypertrophy of the anterior scalene muscle.
- Cervical rib abnormality: causes elevation of the floor of the scalene triangle with a decrease in the costoclavicular space.
- Abnormality of the scalenus minimus muscle, which extends from the transverse process of the seventh cervical vertebra to the first rib, with insertion between the subclavian artery and brachial plexus.
- Anomalous first rib, which causes narrowing of the costoclavicular space.

42. List the acquired causes of TOS.

- Fracture of the clavicle or first rib with nonanatomic alignment or callus formation
- Muscular body habitus
- Slender body habitus with long neck and sagging shoulders.

43. How do you diagnose TOS that causes venous occlusion or thrombosis?

Good history and physical examination. Diagnosis can be confirmed with venogarphy in a nonthrombotic occlusion by performing venography in the adducted position of the arm followed by abduction and external rotation (Fig. 7). With the arm adducted, occlusion or narrowing may or may not be seen. Positioning the arm in abduction and external rotation shows the occlusion or narrowing of the venous flow. In patients with evidence of thrombus, thrombolysis can be performed first; once the thrombus is cleared, the above maneuvers can be performed to confirm the diagnosis.

44. Describe the management of TOS causing venous occlusion or thrombosis.

Immediate treatment with IV heparin and local, mechanical, and/or catheter-directed thrombolysis in the acute phase is now the most effective modality for achieving vein patency. After thrombolysis therapy is concluded, anticoagulation with oral warfarin for 3 month is widely used.

45. What is the success rate of mechanical and/or catheter-directed thrombolysis?

The success rate ranges from 69% to 94%. The time from symptom onset to beginning of thrombolysis, however, affects the success rate. The greatest success is achieved when throm-

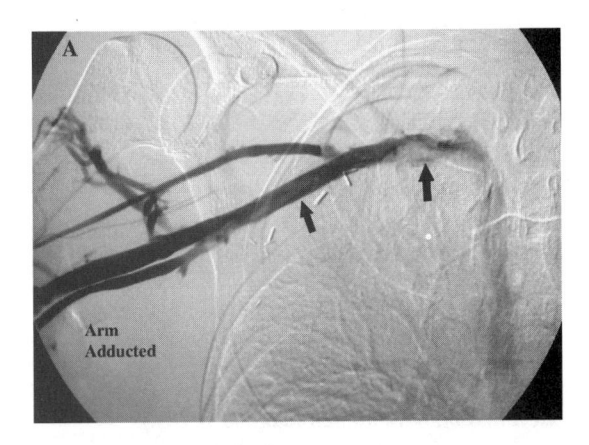

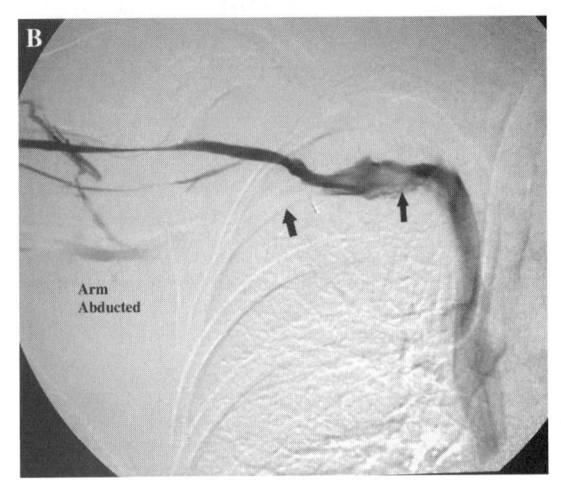

FIGURE 7. A 30-year-old woman presented with right upper extremity swelling. **A,** Venogram of the right upper extremity reveals minimal stenosis at the right subclavian-brachiocephalic junction. **B,** Abduction of the right arm leads to complete collusion of the right subclavian vein. This scenario is consistent with Paget-von Schrotter syndrome.

bolysis is begun within about 7 days of symptom onset, although initiating thrombolysis up to 10–14 days after onset is reasonable.

46. Describe the post-thrombolysis management of TOS causing venous occlusion or thrombosis.

The goal of post-thrombolysis management is to treat the cause by surgical decompression.

BIBLIOGRAPHY

1. Frisoli JK, Sze D: Mechanical thrombectomy for the treatment of lower extremity deep vein thrombosis. Tech Vasc Intervent Radadiol 6:49–52, 2003.
2. Hansch EC, Razavi MK, Semba CP, et al: Endovascular strategies for inferior vena cava obstruction. Tech Vasc Intervent Radiol 3:40–44, 2000.
3. Lang EV, Farrell T, Varchliotis TG, et al: Sharp recanalization for chronic central venous occlusion. Tech Vasc Intervent Radiol 3:21–28, 2000.
4. Mewissen MW: Catheter-directed thrombolysis for lower extremity deep vein thrombosis. Tech Vasc Intervent Radiol 4:111–114, 2001.
5. Sebma CP: Venous thrombolysis in the post-urokinase era. Tech Vasc Intervent Radadiol 3:2–11, 2000.
6. Sze DY, Shifrin RY, Semba CP: Current diagnostic and therapeutic strategies for effort vein thrombosis. Tech Vasc Intervent Radiol 3:12–20, 2000.
7. Vedantham S: Endovascular strategies for superior vena cava obstruction. Tech Vasc Intervent Radiol 3:29–39, 2000.

24. PULMONARY ANGIOGRAPHY AND INTERVENTION

Bulent Arslan, MD

1. What are the indications for a pulmonary angiogram?
In our institution the current indications are evaluation of suspected pulmonary embolus in patients with an indeterminant ventilation-perfusion (V/Q) scan or an equivocal computed tomography (CT) scan and guidance for interventions such as pulmonary embolization of an arteriovenous malformation (AVM), foreign body removal, and pulmonary embolectomy. With the advances in CT imaging pulmonary the angiogram is used less often.

2. List the diagnostic studies used for evaluation of pulmonary embolism (PE).
- Chest x-ray
- D-dimer level
- V/Q scan
- CT angiogram
- Magnetic resonance (MR) angiogram
- Pulmonary angiography
- Lower extremity ultrasound

3. What causes PE?
Detachment of thrombus from lower extremity deep venous thrombosis (70–80 % from the femoropopliteal vein and 10–15% from the iliac vein) is the main cause of PE. Amniotic fluid, fat, air, tumor, and parasites are rare causes.

4. List risk factors for development of DVT.
- Venous stasis (surgery, prolonged bed rest, limb paralysis, and long distance air travel)
- Venous injury (e.g., trauma, intravenous cannulation)
- Increased coagulability (e.g., malignancy, oral contraceptives)
- Inherited coagulation defects (antithrombin III, protein C, or protein S deficiency)
- Increasing age

5. What is the clinical significance of PE?
Approximately 120,000–150,000 people die from PE every year in the United States. Another 700,000 people experience significant PE each year.

6. List the common clinical symptoms of PE.
Dyspnea, pleuritic chest pain, anxiety, and cough are nonspecific symptoms of PE.

7. List the clinical signs of PE.
Tachypnea and rales are common, nonspecific signs.

8. Why is early diagnosis crucial in the management of PE?
With early diagnosis and treatment, the mortality rate has been shown to decrease to less than 8% in comparison with 30% when PE is not treated.

9. Discuss the preprocedural steps before a pulmonary angiogram is performed.
In addition to evaluation of the patient's renal function and history of contrast allergy, an electrocardiogram (ECG) should be obtained to exclude a left bundle-branch block (LBBB). If LBBB

is present, a temporary pacer should be applied before the procedure to prevent induction of a complete heart block. In addition, once the pulmonary artery is catheterized, pulmonary arterial pressures should be measured to exclude severe pulmonary arterial hypertension (> 70 mmHg). In the setting of severe pulmonary arterial hypertension, selective pulmonary angiogram of the suspected branches may be obtained.

10. How does low-osmolarity, nonionic contrast injection affect pulmonary arterial pressure?

According to a study published by Smith et al., there is a small but statistically significant rise in pulmonary artery pressure after injection of low-osmolarity, nonionic contrast material for pulmonary angiography; it is unlikely to be of clinical significance.

11. Describe the angiographic findings of pulmonary hypertension.

Enlarged main pulmonary arteries and pruning of the peripheral branches. The same findings can be appreciated on a frontal chest x-ray and a contrast CT scan of the chest.

12. Describe the technique for performing a pulmonary angiogram.

Brachial/basilic, jugular, or preferably femoral vein access should be obtained by modified Seldinger technique. Depending on the catheter type, a 6- or 7-French sheath should be placed. Grollman and AP2 are two of the catheters that have the curvature to provide an easy access to the right ventricle from the right atrium. A J wire or a Benzton wire can also be used to guide the catheter into the right ventricle. During this step of the study continuous heart monitoring should be performed to check for irregularities in the heart rhythm. If premature ventricular contractions (PVCs) are seen, immediate removal of the catheter from the right atrium until rhythm returns to normal is crucial. Once access is gained into the pulmonary arteries, pulmonary arterial pressures should be obtained prior to contrast injection. Then a bilateral, unilateral, or selective pulmonary angiogram can be obtained as planned. Injection of contrast at 15–25 ml/sec with a total dose of 30–50 ml is required for optimal images. Two views should be obtained for each lung, usually the anteroposterior (AP) and ipsilateral oblique views. Fast filming is also important (6 frames/sec) during breath holding.

13. How often does PE result in infarction?

In less than 10% of cases. Retrograde pulmonary venous flow and collateral bronchial arterial flow prevent infarction in most cases.

14. Describe the chest x-ray findings of PE.

Most commonly the chest x-ray is normal. In patients with pulmonary embolism with infarction, there may be a small pleural effusion with a pleural-based, wedge-shaped opacity, known as Hampton's hump.

The most common chest-x-ray finding of a PE without infarction is Westermark's sign, which is localized peripheral oligemia with or without distended proximal vessels.

15. What are the PIOPED criteria?

The Prospective Investigation of Pulmonary Embolism Diagnosis (PIOPED) developed a set of criteria for interpreting the results of V/Q scans:

1. V/Q imaging demonstrating two or more large (> 75% of a segment) mismatched segmental defects is a **high-probability** study. (Two moderate defects = one large defect.)

2. A study is considered **intermediate** if mismatched segmental defects total less than two large defects, if the study is difficult to categorize as high or low probability, or if the study does not meet the criteria for either high or low probability.

3. A study with nonsegmental perfusion defects, matched defects, small subsegmental defects and a small perfusion defect with a large corresponding radiographic defect is considered **low probability**.

16. Describe the CT findings of acute PE.
A filling defect, usually cresecent-shaped, is visible within the pulmonary arteries (Fig. 1).

17. Describe the CT findings of chronic PE.
A chronic PE is usually adherent to vessel wall. Central pulmonary arteries are usually enlarged due to pulmonary hypertension. Calcifications at the vessel walls may also be seen in chronic PEs.

18. What are the sensitivity and specificity of CT for PE?
Sensitivity and specificity are 100% for PE in the main pulmonary artery. Sensitivity is about 90–95% for segmental branches and considerably lower for subsegmental branches.

19. Describe the angiographic findings of PE.
Intraluminal filling defect or demonstration of the trailing end of an occluding thrombus by outlining contrast are the angiographic findings of PE (Fig. 2).

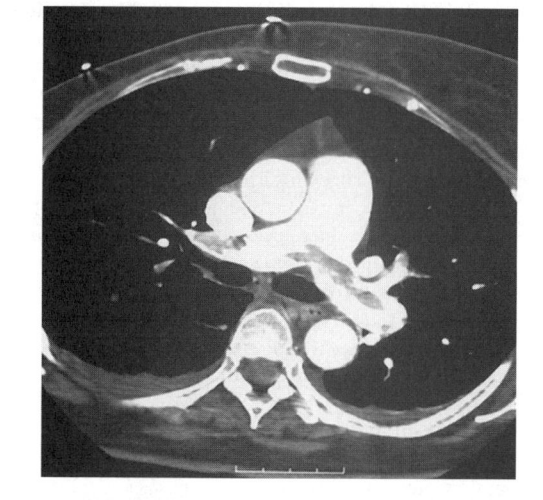

FIGURE 1. CT scan demonstrates central pulmonary embolism.

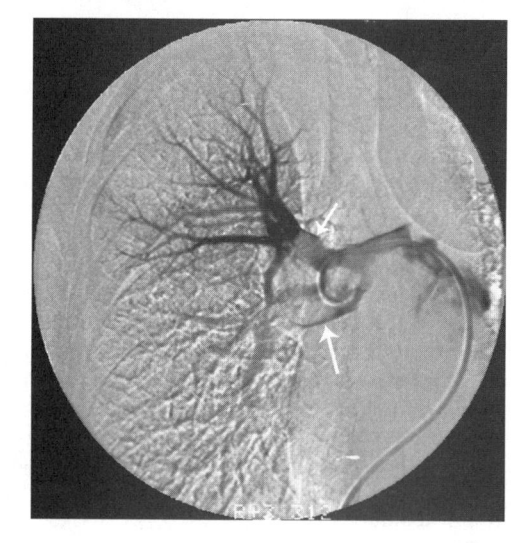

FIGURE 2. Right pulmonary angiogram. Two white arrows show filling defect in both upper lobe and lower lobe branches, representing embolus in a patient with deep venous thrombosis.

20. What are the sensitivity and specificity of pulmonary angiograms for PE?

Sensitivity of approximately 98% and specificity of approximately 99% are shown when angiograms are correlated with clinical follow-up.

21. How is PE treated?

If there are no contraindications, anticoagulation is the treatment. It usually starts with IV heparin with a bolus dose. After 2–3 days of heparin therapy oral warfarin can be started and should be taken for 6 months. Warfarin levels are adjusted to keep the INR around 2. In patients with absolute contraindication to anticoagulation, placement of an inferior vena cava filter is an alternative to prevent subsequent PEs. Systemic thrombolysis is reserved for massive PE.

22. What are the treatment options for life-threatening massive PE that does not respond to systemic thrombolysis?

In massive PEs immediate intervention to decrease thrombus burden may be life-saving. Catheter-directed thrombolysis should be the first approach if there are no contraindications. If thrombolysis fails, embolectomy should be performed.

The traditional method of embolectomy for massive PEs used to be thoracotomy, which has high morbidity and mortality rates (10–40%). The procedure requires general anesthesia and cardiopulmonary bypass. With the advance of catheter-directed treatments, the transvenous approach for pulmonary embolectomy has become the treatment of choice for embolectomy. Greenfield and colleagues used the Greenfield embolectomy device with lower mortality rates than surgical embolectomy.

23. What are the diagnostic tests for DVT?

Currently the test of choice is Doppler ultrasound for initial evaluation of DVT. It is highly sensitive and specific. Lower extremity venogram, which used to be the gold standard for evaluation of DVT, is currently rarely used.

24. What are the ultrasound criteria for diagnosis of DVT?

Compressibility, complete filling of the vein with color flow imaging, augmentation, and respiratory phasicity are characteristics of a normal vein. If a vein is not compressible or contains a filling defect in color flow imaging, DVT is the diagnosis. Also lack of augmentation and loss of respiratory phasicity are suggestive of proximal occlusion.

25. How is DVT treated?

The usual treatment is 3–6 months of anticoagulation with warfarin. If anticoagulation is contraindicated, an IVC filter placement is an alternative to prevent PEs.

26. What are the clinical signs and symptoms of pulmonary AVMs?

Epistaxis, hemoptysis, hemothorax, shortness of breath, cyanosis, and clubbing are common signs and symptoms.

27. Describe common locations of pulmonary AVMs.

Pulmonary AVMs are most commonly located in lower lobes (see Fig. 3B), then in middle lobe and lingually. They are least commonly found in the upper lobes.

28. Explain the two types of pulmonary AVMs.

Simple AVMs (see Fig. 3F) are a direct communication between a single pulmonary artery and pulmonary vein with dilatation of the vein. **Complex AVMs** have more than one feeding artery and frequently multiple draining veins. More than 80% of pulmonary AVMs are simple.

29. Describe the treatment of pulmonary AVMs.

Embolization with coils or detachable balloons can be curative. Coil embolization is the commonly performed technique in the United States (Fig. 3) since detachable balloons are not yet

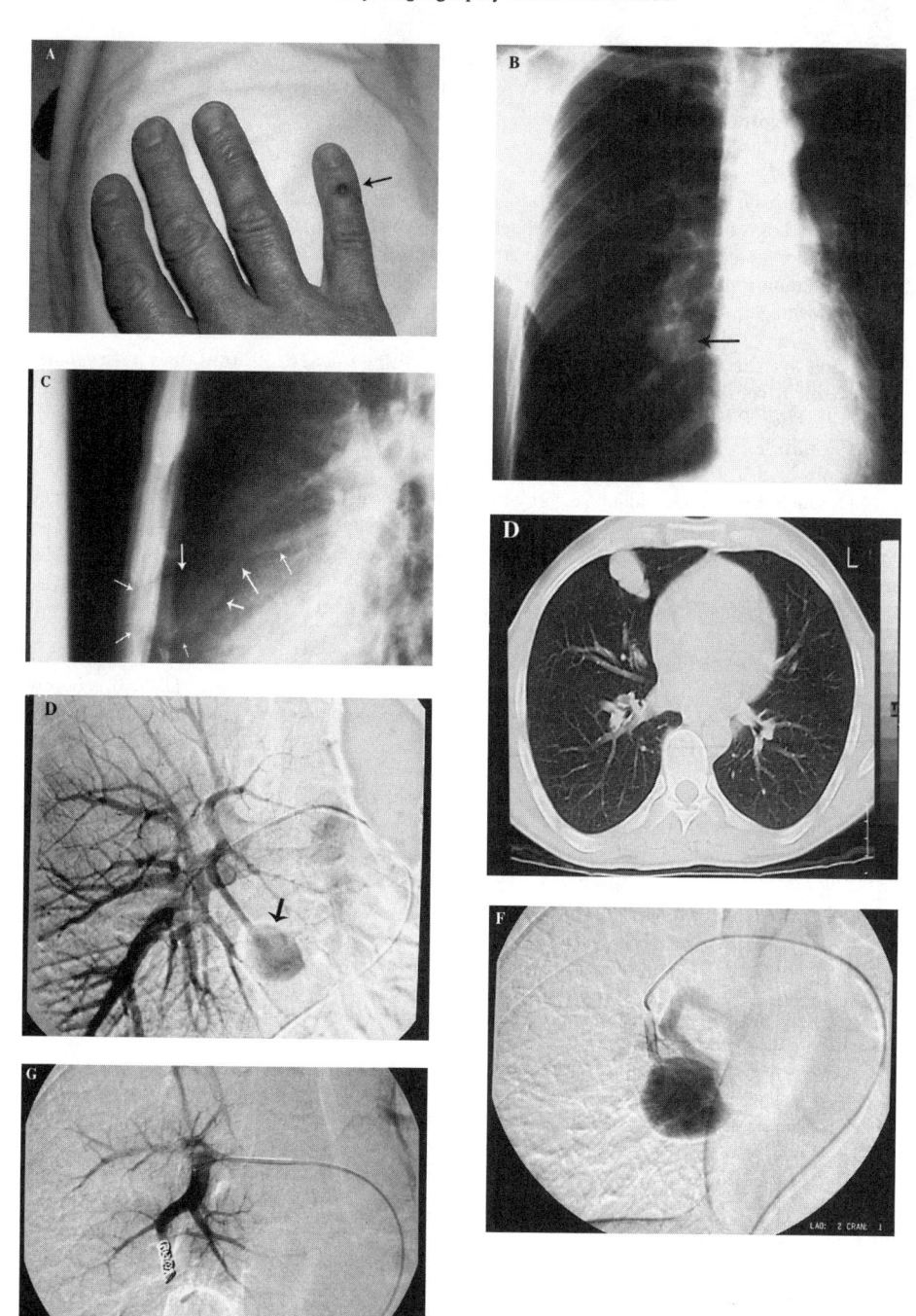

FIGURE 3. A cutaneous lesion in a patient with dyspnea on exertion was identified as telangiectasia (**A**). Chest x-rays (**B** and **C**) demonstrated a mass in the right lower lobe (arrows). A CT scan (**D**) confirmed the mass. Angiograms (**E** and **F**) confirmed the suspicion of a pulmonary AVM. This simple AVM has a single feeding artery that empties into a bulbous, nonseptated aneurismal segment with a single draining vein. The AVM was successfully embolized with multiple coils (**G**). The clinical and imaging findings in this patient are consistent with Osler-Weber-Rendu syndrome.

available. In Osler-Weber-Rendu syndrome, pulmonary AVMs are usually multiple and may require several sessions of embolization. During the procedure initially a pulmonary angiogram is obtained to localize the AVM(s) (Fig. 4). Then, after localizing the feeding artery by small amounts of contrast injection while cannulating different arteries, a selective pulmonary angiogram should be obtained using wire and catheter guidance.

30. Identify a devastating complication of pulmonary AVMs.
A brain abscess or infarct (see Fig. 4) due to a paradoxical embolism. This complication is more commonly seen in children.

31. What is the most common cause of foreign bodies in pulmonary arteries?
Broken catheter fragments.

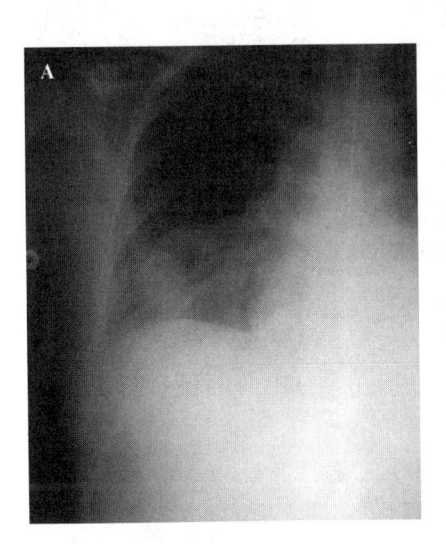

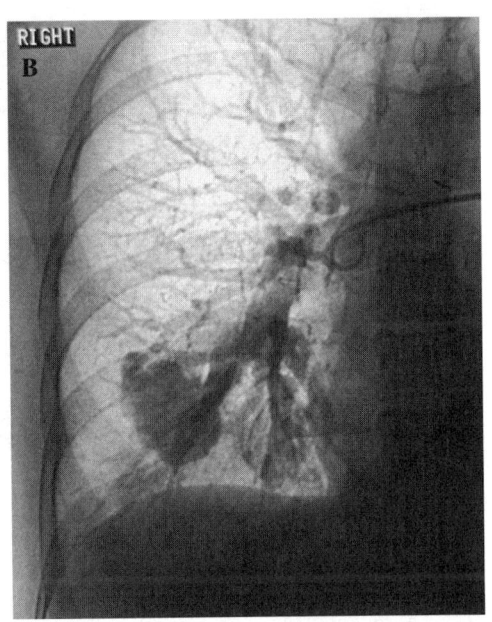

FIGURE 4. A 33-year-old woman with shortness of breath while climbing stairs in the house presented to the pulmonologist for work-up of her symptoms. Detailed history revealed that she has a 7-year-old boy who also has shortness of breath after riding his bike for a short distance. Clinically Osler-Weber-Rendu syndrome was suspected. Chest x-ray (**A**) demonstrated a mass in right lower lobe highly suspicious of pulmonary AVM. Pulmonary angiogram (**B**) confirmed the findings of two AVMs in the right lower lobe. The treatment plan was to embolize the AVMs. Selective right lower lobe pulmonary angiogram demonstrated a complex AVM supplied by two arteries with a single large draining vein. One of the arteries supplying the AVM was embolized with multiple coils after administering 5000 units of heparin IV (**C**). Just before the onset of embolization of the second arterial feeder, the patient developed hemoptysis and was noted to have left hemiparesis. Immediate embolization of the second arterial feeder was performed, and in the process thrombus was noted in the AVM (**D**) with a patent large draining vein (**E**). Part of the thrombus had embolized to the brain via the draining pulmonary vein " left atrium " left ventricle " aorta " innominate artery " right common carotid artery " right internal carotid artery " right middle cerebral artery. Successful embolization was performed of both arterial feeders. A second AVM noted in the right lower lobe (**F**) was not embolized at the time. Due to the left hemeperesis, a right internal carotid artery angiogram was performed and demonstrated acute termination secondary to thrombus in the right middle cerebral artery (**G**). This lesion was successfully thrombolysed with catheter-directed thrombolysis (**H**). The patient clinically recovered all functions except for mild paraesthesia in the left hand.

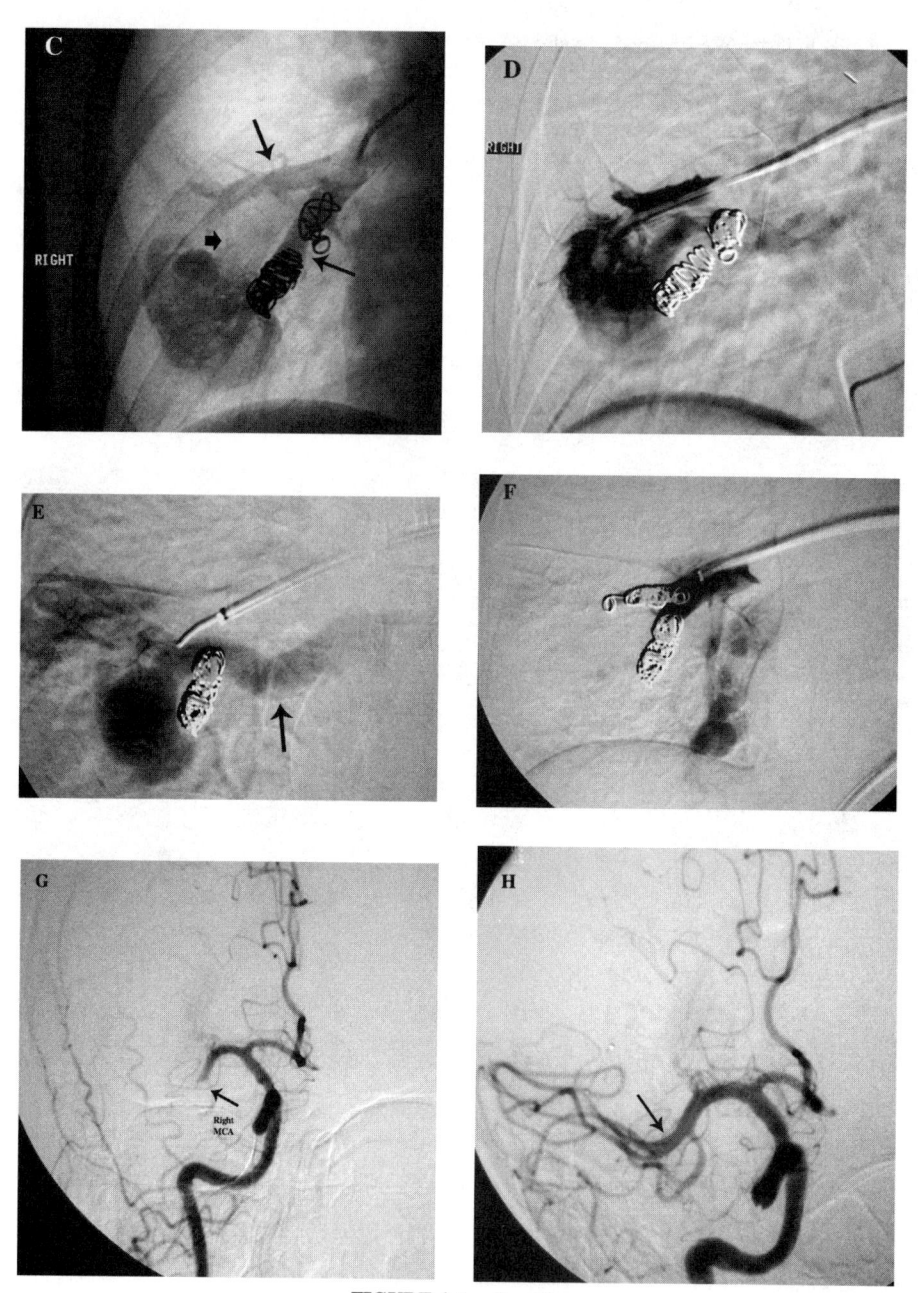

FIGURE 4. (continued)

32. Describe the endovascular technique for removal of a foreign body from pulmonary arteries.

Preferably femoral or jugular venous access should be obtained. A commercially available snare device is advanced through a large (preferably 8-French) sheath, and the foreign body is encased by the snare. Then the snare should be tightened around the catheter fragment by advancing the outer sheath of the snare over the wire component. Subsequently foreign body and snare should be removed together from the sheath.

BIBLIOGRAPHY

1. Bookstein JJ, Silver TM: The angiographic differential diagnosis of acute pulmonary embolism. Radiology 110:25–33, 1974.
2. Drucker EA, Rivitz SM, Shepard JA, et al: Acute pulmonary embolism: Assessment of helical CT for diagnosis. Radiology 209:235–241, 1998.
3. Edwards CRW, Bouchier IAD, Haslett C, Chilvers ER (eds): Davidson's Principles and Practice of Medicine. 17th ed. New York, Churchill Livingstone, 1996.
4. Greenfield LJ, Proctor MC, Williams D, Wakefield T: Long-term experience with trans-venous catheter pulmonary embolectomy. J Vasc Surg 18:450–457, 1993.
5. Greenfield LJ, Reif M, Guenter C: Trans-venous pulmonary embolectomy by catheter device. Ann Surg 174:881–886, 1971.
6. Killewich LA, Nunnelee JD, Auer AI: Value of lower extremity venous Doppler examination in the diagnosis of pulmonary embolism. J Vasc Surg 17:934–939, 1993.
7. Laberge JM, Gordon RL, Kerlan RK Jr, Wilson MW (eds): Interventional Radiology Essentials. Philadelphia, Lippincott Williams & Wilkins, 2000.
8. Perler BA, Becker GJ (eds): Vascular Intervention: A Clinical Approach. New York, Thieme, 1998.
9. PIOPED investigators: Value of the ventilation/perfusion scan in acute pulmonary embolism. JAMA 263(20):2753–2759, 1990.
10. Smith TP, Lee VS, Hudson ER, et al: Prospective evaluation of pulmonary artery pressures during pulmonary angiography performed with low-osmolar nonionic contrast media. J Vasc Intervent Radiol 7:207–212, 1996.
11. Urokinase Pulmonary Embolism Trial: A national cooperative study. Circulation 47:1–108, 1973.
12. Zuckerman DA, Sterling KM, Oser RF: Safety of pulmonary angiography in the 1990s. J Vasc Intervent Radiol 7:199–205, 1996.

25. INFERIOR VENA CAVA INTERRUPTION

Nikhil C. Patel, MD

1. Give the fatal and nonfatal incidence of pulmonary embolism (PE) in the United States per year.

The nonfatal incidence of PE ranges from 400,000 to 630,000 cases per year; from 50,000 to 200,000 fatalities per year are directly attributable to PE.

2. What is the preferred treatment for deep vein thrombosis (DVT) and PE?

In a patient who has no contraindication, anticoagulation is the treatment of choice. However, as many as 20% of patients treated with anticoagulation have recurrent PE.

3. What preventive method was initially used for PE?

Armand Trousseau first proposed interruption of the inferior vena cava (IVC) for the treatment of PE in 1868. IVC interruption with surgical ligation was first performed in 1893. Over the years, surgical interruption took many forms, such as ligation and placation with external clips or staples. Thrombosis was a frequent complication after these procedures. In 1967, the endovascular approach became reality with the introduction of the Mobin-Uddin filter.

4. List criteria used in choosing the appropriate filter.
- Clot-trapping efficiency
- Occlusion rate of IVC and access vein
- Risk of filter migration
- Filter embolization
- Structural integrity of the device
- Precise placement

5. List important characteristics to look for in an IVC cavagram before placing a filter.
- Infrarenal IVC length and diameter
- Location and number of renal veins, including presence of circumaortic left renal vein.
- IVC anomalies such as duplicated IVC (Fig. 1)
- Intrinsic IVC disease such as pre-existing thrombus or extrinsic compression.

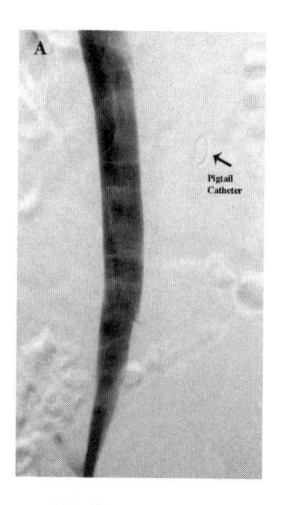

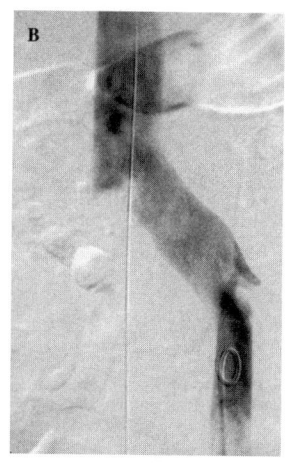

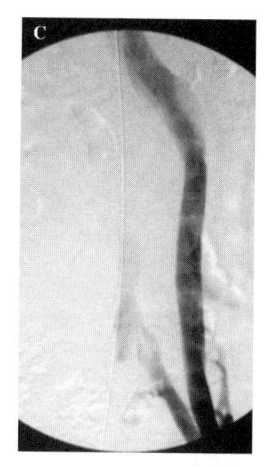

FIGURE 1. A, B, and **C,** Inferior vena cava (IVC) cavagrams demonstrate duplicated IVC.

6. **Describe the ideal placement of a filter for prevention of lower extremity and pelvic venous thromboembolism.**

The ideal placement of an IVC filter is at the infrarenal IVC. The apex of any filter device should be at the level or immediately inferior to the lowest renal vein.

7. **What other sites have been used for IVC filter placement for different causes?**
   - Iliac veins
   - Superior vena cava
   - Suprarenal IVC (Fig. 2)

   Limited data are available for use of the above sites for IVC filter placement.

8. **Define filter migration.**

Filter migration is defined as a change in filter position of more than 2 cm (compared with the deployment position), as documented by plain film imaging, CT, or venography.

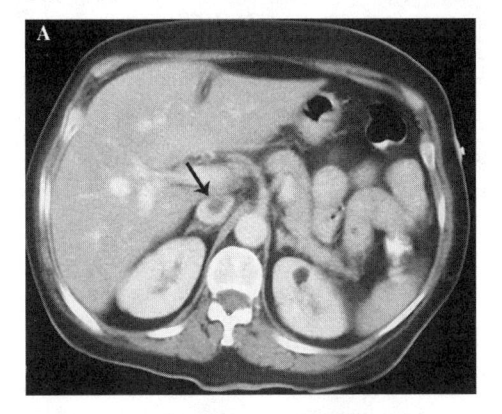

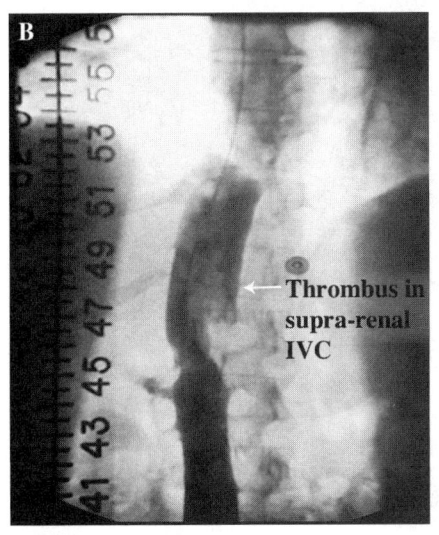

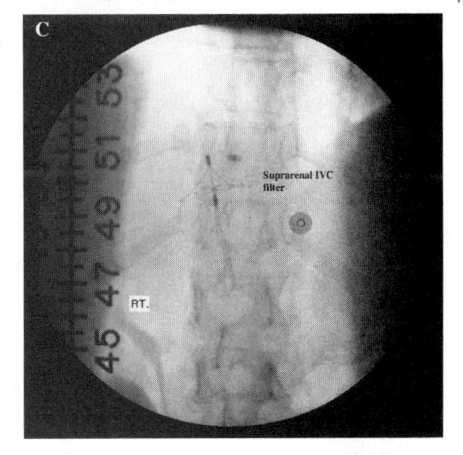

FIGURE 2. A, CT scan of abdomen demonstrates thrombus of the inferior vena cava (IVC) at and above the level of the renal veins *(arrow)*. The fatty lesion in the left kidney is consistent with angiomyolipoma, an incidental finding. **B,** IVC cavagram confirms the position of the thrombus. **C,** A suprarenal IVC filter was placed.

9. Define filter penetration of the IVC.

The filter is said to penetrate the IVC if the filter's strut or anchor devices extend more than 3mm outside the wall of the IVC.

10. At what angle is the filter tilt considered significant?

More than 15° from the IVC axis is considered a significant filter tilt.

11. List the accepted indications for infrarenal IVC filter placement.

1. Patients with PE or IVC thrombus and iliac vein thrombus or femoral-popliteal DVT with one or more of the following:
   - Contraindication to anticoagulation (Fig. 3)

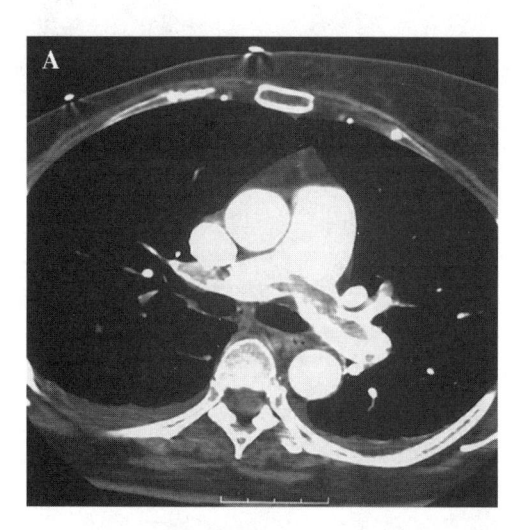

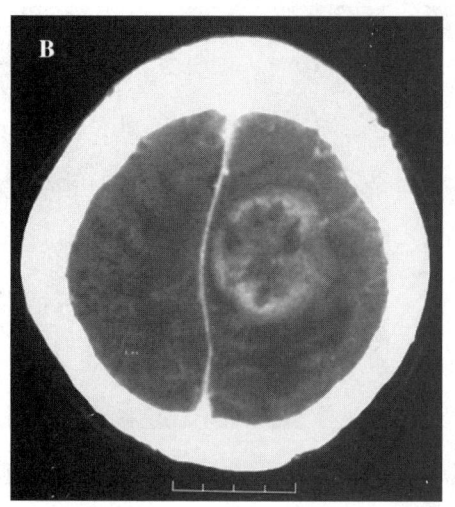

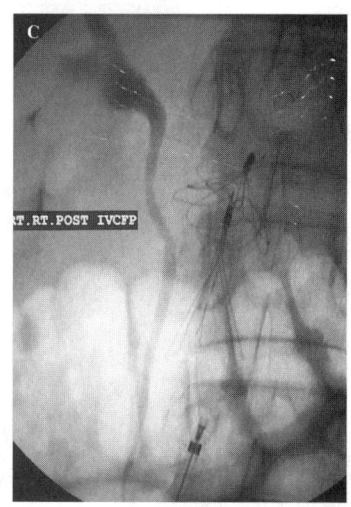

FIGURE 3. A 39-year-old woman with a history of breast cancer presented to the emergency department with shortness of breath and confusion. **A,** CT confirms clinical suspicion of pulmonary embolism. **B,** CT of the brain revealed intracranial enhancing lesion thought to be metastasis of breast cancer. **C,** An inferior vena cava filter was placed because the patient was not a candidate for anticoagulation due to metastatic disease to the brain.

- Complication of anticoagulation
- Failure of anticoagulation, such as recurrent PE despite adequate therapy, or inability to achieve adequate anticoagulation

2. Massive pulmonary embolism with residual deep vein thrombosis in patient with risk of further PE
3. Free-floating IVC or iliofemoral thrombus
4. Severe cardiopulmonary disease such as cor pulmonale or pulmonary hypertension with DVT
5. Poor compliance with anticoagulation medications

12. What are the other indications for IVC filter placement for selected patients?
- Severe trauma without documented PE or DVT. Severe trauma includes head injury, spinal cord injury, or multiple long bone or pelvic fractures.
- High-risk patients, such as immobilized, intensive care patients. Prophylactic preoperative placement may be used in patients with multiple risk factors for venous thromboembolism.

13. List the indications for suprarenal filter placement.
- Renal vein thrombus
- IVC thrombosis extending above the renal veins (Fig. 4)
- Thrombus extending above previously placed infrarenal filter
- Anatomic variant such as duplicated IVC and low insertion of renal veins
- PE after gonadal vein thrombosis
- Filter placement during pregnancy (Suprarenal placement is also appropriate in women of child-bearing age.)

14. What are the relative contraindications for an IVC filter placement?
- Uncorrectable severe coagulopathy
- Patients with the bacteremia or untreated infection (Clinical judgment should be applied in this situation.)
- Pediatric or young adult patients (The indication for filter placement should be strict due to the long-term effect; in addition, the durability of the device is not precisely known.)

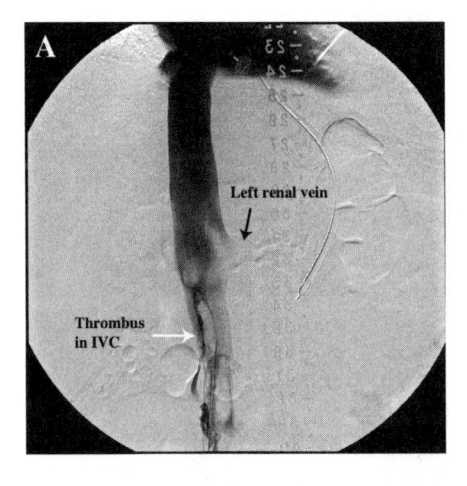

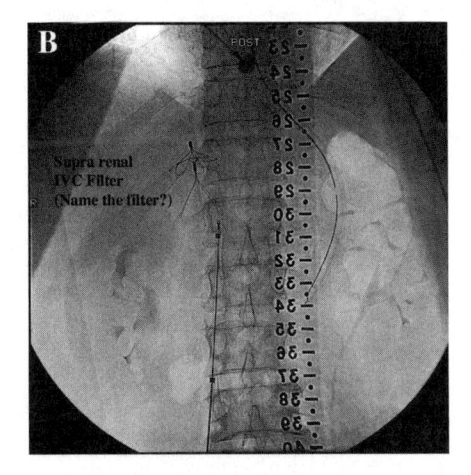

FIGURE 4. A 34-year-old man involved in a motor vehicle accident suffered cervical spine injury and was scheduled for prophylactic placement of an inferior vena cava (IVC) filter. **A,** IVC cavagram demonstrates large, free-floating thrombus (white arrow) extending to the level of the left renal vein (black arrow). Ideally, the filter should be placed from the internal jugular approach, but the patient's spine injury required a cervical collar that could not be removed. **B,** As a result, the filter sheath was gently manipulated past the thrombus, and a suprarenal IVC filter (Simon Nitinol filter) was placed.

15. List the complications of IVC filter placement along with their incidence.

Complication rates are highly variable, depending on the filter used. Considered as a group, the following complication rates have been reported:
- Death (less than 1%)
- Recurrent clinical PE (2–5%)
- IVC occlusion (2–30%)
- Filter embolization (2–5%)
- Access site thrombosis (0–6%)
- IVC penetration (0–41%)
- Migration (0–18%)
- Filter fracture (2–10%)

16. At what level does the right renal vein join the IVC?

The right renal vein joins the IVC at the level of the lower first lumbar vertabrae.

17. What percentage of the population is reported to have multiple right renal veins?

28%.

18. Describe the normal pattern of passage of the left renal vein before it joins the IVC.

The usual pattern is to pass anterior to the aorta and under the superior mesenteric artery before joining the IVC.

19. What percentage of the population has a retroaortic left renal vein?

3%.

20. Define circumaortic left renal vein.

Circumaortic vein consists of two left renal veins with one passing anterior to the aorta in the usual position. The additional renal vein passes posterior to the aorta, joining the lower IVC or the iliac vein. Circumaortic renal vein is more common than retroaortic left renal vein. Its incidence has been at 8–17% of the population.

21. Describe the two variations seen with circumaortic renal vein.

In the most common variation (75% of cases), a single renal vein bifurcates at the renal hilum. In the less common variation, two renal veins originate at the renal hilum.

22. The use of IVC filter is associated with what percentage of reported reduction in PE mortality?

The reported rate of PE mortality with use of the IVC filter is less than 4%. Since the mortality rate for untreated cases is 30%, IVC filter use results in a 24% reduction.

23. What type of traumatic injury is an indication for prophylactic placement of a vena cava filter?

Patients who cannot receive anticoagulation and have one or more of the following injury patterns:
- Recent brain injury
- Incomplete spinal cord injury with para- or quadriplegia
- Complex pelvic fractures with associated long bone fractures
- Multiple long bone fractures
- Major eye injury

24. What are the rates of recurrent PE and caval penetration when Greenfield filters are used?

The recurrent PE rate is 3–5%, and the caval penetration rate is 2%.

25. Prophylactic IVC filter placement in trauma patients has been projected to result in what percentage of reduction of PE-related mortality?
A reduction rate of 66% in PE-related mortality has been reported.

26. Explain the IVC size criteria for filter placement.
For most filters, the maximum acceptable size of the IVC for filter placement is 28 mm. Exceptions are Trapease filters, for which the maximum size is up to 30 mm, and birds' nest filters, for which the maximum size is 40 mm.

27. Define megacava.
An IVC bigger than 30 mm.

28. What filters can be placed in an IVC larger than 30 mm?
Ideally a birds' nest filter (Fig. 5). If the centers does not carry birds' nest filters, any filter can be placed in bilateral iliac veins (Fig. 6).

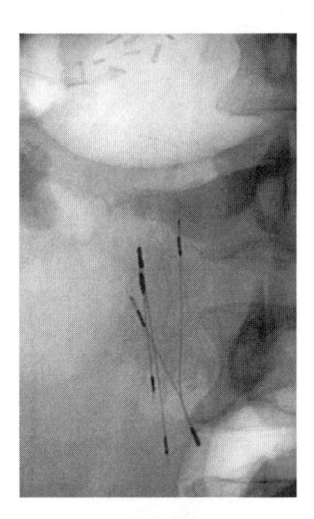

FIGURE 5. Bird's nest filter (BNF) with wire prolapse beyond the struts *(arrow)*. Wire prolapse has been reported but does not affect the clot-trapping ability of the BNF. Inferior vena cava thrombosis has been reported at a rate of 2.9%. The rate of confirmed pulmonary embolus is 1%, and the rate of suspected recurrent pulmonary embolus is 3%.

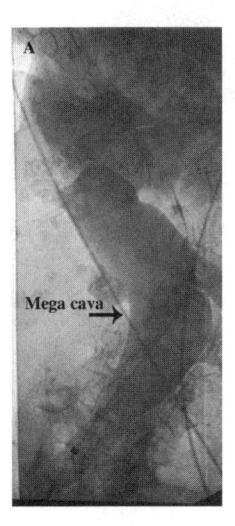

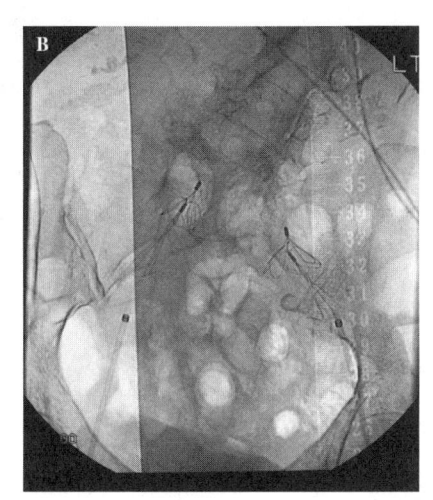

FIGURE 6. A patient with ovarian cancer and deep venous thrombosis presented for placement of an inferior vena cava (IVC) filter. **A,** IVC cavagram demonstrates megacava as well as significant curvature due to scoliosis. **B,** Bilateral Simon Nitinol filters were placed in the iliac veins because bird's nest filter was not available at the time.

29. Describe temporary and optional retrievable filters.

Temporary filters have to be removed within a certain time frame, usually 2 weeks. **Optional retrievable filters** can be removed within a certain time frame (usually 2 weeks) or left in place permanently.

30. List the indications for temporary or optional retrievable filters.
- Protection during thrombolytic therapy for DVT
- Prophylaxis in trauma patients (Fig. 7)
- Patients with a short-term contraindication to anticoagulation or with free-floating iliac vein or IVC thrombus

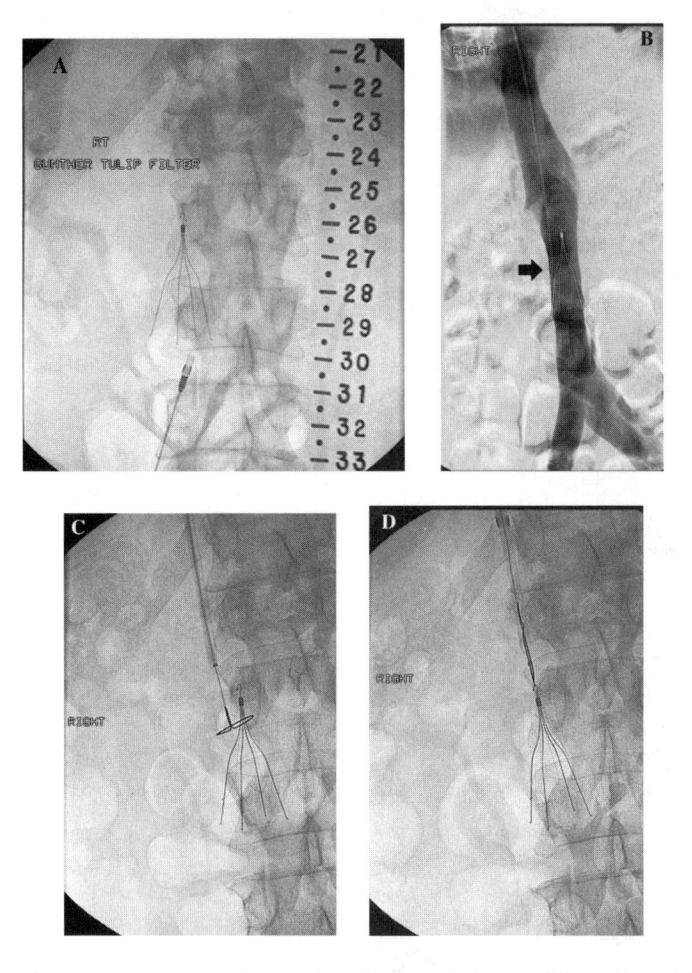

FIGURE 7. A 32-year-old man involved in a motor vehicle accident suffered femoral and pelvic fractures and presented for placement of an optional filter as a prophylactic measure for pulmonary embolism. **A,** A tulip filter was placed via the right common femoral vein approach. **B,** A cavagram documented absence of any thrombus caught by the filter before it was removed on the eleventh day. **C,** A 10-mm gooseneck snare was introduced and passed over the top of the filter to collapse the filter. **D,** The hook was snared. **E,** The sheath was advanced over the filter to collapse the filter. **F,** The filter was pulled into the sheath. **G,** The filter was then removed through the guiding sheath.

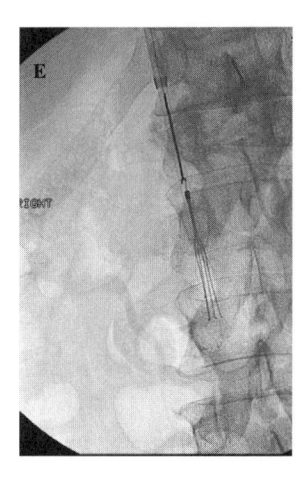

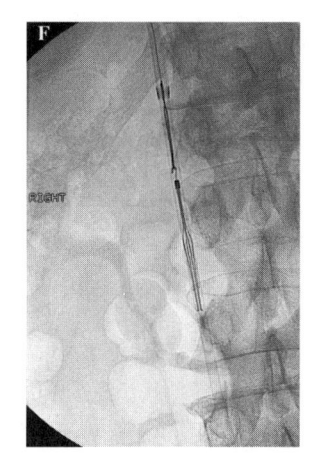

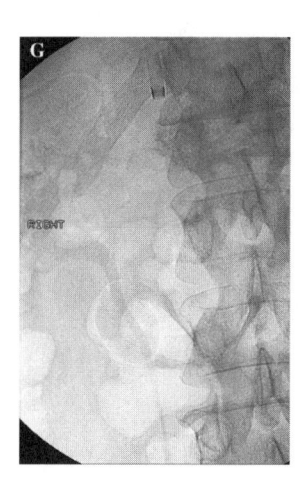

FIGURE 7. (continued)

31. What types of filters are currently available?
Permanent filters and optional retrievable filters (Fig. 8). See Table 1 for details.

32. What contrast agents and modalities can be used for filter placement?
- Fluoroscopy using iodinated contrast, gadolinium, or carbon dioxide (Fig. 9)
- Selective catherization of renal veins without contrast injection. The level of renal veins is used as the landmark. This modality cannot assess the size or evidence of thrombus in IVC.
- Bony landmark at the L1-L2 level. This modality cannot assess the size or evidence of thrombus in IVC.
- Intravascular ultrasound

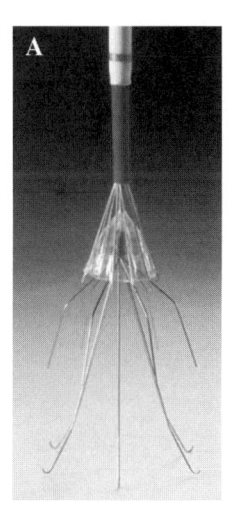

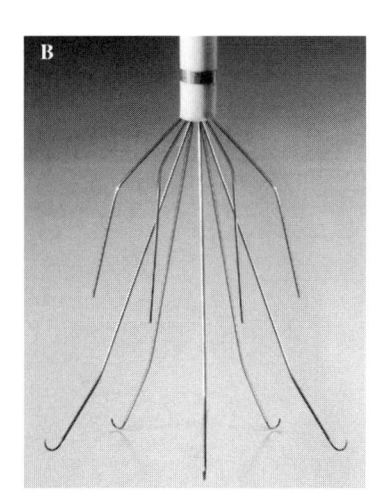

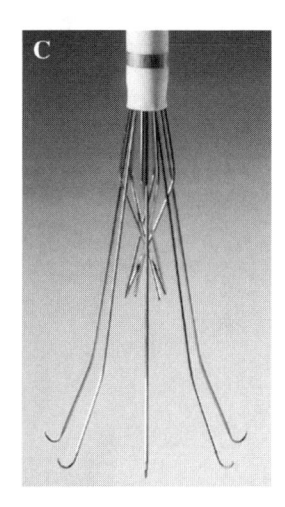

FIGURE 8. Recovery filter made by Bard. **A, B,** and **C** show the filter as well as the recovery cone, which is used to retrieve the filter (Courtesy of Bard, Inc.). The Bard recovery filter is the only currently available filter with "open-ended recoverability" (i.e., the filter can be retrieved at any time). To date the recovery filter has been left in place for as long as 286 days. The filter can be removed only via the jugular, subclavian, or upper extremity veins. Optional tulip filters, made by Cook, are also available but must be removed before 12–14 days via the jugular approach. The optional OptEase filter, made by Cordis, must be removed before 12–14 days via the femoral approach.

Table 1. Types of Permanent and Optional Retrievable Filters

NAME OF FILTER	COMPANY	MATERIAL	FILTER CATHETER CARRIER SIZE	INTRODUCER SHEATH SIZE	MAXIMUM ACCEPTABLE IVC SIZE	LENGTH OF FILTER	PERMANENT OR OPTIONAL RETRIEVABLE
Original Greenfield filter	Meditech	Stainless steel	24 Fr	29 Fr (OD)	28 mm	41 mm	Permanent
Titanium Greenfield filter	Meditech	Titanium	12 Fr	14.3 Fr (OD)	28 mm	41 mm	Permanent
12-F Stainless steel Greenfield filter	Meditech	Stainless steel	12 Fr	14 Fr (OD)	28 mm	41 mm	Permanent
Gianturco-Roehm Bird's Nest	Cook Inc.	Stainless steel	11 Fr	12 Fr (OD)	40 mm	70 mm	Permanent
Vena Tech	Braun/Vena Tech	Phynox (a non-ferromagnetic alloy)	7 Fr (ID)	9 Fr (OD)	30 mm	43 mm	Permanent
TrapEase	Cordis	Nitinol		6 Fr (OD)	30 mm	50–65 mm	Permanent
Simon Nitinol	Bard	Nitinol	7 Fr	9 Fr (OD)	28 mm	45 mm	Permanent
OptEase	Cordis	Nitinol		6 Fr (OD)	30 mm	50–65 mm	Optional retrievable (received FDA approval on 3/30/04)
Gunther Tulip	Cook	Metallic alloy	8.5 Fr	10 Fr (OD)	30 mm	45 mm	Optional retrievable
Recovery	Bard	Nitinol	7 Fr	9 Fr (OD)	28 mm	45 mm	Optional retrievable

OD = outer diameter, Fr = French, FDA = Food and Drug Administration, ID = inner diameter.

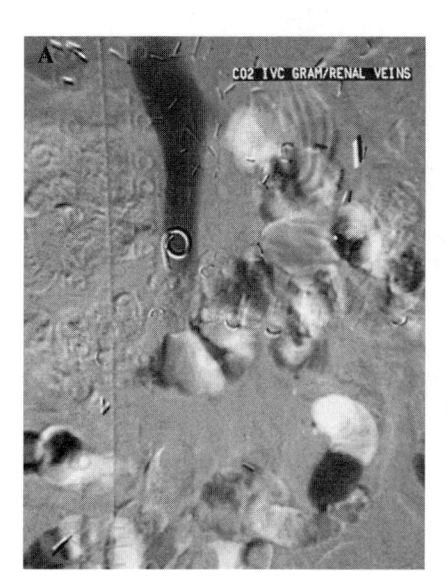

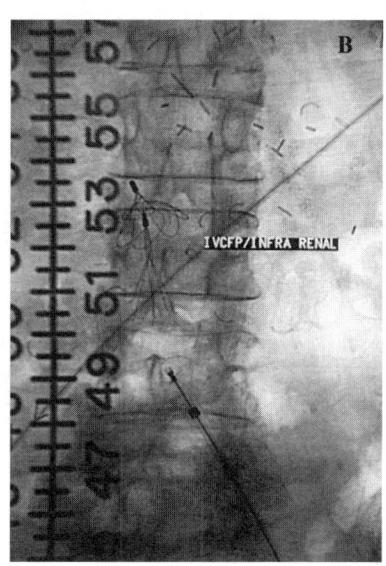

FIGURE 9. A, Inferior vena cava cavagram in a patient with iodinated contrast dye and prednisone allergy. **B,** The filter is placed using carbon dioxide as the contrast agent.

BIBLIOGRAPHY

1. Bick RL, Haas S: Thromboprophylaxis and thrombosis in medical, surgical, trauma and obstetric/gynecologic patients. In Hematology Oncol Clin North Am 17(1), 2003.
2. Cogo A, Bernardi E, Prandoni P, et al: Acquired risk factors for deep-vein thrombosis in symptomatic outpatients. Arch Intern Med 151:164–168, 1994.
3. Dalen JE, et al: Natural history of PE. Prog Cardiovasc Dis 17:257–270, 1975.
4. de Weber K: Effort thrombosis with sepsis. Physician Sportmed 27(5), 1999.
5. Hill SL, Holtzman GI, Martin D, et al: Selective use of the duplex scan in the diagnosis of deep venous thrombosis. Surg 170:201–205, 1995.
6. Hirsh J, Hoak J: Management of deep vein thrombosis and pulmonary embolism. A statement for healthcare professionals. Council on Thrombosis (in constitution with the Council on Cardiovascular Radiology), American Heart Association. Circulation 93:2212–2245, 1996.
8. Lensing AWA, Hirsh J, Buller HR: Diagnosis of venous thrombosis. In Colman RW, Hirsh J, Marder VJ, et al (eds): Hemostasis and Thrombosis: Basic Principles and Clinical Practice, 3rd ed. Philadelphia, J.B. Lippincott; 1994, pp 1297–1321.
9. Menzoian JO, Doyle JE: Venous insufficiency of the leg. Hosp Pract 24:109, 1989.
10. Milne AA, Stonebridge PA, Bradbury AW, et al: Venous function and clinical outcome following deep vein thrombosis. Br J Surg 81:847–849, 1994.
11. Roberts AC: Endovascular Today. Available at http://www.evtoday.com/o3_archive/0103/061.html.
12. Zamorski MA, Opdycke RA: Advances in the prevention, diagnosis, and treatment of deep venous thrombosis. Am Fam Physician 47:457–469, 1993.

26. VARICOSE VEINS AND ENDOVASCULAR MANAGEMENT

Wael E. A. Saad, MBBCh

1. **How common is insufficiency of the superficial venous system?**
   Insufficiency of the superficial venous system of the lower extremity is common. Up to 25% of women and 15% of men suffer from varicose veins.

2. **List the anatomic components of the draining venous system of the lower extremity.**
   Deep venous system: popliteal, superficial femoral, and common femoral veins
   Superficial venous system: greater and lesser saphenous veins.
   Perforator (communicator veins)

3. **How does the normal venous drainage of the legs flow?**
   The perforator veins communicate between the superficial and deep venous system. Valves at the saphenofemoral junction, at the saphenopopliteal junction, and within perforating veins direct blood flow from the superficial to the deep venous systems. The whole system (venous flow antegrade to gravity) moves by muscle contractions in the calves. Reversal of flow is normally prevented by competent unidirectional valves.

4. **What is the calf muscle pump?**
   The calf muscle contractions squeeze the veins and propel venous flow upward against gravity. The main muscle to do so in the lower extremity is the soleus muscle—not the gastrocnemius muscles.

5. **Discuss the theories behind the pathophysiology of varicose veins.**
   Many theories about the nature of varicose veins have been proposed. One hypothesis divides varicose veins into primary and secondary types.
   Primary varicose veins: congenital weakness in the vein walls and/or valve cusps (or deficiency in the number of valves). The primary abnormality leads to luminal distention and further valvular incompetence, resulting in venous reflux.
   Secondary varicose veins: result of a prior episode of venous thrombosis. Subsequent recanalization and inflammation lead to valvular damage and subsequent venous reflux.

6. **List the predisposing factors for development of varicose veins.**
   Females > males (hereditary), pregnancy, hormones, aging, obesity, constipation, prolonged standing, and leg trauma.

7. **List the symptoms associated with varicose veins.**
   Leg pain, night cramps, fatigue, heaviness, symptoms that worsen with prolonged standing, and symptoms of chronic venous insufficiency and venous hypertension (swelling, eczema, pigmentation, venous ulceration).

8. **List the noninvasive modalities used to evaluate for varicose veins.**
   Doppler/duplex ultrasound, continuous-wave Doppler, and photoplethysmography.

9. Explain the goals of noninvasive testing in the evaluation of varicose veins.

The primary goal is to construct a precise layout of the pathways of venous incompetence, including sources of reflux between the superficial and deep venous systems and the distribution of abnormal venous tributaries. Anther goal is to determine the size and morphology of abnormal veins.

10. Describe the common variations in venous anatomy.
- Duplicated great saphenous vein
- Aberrant termination of the lesser saphenous vein (20–40% of population)
- Variable communicators between the lesser saphenous and the gastrocnemial veins

11. List the common patterns of venous reflux in the lower extremity.
- At the saphenopopliteal junction
- At the saphenofemoral junction
- Incompetent anterolateral tributary of the greater saphenous vein
- Reflux in the greater saphenous vein from pudendal varices, gluteal varices, epigastric tributaries, and various perforator veins

12. What are the advantages of duplex ultrasound over other noninvasive tests?

Duplex ultrasound is invaluable for evaluating patients with nonconventional reflux patterns and with variable or anomalous venous anatomy.

13. In what position is the patient with varicose veins placed during physical and/or duplex examination?

Duplex and physical exams should be performed with the patient standing because this is the position in which abnormalities of the superficial venous system are most evident.

14. Describe the mechanism of action of sclerosants in varicose vein sclerotherapy.

Sclerosants cause endothelial and vein wall damage, resulting in fibrosis and eventual resorption of the sclerosed/fibrosed varicose vein.

15. What are the indications for varicose vein sclerotherapy?
- Telangiectasia and feeding reticular veins
- Varicose tributaries with normal saphenous veins
- Residual or recurrent varicosities after surgery
- Varicosities due to incompetent perforator veins

16. List the contraindications for varicose vein sclerotherapy.

Inability to ambulate, (DVT), hypercoagulable states, allergic reaction to sclerosants, and general poor health.

17. Describe the general technique in treating varicose veins with sclerotherapy.

1. Move from the highest to the lowest level of venous reflux and from the largest to the smallest veins

2. Injections are usually performed with the patient in the supine position. A direct percutaneous needle insertion into the target vein is made at an angle of 15–30°. Sclerosants are then injected directly into the varicose vein

2. After each sclerosing session, compression bandages are worn for 3–14 days.

18. List the adverse reactions encountered after varicose vein sclerotherapy.

Serious complications are rare in good hands, but potential complications include cutaneous ulcerations, allergic reactions, arterial injection, and DVT.

Transient (self-limiting within 3 months) hyperpigmentation and/or telangiectasia may be experienced

19. Explain the strategy of treating varicose veins by obliterating the reflux point between the superficial and deep venous systems.

Obliterating the major sources of reflux between the two systems reduces the pressure in the superficial venous system and thus allows the varicose veins to decompress. The greater saphenous vein is often the underlying cause of varicose veins, and the most common site of reflux is at the saphenofemoral junction.

20. List the treatment options for varicose veins that obliterate reflux points and/or the greater saphenous vein.

Surgical options: ligation and saphenous vein stripping, subcutaneous endoscopic ligation and stripping.
Endoluminal options: endoluminal electrocoagulation, ultrasound-guided sclerotherapy, bipolar radiofrequency ablation, laser ablation.

21. Compare the results of endoluminal treatment using radiofrequency ablation (RFA) with saphenous vein stripping.

The recurrence rates of varicose veins after ligation and stripping and after ligation only are 18–29% and 45–71%, respectively. The recurrence rate of varicose veins after surgical ligation and saphenous RFA is 5%. The recurrence rate after saphenous vein RFA only is 10–13%.

22. List the complications sustained after endoluminal RFA.

Parathesias (9% in thigh, 51% in the leg), skin burns (3–5%), DVT (3–5%), and pulmonary emboli (1–2%)

23. What are the advantages of endoluminal laser therapy compared with other endoluminal techniques?

- Small-caliber fibers, minimizing access site size and widening the range of treatable veins
- Reduced depth of penetrating laser energy, resulting in less damage to surrounding structures
- Patients with pacemakers are not excluded (a problem with RFA)

24. List the technical steps involved in endovenous laser therapy of varicose veins.

1. Begin with duplex mapping of the greater saphenous vein.
2. Choose a percutaneous access site—usually the minimal accessible diameter of the vein perceived by the operator.
3. Obtain access with ultrasound guidance to the greater saphenous vein in an antegrade approach (toward the groin) and place a 5-French sheath (45 cm long).
4. Introduce a laser fiber probe with a diameter of 600 micrometers through the sheath, exposing 1–2 cm of the distal filter tip.
5. Position the laser tip 5mm below the saphenofemoral junction. The positioning is confirmed by direct visualization of the red aiming beam of the laser probe through the skin.
6. Administer tumescent (infiltrative) 0.25% lidocaine anesthesia along the course of the greater saphenous vein.
7. Deliver diode laser energy with wavelength of 810 nanometers endovenously as the laser tip is pulled back at a rate of 3–5 mm/second.

25. Explain the threefold function of tumescent/infiltrative lidocaine anesthesia.

1. Anesthesia
2. Perivenous compression, which reduces the saphenous vein diameter to provide improved vein wall apposition around the fiber tip, optimizing vein wall coagulation and subsequent fibrosis
3. Provision of a heat sink, reducing heat-related damage in the adjacent tissues

26. Discuss the post-laser therapy instructions/recommendations.
- Immediate class II (30–40 mmHg) graduated compression stockings should be worn for 1 week after treatment.
- Instruct the patient to ambulate and to continue normal daily activities.
- Instruct the patient to avoid vigorous exercise.
- Residual venous tributaries can be treated with sclerotherapy 4 weeks after the laser treatment session.

27. What symptoms and patient complaints may be expected after laser treatment?
- Bruising at the percutaneous access site
- Mild-to-moderate lower extremity discomfort
- Tightness or pulling sensation, peaking at 5–7 days after laser therapy

The above three complaints resolve within 1–3 weeks and are very common if not universal. Thigh tenderness and fever (superficial thrombophlebitis) may be seen in up to 8% of patients.

28. Summarize the results of endovenous laser therapy of the greater saphenous vein.
- 97% of patients have obliterated greater saphenous veins (no flow by Doppler ultrasound)
- 98% of patients have no evidence of reflux by at least 3 months
- The recanalization rate is 2–3%.

29. Describe the subacute histopathologic changes that the laser ablated vein undergoes.
Subacute histopathologic changes include denudation of the endothelium and carbonization and intensive vascularization of the intima and inner media. The ablated vein progressively decreases in diameter for at least 3 months after the laser ablation session. The reductions in diameter of the ablated veins at 1 month and 3 months after therapy are 48–56% and 27–33%, respectively.

30. What are the endpoints of venous laser ablative therapy?
- Elimination of the highest point of reflux
- Ablation of the incompetent venous segment

BIBLIOGRAPHY

1. Callam MJ: Epidemiology of varicose veins. Br J Surg 81:167–173, 1994.
2. Cotton LT: Varicose veins: Gross anatomy and development. Br J Surg 48:589–598, 1961.
3. Min RJ, Khilnani NM: Lower-extremity varicosities: Endoluminal therapy. Semin Roentgen 37:354–360, 2002.
4. Min RJ, Navarro L: Transcatheter duplex ultrasound-guided sclerotherapy for treatment of greater saphenous vein reflux: preliminary report. Dermatol Surg 26:410–414, 2000.
5. Oh CK, Jung DS, Jang HS, Kwon KS: Endovenous laser surgery of the incompetent greater saphenous vein with a 980-nmfiode laser. Dermatol Surg 29:1135–1140, 2003.
6. Rautio TT, Perala JM, Wiik HT, et al: Endovenous obliteration with radiofrequency-resistive heating for greater saphenous vein insufficiency: A feasibility study. JUR 13:569–575, 2002.
7. Weiss RA, Weiss MA: Controlled radiofrequency endovenous occlusion using a unique radiofrequency catheter under duplex guidance to eliminate saphenous varicose vein reflux: a 2-year follow-up. Dermatol Surg 28:38–42, 2002.

27. VARICOCELES AND TESTICULAR VEIN EMBOLIZATION

Wael E. A. Saad, MBBCh, and Labib H. Sayed, MD

1. **Name the most common clinical indication for testicular vein embolization (TVE).**
   Varicocele(s) (VCs).

2. **What are VCs? How are they formed?**
   VCs are abnormal dilatations and tortuosity of the veins of the pampiniform plexus (PP). They are formed in response to increased pressure in any of the outflow pathways.

3. **How common are VCs?**
   VCs affect pproximately 10% of the male population, most commonly on the left side.

4. **Describe the outflow pathways of the PP.**
   The PP drains into three groups of veins: the internal, middle and external spermatic veins. The **internal spermatic vein** drains into the renal vein on the left side and directly into the vena cava on the right side. **The middle spermatic vein** drains into the internal iliac vein. The **external spermatic vein** drains into the external iliac vein.

5. **What is the most common treatable cause of male infertility?**
   VC.

6. **The sudden onset of VC after age 30 should start a work-up for what condition?**
   Hydronephrosis or a renal tumor.

7. **What sperm characteristics are most suggestive of VC?**
   Abnormal morphology with a decrease in sperm motility; also a minimal decrease in sperm count.

8. **How are VCs diagnosed?**
   Most VCs are palpable as a mass during routine scrotal examination. Doppler sonography is used to confirm physical findings and may also detect subclinical VCs.

9. **List the indications for TVE.**
   - Scrotal pain and edema
   - Recurrent VC after surgical treatment and failure of semen analysis to improve 3 months after therapy
   - Testicular atrophy in a pediatric patient with a large VC on physical exam

10. **List the contraindications to TVE.**
    - Severe abnormality of the coagulation system
    - Demonstrated severe prior contrast reaction

11. **What preprocedural preparation is required for TVE?**
    - Standard pre-angiography work-up
    - Lab tests: hemoglobin/hematocrit, platelet count, prothrombin time (PT), partial thromboplastin time (PTT), blood urea nitrogen (BUN), creatinine
    - Lead shielding to protect testicles from radiation

12. During TVE when should the testicles and PP be visualized by fluoroscopy or seen on film?
Never.

13. What type of sheath should be used for TVE?
An 8-French arterial sheath with infusion of heparinized saline in the sideport.

14. Where should the catheter tip be placed?
In the renal vein beyond the spermatic vein ostium.

15. Why is a left renal venogram performed after catheter placement?
The venogram is performed to demonstrate reflux down the spermatic vein. Collaterals that originate from the renal hilum or paralumbar region may be noted.

16. What is the patient required to do during the left renal venogram?
Valsalva maneuver.

17. List the four most common methods of embolization.
- Metallic coils (Fig. 1)
- Detachable balloons
- Vein occlusion with hot contrast material
- Sclerosants

18. On average, how many coils may be required?
6–12 coils.

19. Where is the first coil deployed? Why?
Near the superior pubic ramus to ensure that no draining collaterals are present beyond this point.

20. Why are repeated contrast injections required after spermatic vein occlusion?
New collaterals become visible with the higher pressure now present in the occluded spermatic vein. Each of these collaterals must also be coiled.

21. Why must coils be placed with the patient performing the Valsalva maneuver?
The Valsalva maneuver ensures that the maximum radius of the coil is achieved and thus decreases the risk of migration.

22. What are the advantages of detachable balloons?
They can be positioned and then deflated and moved to another location. Procedure time is significantly decreased because only two balloons are required.

23. What type of catheter is used for hot contrast material (sclerotherapy)?
A 7-French headhunter with 6–8 distal sideholes.

24. What is the biggest disadvantage to this procedure?
It is very painful.

25. Where is the catheter placed during sclerotherapy?
At the middle to upper part of the sacroiliac joint.

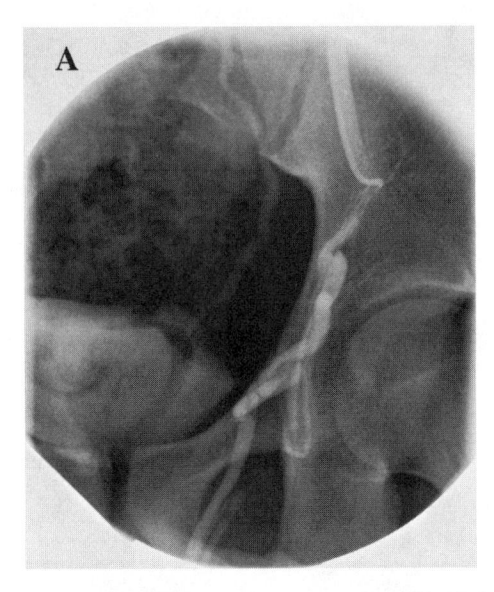

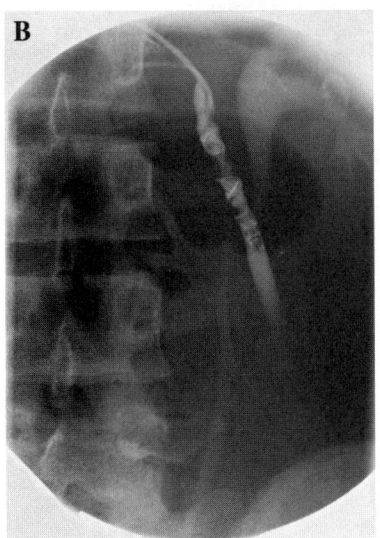

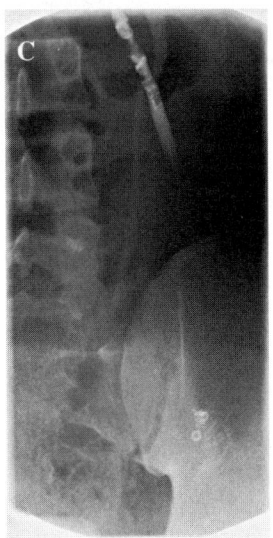

FIGURE 1. Left-sided varicocele (**A**). The vein travels below the inguinal ligament. The varicocele was embolized with coils (**B, C**). It is important to embolize both proximally and distally.

26. Describe standard post procedure management.
   1. Remove all catheters and sheath; attain hemostasis at the puncture site.
   2. Monitor patient recovery for 4 hours.
   3. Evaluate with chest x-ray for any evidence suggestive of migration of coil or balloon to the lung.

27. List the most common complications of coils.
   - Misplacement or migration of coil into central venous circulation
   - Venous perforation, which is usually self-limiting

28. What is the most common complication of balloons?
Migration to the lung, which is usually asymptomatic.

29. List the most common complications of hot contrast.
- Phlebitis of the pampinifrom plexus with testicular atrophy and aspermia
- Thigh anesthesia/paresthesia

30. What is the prevalence of varicoceles in adolescents and young adult men?
Varicoceles are found in 9–14% of young men in the United States and have been described in up to 17% of men in Europe. Up to 39% of infertile/subfertile men may have varicoceles.

31. Describe the clinical picture of VCs.
Signs and symptoms include a dull, dragging pain and oligospermia. Spermatogenesis occurs optimally at a temperature of 34° Celsius. This explains why testicles are found outside the male body in the scrotal sac: to keep them at a lower temperature. VCs cause stasis of venous outflow and raise the temperature in the scrotal sac.

32. On which side are VCs more commonly found? Why?
VCs are found on the left side only in 68–87% of cases; they are bilateral in 11–30% of cases. VCs occur on the right side only in a mere 2% of cases. The exact reason is unknown. However, the difference between the gonadal vein drainage on the left and right is usually implicated. The right gonadal vein usually drains directly (unimpeded) into the inferior vena cava (IVC) and has a higher rate of collaterals (30%). The left gonadal vein usually drains into the left renal vein (indirectly into the IVC via the left renal vein) and has less collateralization (9–10%).

33. List the venous collaterals that the gonadal vein makes.
- Paralumbar/paravertebral collaterals
- Renal capsular veins
- Splenic veins (0–2%) in left VCs
- Inferior mesenteric vein (IMV) tributaries (9%) in left VCs
- Superior mesenteric vein (SMV) tributaries (30%) in right VCs

Eighty percent of patients have venous collaterals communicating with the caudal (inferior) two-thirds of the gonadal vein.

34. What should be done when a man over 40 years old presents with new-onset VCs or if a younger patient presents with extensive unilateral right-sided VCs?
VCs are classified as primary or secondary. **Primary VCs** are more common on the left and in young men. New-onset VCs in older men and extensive VCs on the right side only should raise the possibility of **secondary VCs** and require a work-up. Causes of secondary VCs include renal vein thrombosis, retroperitoneal masses, and renal cell carcinoma.

35. Where does the left gonadal vein insert into a circumaortic left renal vein?
Circumaortic renal veins occur in 2–11% of the population. The left gonadal vein commonly (70% of cases) inserts into the inferior limb of the circumaortic renal vein; less commonly (30% of cases) it inserts into the proximal (main) left renal vein before it bifurcates around the aorta. Rarely if ever does it insert into the superior limb of the circumaortic renal vein.

36. Describe the imaging findings consistent with the diagnosis of testicular VCs.
Doppler ultrasound: dilated veins in the scrotal sac measuring more than or equal to 3 mm in diameter. Diameter increases with the Valsalva maneuver.

Endoluminal venography: gentle hand injection of 2–3 ml of contrast into a cannulated gonadal vein during the Valsalva maneuver. Contrast that travels retrograde (inferiorly) to the level of the inguinal ligament indicates VC.

37. Where should endoluminal therapy be administered in the gonadal vein?
Endoluminal therapy should be started as low as possible and along the entirety of the gonadal vein. This technique reduces the failure rate of endoluminal therapy due to collateral circulation, which is more common caudally than cranially. When endoluminal sclerotherapy is started cranially (high up), the failure rate (32%) is twice as high as when it is administered caudally (16%).

38. What are the technical success rates of endoluminal therapy for VCs?
The technical success rate is 80–90% but has been described as low as 29% in one study.

39. List the causes of failed attempts.
1. Difficult anatomy (venous tortuosity and collateralization): 67–70% of failures
2. Venous spasm: 30–33% failures
3. Prior surgical ligation: 21% of technical failures in one study. However, in another study there was no statistically significant difference in the technical success of patients with prior surgical ligation compared with patients without surgical ligation.

40. Summarize the rates of varicocele persistence/recurrence after endoluminal therapy.
- Metal coils: 4–13%
- Sclerotherapy: 2–16%
- Balloon occlusion: 2–11% (up to 27%)

The overall intention to treat (factoring both technical success and clinical failure) success rate is: 80–83%.

41. Why should coils be oversized when the gonadal vein is embolized?
With the Valsalva maneuver and daily activity, the gonadal vein engorges and widens. Coils should be oversized to accommodate the variations in diameter of the gonadal vein.

BIBLIOGRAPHY

1. Benea G, Galeotti R, Tartari S, Manella P: Percutaneous therapy of primary varicocele: 6 years experience. Radiol Med (Torino) 76:458–465, 1988.
2. Bigot JM, LeBlanche AF, Carrette MF, et al: Anastomoses between the spermatic and visceral veins: A retrospective study of 500 consecutive patients. Abdomen Imag 22:226–232, 1997.
3. Fobbe F, Hamm B, Sorensen R, Felsenberg D: Percutaneous transluminal treatment of varicoceles: where to occlude the internal spermatic vein. Am J Roentgenol 149:983–987, 1987.
4. Pieri S, Minucci S, Morucci M, et al: Percutaneous treatment of varicocele: 13-year experience with the transbrachial approach. Radiol Med (Torino) 101:165–171, 2001.
5. Reyes BL, Trerotola SO, Venbrux AC, et al: Percutaneous embolotherapy of adolescent varicocele: Results and long-term follow-up. J Vasc Intervent Radiol 5:131–134, 1994.
6. Tay KH, Martin ML, Mayer AL, Machan LS: Selective spermatic venography and varicocele embolization in men with circumaortic left renal veins. J Vasc Intervent Radiol 13:739–742, 2002.

28. PORTAL HYPERTENSION AND TIPS

Wael E.A. Saad, MBBCh

1. **Define the term *portal circulation*.**
   All of the body systems—with the exception of two—are vascularly connected to the heart in parallel to one another. The two exceptions are the portal circulations of the body, in which one organ is connected with at least one other organ in series. The connecting vessel(s) between the two organs are referred to as the portal circulation.

2. **Name and describe the two portal circulations of the body.**
   Hepatic portal circulation: the venous drainage system of the intestines (superior mesenteric vein [SMV] and inferior mesenteric vein [IMV]) merges with the splenic vein and the left gastric vein (coronary vein) to form the portal vein, which empties into the liver.
   Hypophyseal portal circulation: capillary portions of the superior hypophyseal artery drain from the hypothalamus, the median eminence, and the superior portions of the pituitary stalk into the anterior pituitary gland via the hypophyseal portal system.

3. **What is the key hemodynamic feature of portal circulations?**
   Portal blood pressure is low relative to systemic arterial pressure because the blood has already passed through the high-resistance capillary beds of the more proximal organ. As a result, the organ on the receiving end of the portal circulation (e.g., the liver) should offer little hemodynamic resistance so that blood from the portal circulation can pass through it. In the case of the hepatic portal circulation, this feature is attributed to the liver's unique histologic architecture, by which blood passes through the sinusoids (blood lakes) instead of capillaries.

4. **Why is the liver connected in series (downstream) to the gastrointestinal tract (GIT)?**
   One of the major roles of the liver is to filter, process, and metabolize toxins and to regulate diet products that are digested by the GIT. It is vital to do so before the blood draining the GIT is given access to the systemic circulation. This task is carried out by the functional unit of the liver: the hepatocytes. The vast majority (if not all) of the hepatocytes have a biliary ductule and a blood sinusoid adjacent to them. This direct access to bile and blood is vital to hepatocyte function and thus to the overall function of the liver. This is a feature of the unique histologic architecture of liver.

5. **What is the normal portal venous pressure?**
   5–10 mmHg. Any value above 12 mmHg is considered portal hypertension.

6. **How much of the hepatic blood supply is supplied by the portal circulation?**
   The liver has a dual blood supply (hepatic arteries and portal circulation). Seventy percent of the liver's blood supply and less than 50% of the liver's oxygen supply is provided by the portal circulation. Approximately 1000 ml of blood pass through the liver via the portal circulation (17–19% of the cardiac output) at any given minute.

7. **Describe the pathogenesis of portal hypertension.**
   According to Ohm's law, portal pressure (delta P) is the result of the product of flow (Q) and hepatic hemodynamic resistance (R):
   $$\text{Delta } P = Q \times R$$
   In almost all cases of portal hypertension an element of both components is involved:
   Portal hypertension = increased liver resistance × increased portal flow
                 (backflow theory)   (hyperdynamic theory).

8. **What are the pathologic causes of increased liver resistance?**
   - Vascular distortions
   - Infiltrative process impinging on the intravascular spaces
   - Architectural changes

9. **What are the pathologic causes of increased portal flow?**
   - Circulating vasodilators (liver failure)
   - Splenomegaly
   - Idiopathic gastrointestinal hyperemia
   - Arterialization of the portal circulation due to arteriovenous (AV) fistula

10. **List the causes of portal hypertension:**
    Prehepatic
    - Splenic AV fistula
    - Splenic or portal vein thrombosis
    - Massive splenomegaly

    Intrahepatic
    - Sarcoidosis
    - Schistosomiasis
    - Nodular regenerative hyperplasia
    - Congenital hepatic fibrosis
    - Idiopathic portal fibrosis
    - Early primary biliary cirrhosis
    - Chronic active hepatitis
    - Myeloproliferative disorders
    - Graft vs. host disease
    - Established cirrhosis
    - Alcoholic hepatitis
    - Alcoholic terminal hyaline sclerosis
    - Venoocclusive disease involving the central veins of the lobules

    Posthepatic
    - Budd-Chiari syndrome
    - Membranous inferior vena cava (IVC) web
    - Right heart failure
    - Constrictive pericarditis

11. **What is the most common cause of portal hypertension in children?**
    Portal venous thrombosis accounts for more than 50% of portal hypertension in children.

12. **What are the more common causes of hepatoportal AV fistulas?**
    1. **Vascular injury**
       - Blunt and penetrating trauma (number one cause)
       - Iatrogenic liver needle biopsy.(number two cause)
       - Iatrogenic postoperative complication from pancreaticoduodenal surgery.
    2. **Infection/inflammation**
       - Pancreatitis
       - Cholangitis
       - Postoperative infection

13. **Where are most hepatoportal AV fistulas located?**
    Most AV fistulas (up to 75%) are intrahepatic; a minority of AV fistulas are extrahepatic. Extrahepatic AV fistulas cause portal hypertension.

14. Define liver cirrhosis.
Liver cirrhosis is loss of the unique hepatic architecture, which is vital for reducing the liver's vascular portal resistance (see question 3) and for proper functioning of the liver (see question 6). Liver cirrhosis is not liver fibrosis, although elements of liver fibrosis are seen in liver cirrhosis.

15. What are the two pathologic classifications of cirrhosis?
- Micronodular (e.g., Laennec [alcohol-induced] cirrhosis)
- Macronodular (e.g., posthepatic cirrhosis, primary biliary cirrhosis)

16. Describe the sinusoidal classification of portal hypertension.
The site/level of increased perihepatic resistance in relation to the hepatic sinusoids is subdivided into presinusoidal, sinusoidal, and postsinusoidal. The categorization of the disease process according to the level of the perihepatic resistance varies from one text to the other, especially between the presinusoidal and sinusoidal categories. The level of increased resistance is controversial and probably varies according to the stage and/or severity of the disease process.

For example, early in its course primary biliary cirrhosis is presinusoidal; later in the disease, sinusoidal resistance predominates. Laennec's cirrhosis, on the other hand, is postsinusoidal early in its course; later in its course, sinusoidal resistance predominates.

17. Why is the sinusoidal classification of portal hypertension important?
This histopathologic classification is a prognostic indicator and predicts response to shunting procedures. For example, presinusoidal disease, in which hepatocellular function usually is preserved, responds well to portosystemic shunts. Ascites occurs mostly in sinusoidal and postsinusoidal pathology.

18. Define Budd-Chiari syndrome.
Budd-Chiari syndrome is due to hepatic venous outflow obstruction. It is classified as postsinusoidal.

19. List the general causes of Budd-Chiari syndrome.
- Idiopathic origin
- Hypercoagulable states
- Injury to venous outflow (e.g., radiation treatments, chemotherapy, trauma, pyrolizidine alkaloids [Jamaican tea])
- Tumor thrombosis (renal cell carcinom, hepatoblastoma and primary leiomyosarcoma of the IVC)
- Membranous suprahepatic IVC
- Right atrial tumor (myxoma or angiosarcoma)
- Constrictive pericarditis
- Severe right heart failure

20. What is the most common cause of Budd-Chiari syndrome?
More than 50% of cases are idiopathic.

21. How is Budd-Chiari syndrome classified?
Type I: Level of obstruction mostly at the IVC
Type II: Level of obstruction mostly at the hepatic veins (Fig. 1)
Type III: Level of obstruction at the centrilobar veins
Budd-Chiari syndrome also may be classified as **acute** (less common) or **chronic** (more common).

22. Which hepatic segment is usually spared, if not hypertrophied, in Budd Chiari syndrome? Why?
Segment I, the caudate lobe, because it has direct drainage into the IVC. Relative caudate hypertrophy occurs in chronic Budd-Chiari syndrome.

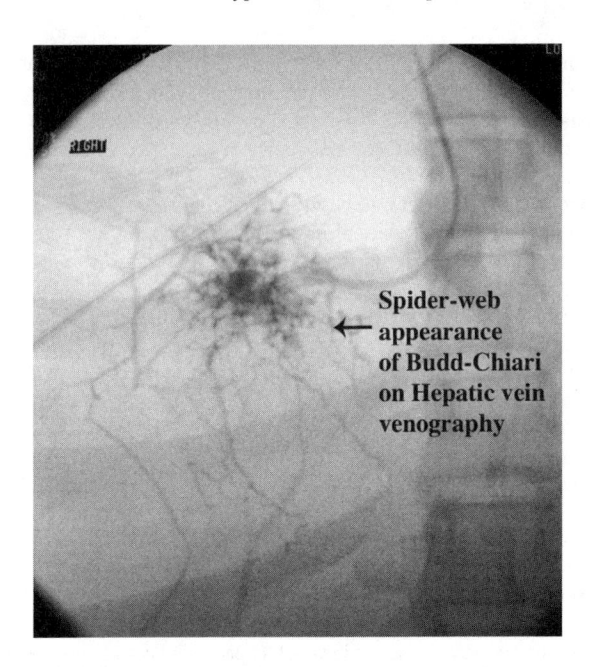

FIGURE 1. Budd-Chiari type II: absence of main hepatic vein with spider web-like appearance of collaterals.

23. List the broad clinical findings of portal hypertension.
1. Liver failure: coagulopathy, edema, and hepatic encephalopathy
2. Gynecomastia in men
3. Splenomegaly
4. Ascites
5. Creation of portosystemic collaterals with potential GI bleeding

24. Name the most important causes of mortality in liver cirrhosis and portal hypertension.
1. Nonhepatic causes (43%)
2. Hepatocellular failure (31%)
3. GI bleeding (15%)
4. Hepatocellular carcinoma (1%)

25. What is the most widely used prognostic classification for patients with liver disease?

Childs-Pugh Classification

CRITERION	1 POINT	2 POINTS	3 POINTS
Ascites	None	Mild	Moderate to severe
Encephalopathy	None I or II	III or IV	
Albumin (gm/L)	> 3.5	2.8–3.5	< 2.8
Bilirubin (mg/dl)	< 2	2–3	> 3
Prothrombin time (secs above normal)	1 to 4	4–6	> 6

Class A: 5–6 points
Class B: 7–9 points
Class C: More than 10 points

Childs-Pugh Class A has the best prognosis for GI bleeding, transjugular intrahepatic portosysemic shunt (TIPS) procedures, surgical portosystemic shunts, and liver transplants. Childs-Pugh Class C has the worst prognosis for GI bleeding, TIPS procedures, surgical portosystemic shunts and liver transplants. Some studies advocate the use creatinine as an additional prognostic indicator. However, creatinine is not included in the Childs-Pugh classification.

26. Why do portosystemic collaterals develop? What is their significance?

As the portal blood pressure rises above 12 mmHg, potential connections (portosystemic anastomoses) between the portal circulation and the systemic venous circulation open up and start shunting blood from the portal circulation to the systemic circulation, thus bypassing the liver. In turn, undetoxified/unmetabolized toxins and poorly regulated digestive products are passed into the system circulation (see question 4). In addition, prominent portosystemic collaterals at certain locations (lower esophagus, gastric fundus, stoma of enterostomies and rectoanal junction) are potential sites for bleeding.

27. Name the portosystemic collaterals that are of clinical significance.

- **Gastroesophageal varices** (ascending varices): connections between the coronary vein (left gastric vein) of the stomach (portal circulation) and the azygos vein tributary (systemic veins). Significance: potential sites for life-threatening upper GI bleed (Fig. 2).

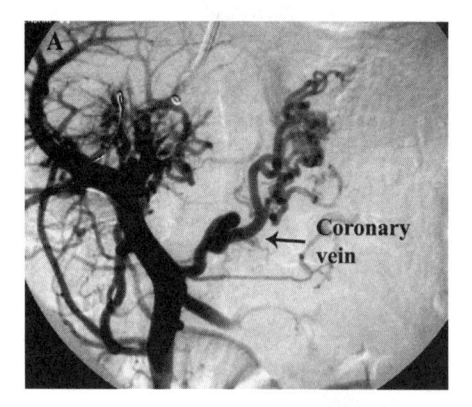

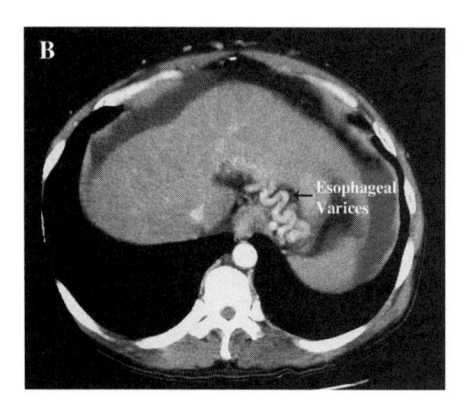

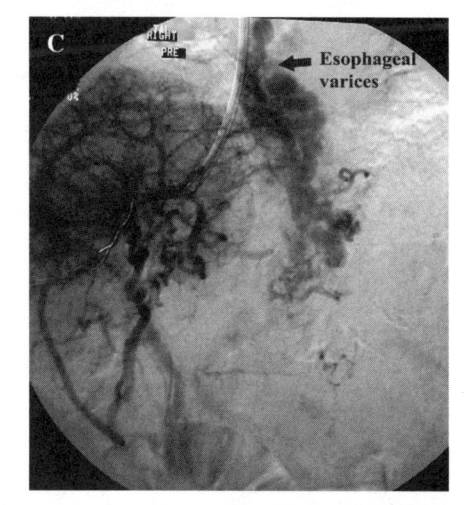

FIGURE 2. Portosystemic collaterals with filling of coronary vein (**A**) and esophageal varices (**B** and **C**).

- **Anorectal varices** (internal hemorrhoids/piles): connections between the middle and superior hemorrhoidal veins of the IMV and the inferior hemorrhoidal vein from the internal iliac vein (systemic circulation). Significance: potential sites for lower GI bleeding.
- **Caput medusae** (Cruveilheir-von Baumgarten syndrome): result of radiating veins from the umbilicus draining a recanalized paraumbilical vein and communicating with the systemic veins of the anterior abdominal wall (Fig. 3). Significance: one of the landmark clinical find-

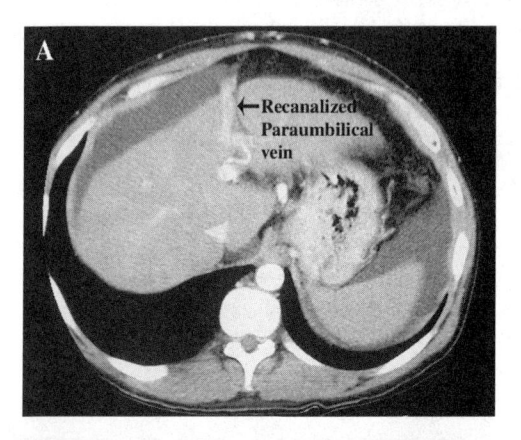

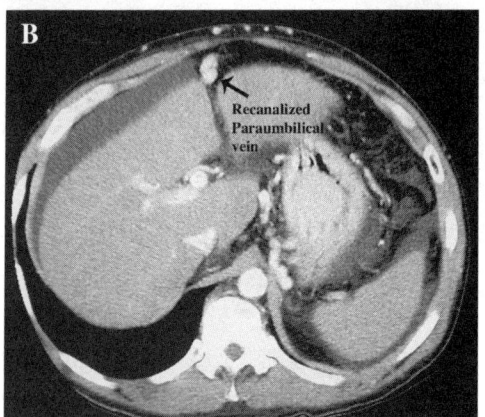

FIGURE 3. Portosystemic collaterals with recanalization of paraumbilical vein (Cruveilhier-von Baumgarten syndrome) originating from left portal vein (**A** and **B**). Caput medusae is seen on computer tomography (**C**).

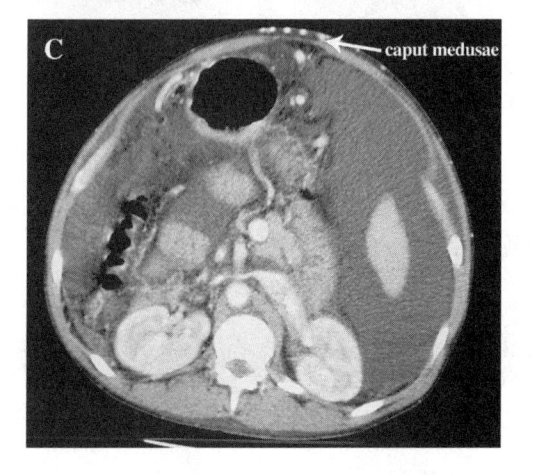

ings of severe portal hypertension. The dilated veins of the anterior abdominal wall are a cause of significant bleeding in abdominal surgeries in patients with uncorrected portal hypertension.

28. Define cavernous transformation of the portal vein.

When the portal vein thromboses, hepatopetal (toward the liver) flow is maintained by serpiginous collaterals that run along the portal vein. It is believed that these collaterals originate from prominent vasa vasorum of the portal vein itself. (Fig. 4).

29. What is the most common cause of upper GI bleeding in portal hypertensive patients?

Portal hypertensive gastropathy (painless)

30. List the other causes of upper GI bleeding in cirrhotic patients.
- Erosive gastritis (pain/dyspepsia)
- Peptic ulcer disease (PUD)
- Gastroesophageal varices (deadliest form of bleeding in cirrhotic patients, representing 30–50% of upper GI bleeding)

31. What is the incidence of gastroesophageal varices in portal hypertensive patients?
- 90% of patients eventually get gastroesophageal varices.
- 30% of those varices eventually bleed.

32. What is the portal venous pressure threshold for formation of gastroesophageal varices?

12 mmHg. However, there is no correlation between the degree of varices and the severity of the bleeding beyond 12 mmHg.

33. What is the first diagnostic study of choice for evaluating upper GI bleeding for varices?

Flexible esophagogastroduodenocscopy (EGD): This study is the first line study for evaluation of upper GI bleeding, regardless of the etiology (portal hypertension or not). It also provides a first-line therapeutic option.

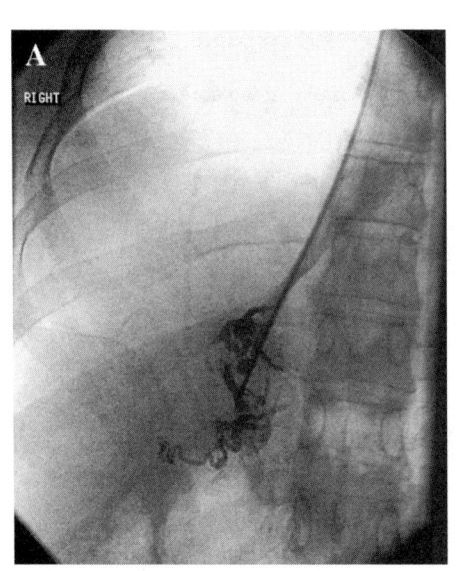

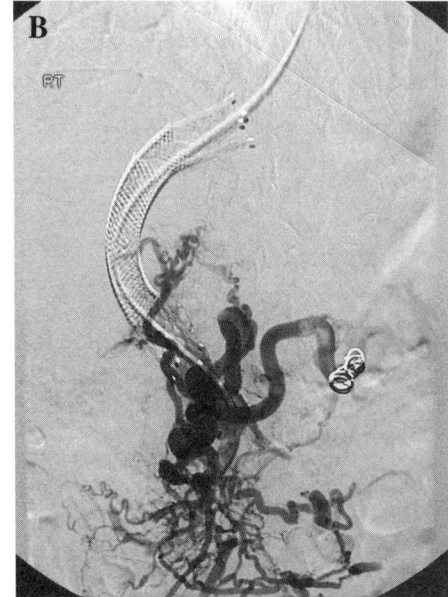

FIGURE 4. Cavernous transformation of portal vein with presence of a racemose conglomerate of collateral veins. Before (**A**) and after (**B**) TIPS.

34. **List the elective/preventive management strategies for gastroesophageal bleeding.**
    - Stop drinking
    - Beta blockers (propranolol and carvedilol)
    - Isosorbide mononitrates (given with beta blockers synergistically)
    - Endoscopic sclerotherapy (3–6 sessions)
    - Elective shunts (surgical vs. TIPS)
    - Liver transplant

35. **List the emergent management strategies for variceal bleeding.**
    - Advanced cardiac life support (ACLS) and volume resuscitation
    - Vasoconstrictive drugs for 24–48 hours (vasopressin and somatostatin)
    - Esophageal balloon tamponades
    - Endoscopic sclerotherapy
    - Emergent surgical portocaval shunts
    - Esophageal transsection and stapling (abandoned in the U.S. and popular in Japan)
    - TIPS
    - Esophageal banding

36. **Explain the mechanism of action of vasoconstrictive drugs.**
    They cause smooth muscle vasoconstriction in the arterial bed and thus reduce the portal flow. However, vasopressin has the same effect on the systemic arteries and splanchnic vessels, causing side effects such as peripheral vascular ischemia, increased cardiac work, and reduced coronary flow. To reduce the side effects, nitroglycerine is given in conjunction with vasopressin. Somatostatin, on the other hand, is more specific for the splanchnic vessels and thus has fewer systemic side effects.

37. **What are the rate of effectiveness and the rate of complication for vasopressin and nitroglycerine combined?**
    - 65% effective in controlling acute bleeding
    - 7% complication rate

38. **How effective is endoscopic sclerotherapy in controlling acute GI bleeding?**
    It is effective in 85–95% of cases.

39. **How effective is esophageal banding? What is the complication rate?**
    - 86% effective
    - 2% complication rate

40. **What are the key complications of esophageal balloon tamponade?**
    - Balloon aspiration with impaction of the larynx, causing suffocation (patient must be intubated to avoid suffocation)
    - Esophageal rupture
    - Esophageal ischemia, leading to necrosis and perforation

41. **What are the key complications of endoscopic sclerotherapy? How common are they?**
    - Chest pain and acute dysphagia
    - Esophageal ulcers and bleeding (sloughing)
    - Esophageal strictures and chronic dysphagia

    The major complications of endoscopic sclerotherapy occur in 20–40% of patients.

42. **What percentage of patients who receive endoscopic treatment eventually require TIPS rescue?**
    12–30% of patients eventually require TIPS rescue.

43. Explain the pathogenesis of ascites.
- Increased sinusoidal and postsinusoidal resistance causes rediversion of splanchnic circulation and transudation of fluids.
- Decreased intravascular volume causes the kidney to respond with sodium and water retention.
- Production of naturitic factors by the liver is reduced (hepatocellular failure).
- Hypoalbuminemia (hepatic failure)

44. What is the most definitive treatment for portal hypertension and liver cirrhosis?
Liver transplant, which had a 1-year survival of 80% and a 5-year survival rate of 60% in the mid 1990s.

45. What is the most common cause of liver transplant in children?
Biliary atresia. Portal venous thrombosis is the most common cause of portal hypertension in children. However, it is not the number-one cause for liver transplant in children.

46. Name the more common surgical portosystemic shunts.
- End-to-side portacaval shunt (Eck fistula)
- Side-to-side portacaval shunt
- Portacaval interposition H shunt
- Mesocaval shunt end to side or interposition graft
- Warren-Salem distal splenorenal shunt plus splenectomy

47. What is the most successful surgical portosystemic shunt?
It depends on what the surgeon is comfortable with. However, in terms of encephalopathy and postoperative quality of life as well as long-term patency (which is usually the trade-off for reduced encephalopathy in selective shunts), the best shunt is the Warren-Salem distal splenorenal shunt, which has a patency rate of more than 90%. It also preserves the hilum for a potential liver transplant.

48. What is the transjugular intrahepatic portosystemic shunt procedure?
TIPS is a percutaneously placed stent connection between a hepatic vein and a portal vein radical. Portal blood flow is directed through the shunt and into the hepatic vein and, in turn, into the right atrium. As a result, blood is diverted away from the liver and the portal circulation is decompressed.

49. List in order the steps involved in the TIPS procedure (Fig. 5).
1. Catheterization of the hepatic veins and hepatic venography.
2. If portal vein thrombosis has not been ruled out, carbon dioxide portography (Fig. 6) should be performed after wedging a 5-French catheter in the hepatic parenchyma.
3. Passage of a long, curved transjugular needle from the chosen hepatic vein through the liver parenchyma into the intrahepatic branch of the portal vein.
4. Direct measurement of the systemic and portal vein pressure through transjugular access.
5. Balloon dilation of the tract between the hepatic and portal vein.
6. Deployment of a metallic stent within the tract to maintain it against the recoil of the surrounding hepatic parenchyma.
7. Angiographic and hemodynamic assessment of the resultant pressure reduction.
8. Serial dilation of the stent until satisfactory pressure levels have been reached.
9. Variceal embolization, when indicated.

50. What is the preferred hepatic vein for creation of a TIPS? Why?
The right hepatic vein, because it is the largest of the hepatic veins and the most predictable anatomically. Its anatomic predictability includes its relationship with bile ducts and hepatic arteries, which are avoided during TIPS.

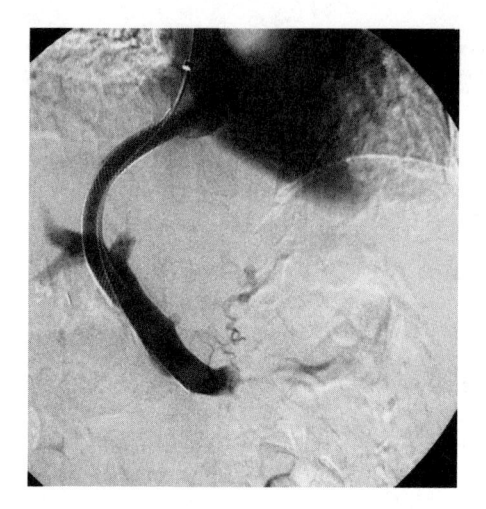

FIGURE 5. Final step of TIPS procedure demonstrating good flow through the shunt without any filling of portosystemic collaterals.

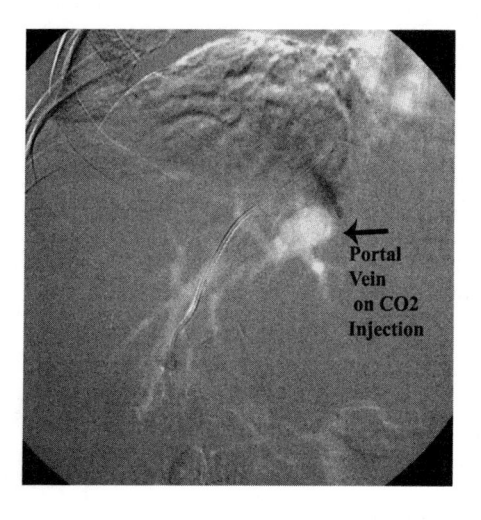

FIGURE 6. Wedge hepatic vein carbon dioxide injection demonstrating the location of the portal vein as a landmark for access guidance.

51. In which direction should you aim the needle to puncture the portal vein and form the right hepatic vein?

Nothing is foolproof: The best way is to start the puncture approximately 1 cm from the confluence of the right hepatic vein with the IVC and direct the needle anteroinferiorly toward or near the portal vein bifurcation, keeping away from the hepatic arteries and bile ducts, which are usually (52%) anterosuperior to the bifurcation. The average length of this tract is 2.7–5.4 cm. (This measurement applies to normal livers; it is shorter in cirrhotic livers.)

From the middle hepatic vein the puncture should be directed posteriorly.

52. What percentage of portal vein bifurcations are intrahepatic?
Approximately 60%.

53. List indications for coronary vein embolization at the end of the TIPS procedure?
- Active bleeding during the procedure
- Persistent visualization of the coronary vein after the TIPS shunt has been established with a portosystemic gradient less than or equal to 12 mmHg has also been included as an indication for embolization of the coronary vein.

54. What is the intraprocedural mortality rate for TIPS? The 30-day mortality rate?
The intraprocedural mortality for TIPS is 0–2%. The 30-day mortality after TIPS is 3–25% (averaging 15%). The 30-day mortality rate depends primarily on the severity of the liver disease (according to Childs-Pugh classification).

55. What are the intraoperative and perioperetive complication rates for TIPS?
The intraprocedural complication rate for TIPS is approximately 7% (3% major, 4% minor). The periprocedural complication rate for TIPS is 10–15%.

56. What is the principal factor determining morbidity and mortality after tips?
Hepatic reserve (Childs-Pugh classification). Childs-Pugh class C has a 30-day mortality rate of 92%.

57. What are the short-term complications of TIPS?
Intra-abdominal bleeding (0.5%), hemolysis, sepsis/fever (2.0%), right heart failure (transient pulmonary edema, 1%), transient renal insufficiency (2%), and stent malposition (1%).

58. What is the rate of encephalopathy after TIPS?
23–29%. Most cases respond to medical therapy. However, 3–5% of patients undergoing TIPS have encephalopathy that is refractory to medical treatment.

59. How can TIPS be considered a procedure that diverts portal blood flow away from the liver when the TIPS stent is actually inside the liver?
Despite the fact that the stent/TIPS shunt is physically inside the liver, it diverts the blood away from the hepatic sinusoids and thus functionally away from the liver.

60. Who created the first transhepatic portosystemic shunts in dogs? In humans?
Dogs: Rosch et al., 1969; **humans:** Colapinto et al., 1982.

61. What must you rule out before or during a TIPS procedure?
Portal vein thrombosis must be ruled out. Portal vein thrombosis was once a contraindication for TIPS shunt. However, mechanical and chemical thrombolysis of the portal vein before or during the TIPS procedure has been reported to be successful.

62. List the various ways of performing a portogram.
- Splenoportography: injecting contrast into the splenic pulp.
- Transhepatic portography: transhepatic injection in the portal radicals.
- Arterial portography: injecting contrast through the SMA or splenic artery.
- Wedge hepatic carbon dioxide portography: injecting approximately 50 ml of carbon dioxide after wedging a 5-French catheter in the hepatic parenchyma.
- CT portography: injecting contrast through the splenic artery while performing a CT scan.
- MR portography.

63. What are the advantages of TIPS over a surgically placed portosystemic shunt?
1. TIPS has the same advantages as any percutaneous procedure, including requiring sedation rather than anesthesia.
2. Morbidity and mortality rates in an emergent setting (e.g., refractory variceal bleeding) are lower with TIPS than with surgically placed portosystemic shunts.
3. In the era of liver transplants, the most important advantage of TIPS over surgical shunt is that the shunt is physically within the liver and is removed with the diseased liver (en bloc) without altering the transplant anastomosis. Surgically placed portosystemic shunts, on the other hand, must be surgically undone befroe the placing the transplant/allograft. This requirement prolongs the transplant surgery and increases morbidity and mortality rates.

64. List the indications for TIPS.
Main indications
- Prophylaxis for recurrent GI bleeding
- Refractory/active variceal bleeding
- Refractory ascites
- Refractory hydrothorax

Less common indications include budd-Chiari syndrome, lower GI or stomal varices, and malignant compression of the hepatic vein or portal veins.

65. Define refractory ascites.
Ascites that is unresponsive to 400 mg of spironolactone (or 30 mg of amiloride) and up to 120 mg of furosemide (Lasix).

66. List the causes of persistent ascites.
- Noncompliance with sodium restriction (a major cause that is often overlooked)
- Spontaneous bacterial peritonitis (SBP)
- Hepatocellular carcinoma (malignant ascites)
- Intrinsic renal pathology

67. Outline the first-line management of ascites.
1. Sodium and water restriction with an aim to decrease the patient's weight by 0.5 kg per day. (If weight loss is more the 0.5 kg per day, there is an increased risk for spiraling renal function.)
2. Potassium-sparing diuretics (spironolactone or the less potent amiloride and triamterene).

68. Why are potassium-sparing diuretics used as the first-line diuretics instead of furosemide?
Hypokalemia and hypokalemic alkalosis are more likely to occur with furosemide and may precipitate encephalopathy or even hepatorenal syndrome.

69. Define spontaneous bacterial peritonitis (SBP) and discuss its prognosis.
SPB is peritonitis (with polymorphonuclear neutrophil [PMN] counts of more than $250/\mu l$) in the absence of a recognizable cause. It is not an uncommon entity and has frequent recurrences. Prophylactic antibiotics (nonabsorbable intestinal antibiotics) reduce recurrence but do not change the prognosis or mortality rate.

70. How do you differentiate between spontaneous bacterial peritonitis and secondary bacterial peritonitis?

	SECONDARY BP	SPONTANEOUS BP
Organism	Multiple	Single (usually *Escherichia coli*)
Protein and ascites	More than 1 gram per deciliter	Less than 1 gm/dl
PMN count response to treatment	Continues to rise despite treatment	Folds exponentially in response to treatment
Culture and sensitivity	Remain positive	Rapidly become sterile

71. Define hepatorenal syndrome. Describe its causes and pathogenesis.
Hepatorenal syndrome is advanced renal failure in patients with severe hepatocellular failure. It usually develops in inpatients; patients are rarely admitted with this diagnosis. The renal histopathology is normal, and if a new liver is transplanted, the kidney resumes normal function.

The exact pathogenesis of this phenomenon is not clearly understood. It is probably due to an imbalance between systemic basal dilators and intrinsic renal circulation control mechanism (i.e., renal intrinsic vasoconstrictors). It is precipitated by diuretic treatment, diarrhea, and/or GI bleeding.

72. Describe the management of hepatorenal syndrome.
Treatment of hepatorenal syndrome is difficult. Other causes of renal failure must be ruled out. The best management is prevention:

- Avoid diuretic overdose.
- Treat ascites slowly.
- Early diagnosis of complications (infection, electrolyte imblance and/or hemorrhage).
- Dialysis does not improve survival.

73. What is the technical and hemodynamic success rate of TIPS?
95%.

74. What is the rate of deterioration of liver function after a TIPS procedure?
10–20% of patients undergoing TIPS experience transient deterioration of liver function. Only 3–8% experience progressive deterioration of liver function.

75. What are the interventional procedural solutions to postoperative TIPS patients with refractory liver failure and/or encephalopathy?
- Permanent embolization with, for example, coils.
- Thrombosis with a balloon occlusion over 12 hours.
- Hourglass balloon stent deployment within the TIPS shunt (artificial stenosis) (Fig. 7).

76. What is the initial success rate of controlling variceal bleeding with TIPS?
91–97% (100% initial success has been reported by Coldwell et al.)

77. What is the 1-year rebleeding rate after TIPS procedure?
17–26%.

78. What finding is almost always associated with rebleeding after a TIPS procedure?
TIPS shunt malfunction—stenosis (Fig. 8) or thrombosis of the TIPS shunt.

79. What are the primary and secondary patency rates of TIPS procedures at 1 year?
- Primary 1-year patency rate: 20–69%.
- Secondary 1-year patency rate: 94–96%.

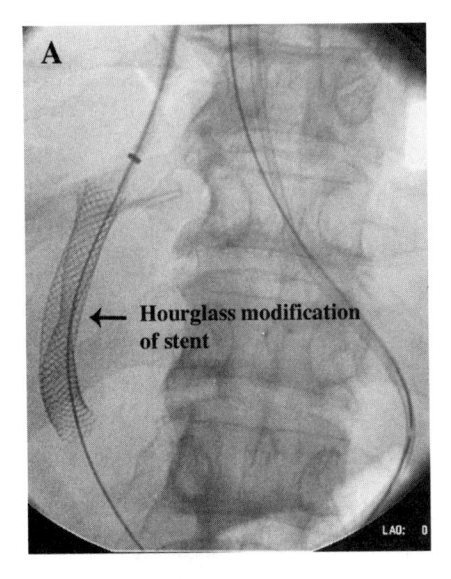

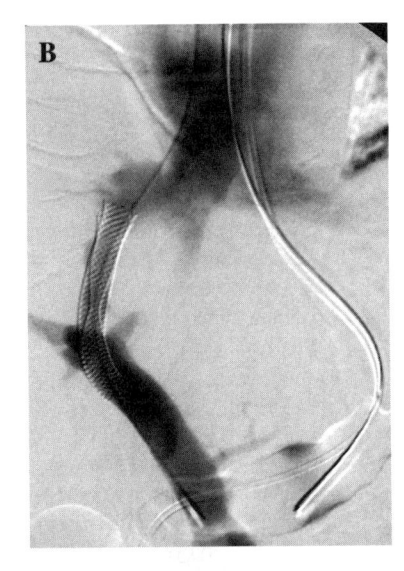

FIGURE 7. Custom-made hourglass stent deployed to reduce portosystemic shunt flow (**A** and **B**).

80. What is the traditional stent used for TIPS procedure?
The Wallstent, a self-expanding stent that has the flexibility to take the C shape of the shunt between the hepatic vein and the portal radical.

81. Explain the theorized pathogenesis of TIPS restenosis.
During the creation of the intrahepatic parenchymal tract, injury of the biliary radicals occurs; thus a bile leak develops in the venous TIPS conduits (biliary venous fistula). The bile causes pseudointimal hyperplasia, which accumulates and causes stenosis.

Increased flow in the hepatic vein outflow of TIPS causes a responsive neointimal hyperplasia (NIH) with subsequent hepatic venous end stenosis.

82. List the causes of TIPS occlusion (thrombosis).
Thrombogenic effect of bile leaks to TIPS fistules (early thrombosis), thrombosis secondary to TIPS stenosis (late thrombosis), stent malposition (early or late thrombosis), propagation of thrombus from portal vein and/or its tributaries (SMV, IMV, splenic vein).

83. What new stents may reduce TIPS restenosis or thrombosis and thus improve patency?
Polytetrafluoroethylene (PTFE) covered stents are theorized to reduce, if not prevent, the bile leak into the venous conduits and thus reduce pseudointimal hyperplasia. PTFE stent grafts improve the primary patency of TIPS by 20–30%.

84. What problems may be posed by the new stent-grafts used to create or revise TIPS?
Obstruction of one of the hepatic veins (partial Budd-Chiari syndrome), which is clinically inconsequential in the long run, and increased incidence of post-TIPS encephalopathy (the jury is still out on this one).

85. How can the patency of TIPS be improved?
By extending the TIPS shunt (with bare stents and/or covered stents) to the hepatic vein to the IVC junction.

86. How do patients with Budd-Chiari syndrome fare after a TIPS procedure?
Patients with Budd-Chiari syndrome (BCS) who undergo TIPS have a higher mortality rate than patients with TIPS performed for other etiologies. However, the prognosis of liver transplants for the treatment of BSC is not as good as for other indications. There are repeated interventions for maintenance of TIPS function in patients with this syndrome.

87. What are the contraindications for TIPS procedure?
Polycystic liver disease, severe hepatic insufficiency, right heart failure, and cavernous portal venous occlusion. **Relative contraindications** include active infection/septicemia and hypervascular hepatic tumors.

88. Why are polycystic liver disease and hypervascular hepatic tumors contraindications for TIPS procedures?
Patients with these conditions are considered to have a high risk of intraperitoneal bleeding. TIPS procedures in cirrhotic patients are tamponaded by near-solid hepatic parenchyma, thus reducing perioperative bleeding. The presence of multiple cysts is theorized to reduce hepatic tamponade and increase the risk for intracystic hemorrhage that may be life-threatening. The theory that polycystic liver disease is a contraindication for TIPS has been challenged in recent years.

89. How is a TIPS shunt followed up?

Patients undergoing TIPS are followed clinically with regard to resolution or recurrence of the clinical indications that instigated the TIPS procedure (e.g., ascites or variceal bleeding).

TIPS shunts are followed with Doppler ultrasound. Doppler ultrasound is usually done within 1 week after TIPS (usually immediately within 24 hours), then at 3 months, and then either at 3-month intervals or as indicated clinically.

90. What are the normal/expected findings by Doppler ultrasound found in TIPS patients?
- High velocity turbulence blood flow throughout the TIPS shunts with a mean peak systolic velocity of 135–200 cm per second
- Hepatofugal flow in the visualized intrahepatic portal radicals
- Increased blood flow in the intrahepatic arteries with increased peak systolic velocity

91. What Doppler findings suggest shunt malfunction and warrant further evaluation of the TIPS shunt?
- No flow in the TIPS shunt
- Low velocity, especially at the portal venous ends of the shunt (less than 60 cm/sec)
- Increase or decrease by 50 cm/sec in the velocity from baseline
- Hepatopetal flow in the portal veins
- Hepatopetal flow in the hepatic veins
- Reappearance of ascites/persistence of ascites by ultrasound

92. Define DIPS. How is the procedure performed?

Direct intrahepatic portosystemic shunt (DIPS) is an intravascular ultrasound (IVUS)-guided puncture of the portal vein directly from the IVC. An IVUS probe is introduced into the IVC from the femoral vein to visualize the portal vein radical. A modified TIPS needle is then advanced down the right internal jugular vein, and the portal radical is punctured through the hepatic parenchyma from the IVC under IVUS visualization.

93. What segments of the liver is punctured in a DIPS procedure?

Segment I, the caudate lobe.

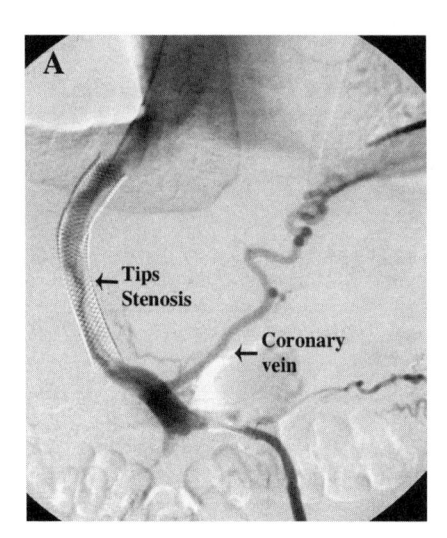

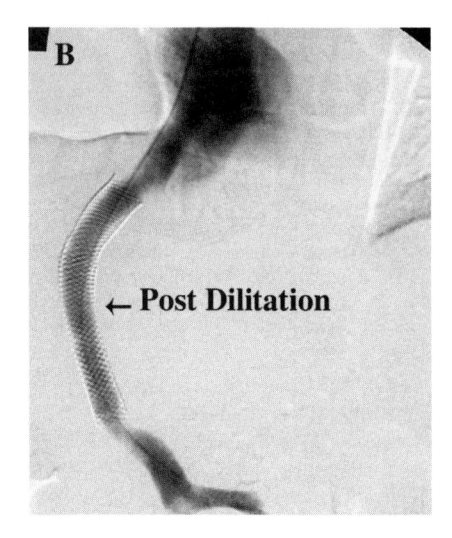

FIGURE 8. Stenosis within the shunt (**A**) with decreased flow and evidence of flow in collaterals. After dilatation (**B**), good flow within the shunt and absence of collaterals indicate decrease in portal pressure.

94. What kind of stent is used in DIPS procedure? What is the diameter of the stent?
It is usually an 8-mm PTFE stent.

95. What are the proposed advantages of DIPS?
Because of visualization of the portal radical and access under image guidance, there is a probable reduction in the number of "sticks" or attempts at accessing the portal radical. This may reduce bleeding as well as the time of the shunt procedure compared with traditional TIPS.

96. What are the technical differences between establishing TIPS shunt in liver transplant recipients and patients with native livers?
The interventionist must be aware of the surgical anatomic variants in the transplant recipient, particularly the venocaval anastomosis, so that a TIPS stent can be placed expeditiously.

97. What are the differences in the follow-up of TIPS in liver transplant recipients and nontransplant patients?
The follow-up should be the same (clinical and Doppler evaluation follow-ups). However, in transplant recipients neurotoxic serum drug levels (cyclosporine and tacrolimus) should be followed after TIPS because they may rise due to the decreased first-path metabolism in the liver and thus may increase the incidence of encephalopathy.

98. What are the long-term results and effects of TIPS shunt in liver transplant recipients?
The long-term results are unknown in liver transplant recipients. However, it is theorized that TIPS shunt in liver transplants may have a higher patency rate due to the effect of cyclosporine on reducing NIH (as it has been proved to do so with coronary stents).

BIBLIOGRAPHY

1. Cejna M, Peck-Radasoljevic M, Schoder M, et al: Repeat interventions for maintenance of transjugular intrahepatic portosystemic shunt function in patients with Budd-Chiari syndrome. J Vasc Intervent Radiol 13:193–199, 2002.
2. Cejna M, Thurnher S, Schoder M, et al: Creation of transjugular portosystemic shunt with stent-grafts: Initial experience with PTFE covered NiTiNOL Endoprosthesis. Radiology 221:437–446, 2001.
3. Clark TW, Agarwal R, Haskal ZJ, Stavropoulos SW: The effect of initial shunt outflow position on patency of transjugular intrahepatic portosystemic shunts. JVIR 15:147–152, 2004.
4. Fanelli F, Marcelli G, Salvatori FM, et al: Prospective analysis of e-PTFE-covered stent grafts vs. conventional bare stents in TIPS: Evaluation of shunt efficacy. JVIR 14(2):S33, 2003.
5. Haskal ZJ, Pentecost MJ, Soulen ML, et al: SIR standards of practice: Quality improvement guidelines for transjugular intrahepatic portosystemic shunts. J Vasc Intervent Radiol 12:131–136, 2001.
6. Hausegger KA, Karnel F, Georgieva B, et al: Transjugular intrahepatic portosystemic shunt creation with the Viatorr expanded polytetrafluoroethylene-covered stent-graft. JVIR 15:239–248, 2004.
7. Menon KV, Kamath PS: Managing the complications of cirrhosis. Mayo Clin Proc 75:501–509, 2000.
8. Otal P, Samyra T, Bureau C, et al: Preliminary results of a new expanded polytetrafluoroethylene-covered stent-graft for TIPS procedures. AJR 178:141–147, 2002.
9. Petersen B: Intravascular ultrasound-guided direct intrahepatic portacaval shunt: Description of technique and technical refinements. J Vasc Intervent Radiol 14:21–32, 2003.
10. Shin ES, Darcy MD: Transjugular intrahepatic portosystemic shunt placement in the setting of polycystic liver disease: Questioning the contraindication. J Vasc Intervent Radiol 12:1099–1102, 2001.

29. VASCULAR INTERVENTION IN RENAL TRANSPLANTATION

Wael E. A. Saad, MBBCh

1. List the arterial complications of renal transplants.
- Transplant renal artery stenosis (TRAS)
- Pseudo-TRAS
- Renal artery dissection
- Renal artery thrombosis
- Renal artery pseudoaneurysms

2. Define pseudo-TRAS.
Pseudo-TRAS (also called proximal TRAS) is stenosis of the iliac inflow to the renal artery and occurs in 0.0–2.4% of renal transplants. It usually is attributed to pre-existing, underlying iliac atherosclerotic disease in the recipient.

3. What is the prevalence of TRAS?
- TRAS affects 1–16% of renal transplants and has been described in up to 23% of renal transplants.
- In most case series the prevalence of TRAS is under 8%.

The wide range is due to varying definitions of "significant TRAS" and the evolving and improving surgical techniques and preoperative work-ups over the years.

4. Which has a higher prevalence of TRAS—cadaveric or live donor renal transplants?
The answer is somewhat controversial. Some authors believe that there is no difference, but most authors believe that the prevalence of TRAS is far less in live donor transplants. They report the following ranges of TRAS:
- Live donor graft: 0.3–5.8%
- Cadaveric graft: 2.0–17.7%

5. How can a lower prevalence of TRAS in live donor allografts be explained?
It can be explained by immunologic factors (including rejection), which cause TRAS and are less prevalent in live donor grafts. In addition, live donor transplants are performed on an elective basis with plentiful anatomic work-ups and planning. Of greater importance, increased cold ischemia time, which does not exist in live donor transplants, adds increased risk of developing TRAS in cadaveric grafts.

6. List the predisposing factors of TRAS.
- Increased cold ischemia time (cadaveric transplants)
- Pulsatile perfusion systems (cadaveric transplants)
- Certain types of perfusion fluids (cadaveric transplants)
- Cyclosporine-related vascular damage
- Immunologic factors
- Rejection, which causes an inflammatory process that can eventually lead to TRAS
- Right renal graft, in which the increased length of the renal artery may cause kinks
- End-to-side vs. side-to-side anastomosis (controversial)
- Flawed surgical techniques
- Cytomegalovirus (CMV) infection

7. **Give the differential diagnosis of the angiographic findings of multiple segmental and subsegmental stenoses in the transplant kidney.**
   - Chronic rejection (Fig. 1)
   - CMV infection
   - Pre-existing disease in the donor graft (e.g., hypertension) (bad work-up)

8. **Can multiple segmental stenoses be treated?**
   If they are caused by CMV, antiviral medication can improve and, in some cases, resolve these stenoses.

9. **List the noninvasive radiologic modalities used for evaluating TRAS.**
   - Doppler ultrasound
   - Magnetic resonance angiography (MRA)
   - Radionuclide renal scan

10. **Why is Doppler ultrasound more effective in detecting arterial stenosis in renal than in hepatic transplants?**
    The arteries involved in renal transplants are larger and more superficial and therefore easier to detect and evaluate. In addition, the anatomy and the variations of surgical anastomoses are simpler in renal transplants.

11. **Discuss the manifestations and consequences of TRAS.**
    Patients exhibit hypertension and renal dysfunction. Patient and allograft survival rates are lower in patients with TRAS than in those without TRAS. In a report by Patel et al., approximately 65% of patients had both hypertension and renal dysfunction and 35% had either with equal prevalence.

12. **How do patients with TRAS present?**
    Within the first week after transplant, patients usually present with anuria and dialysis dependence. They are less likely to present with hypertension because they are not volume-overloaded since they are still on dialysis. Beyond the first week after transplant they usually present with hypertension.

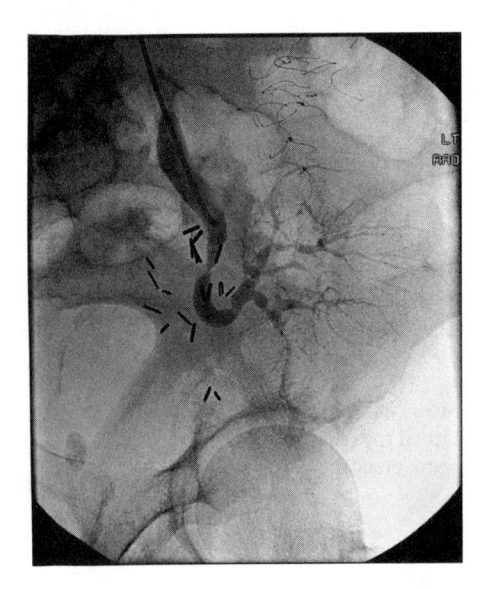

FIGURE 1. Selective renal artery angiogram of the left pelvic renal transplant demonstrates multiple areas of severe stenosis and dilatation, specifically at branch points consistent with chronic rejection.

13. **List the treatment options for patients with TRAS and proximal TRAS.**
    - Surgical revision of anastomotic stenoses
    - Surgical reconstruction using cadaveric iliac artery allografts or synthetic grafts
    - Percutaneous transluminal angioplasty (PTA)
    - Stenting

14. **Which is better—surgery or PTA?**
    The answer is not easy to ascertain from the literature. However, in the best outcome evaluation by Benoit et al., surgery had a better immediate success rate (92.1% vs. 69.0%) and the long-term success rate of surgery was twice that of PTA (81.5% vs. 40.8%).

15. **What is the first line of treatment for patients with TRAS?**
    PTA. Most authors, even Benoit, et al., advocate PTA as the first line of treatment because endoluminal therapy (Fig. 2) is less invasive and does not negate the surgical option if it fails. In addition, the surgical option, although having a better percentage of long-term successes, has devastating complications with a graft loss rate of up to 15% and a mortality rate as high as 5%. In addition, it adds further surgical stress on the patient and has an added risk of perioperative infection and ureteric injury.

16. **Summarize the technical success rate and the long-term clinical outcome of PTA.**
    - The technical success rate is 60–94% with a procedural complication rate of 0–8.3%. Graft loss has been rarely reported.
    - The restenosis rate is 10–12% and has been reported by one article to be above 12% (up to 20%).
    - Immediate control of hypertension is seen in 69–82% of patients; long-term control is seen in 41–67% of patients.
    - Patel et al. documented a mean reduction in the serum creatinine from 2.6 ± 0.5 to 1.7–0.3).
    - The overall graft survival after PTA is 95% at 1 year and 82% at 2 years.

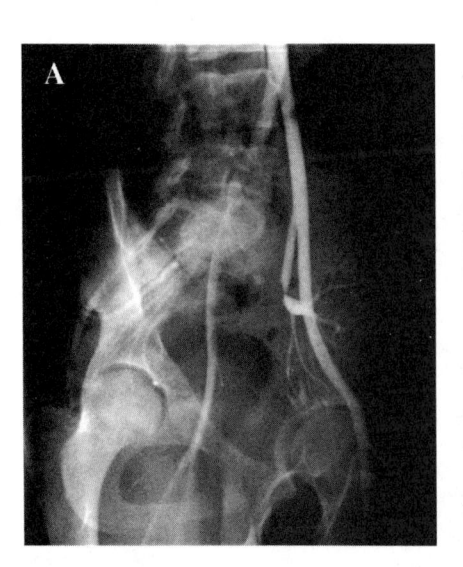

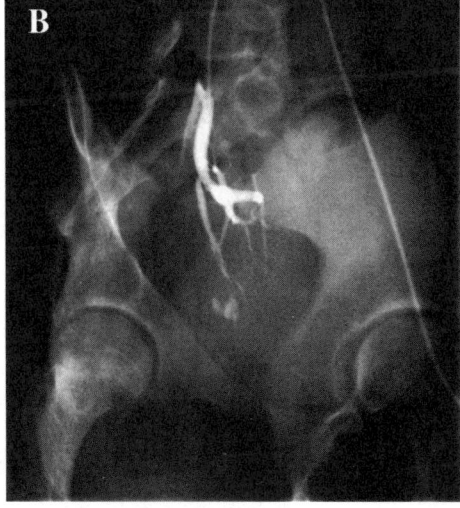

FIGURE 2. In a patient with increasing hypertension, an angiogram demonstrated narrowing of the main renal artery **(A)**, which was treated with angioplasty **(B)**.

17. What are the criteria for improved clinical outcome?

The criteria for improved clinical outcome are arbitrary and thus vary among authors. The clearest criteria were established by Patel et al.:
- 15% reduction in serum creatinine
- 15% reduction in diastolic blood pressure with no reduction in antihypertensive medication
- 10% reduction in diastolic blood pressuer with reduction in antihypertensive medication

18. What findings indicate a poor outcome after PTA?

Higher technical failures and complications have been seen with PTA in association with arterial kinks and end-to-end anastomoses with the internal iliac artery (rarely done now). In terms of clinical outcome, a slow decline in renal function before PTA usually is associated with a less impressive creatinine improvement after PTA compared with reduction in blood pressure.

19. When should renal artery stents be placed?

Some authors believe that stents should never be used because they complicate surgical salvage if anything goes wrong. Those who believe in stent placement recommend the following indications:
- Severe anastomotic stenoses
- Focal iliac disease (in proximal TRAS)
- Repeat restenoses after repeated PTA
- Technical failure of PTA due to elastic recoil or arterial dissection
- Postsurgical arterial dissection

20. What are the known complications of transplant renal artery stent placement?
- Stent occlusion/thrombosis
- Cholesterol/atheromatous emboli
- Restenosis

The reported restenosis rate for stents is 25% (2/8). This rate is probably inaccurate due to the small sample size.

21. Why does endoluminal vascular treatment in transplants (hepatic or renal) carry a high restenosis rate?

The restenosis rates of hepatic artery stents, renal artery PTA, and renal artery stenting are 31%, 10–12%, and 25%, respectively. Almost all restenoses occur within 9 months of the initial intervention. These rates are considered high and may be due to the fact that atherosclerotic disease may be affected in a negative way by immunologic processes or metabolic changes associated with transplantation.

22. How does renal artery dissection occur in renal transplantation?

Renal dissection can be iatrogenic (after PTA) or spontaneous, usually occurring within 1 week after renal transplant. Either type is treated with renal artery stenting. Renal artery dissection can lead to renal artery thrombosis (RAT) and even renal vein thrombosis (RVT).

BIBLIOGRAPHY

1. Benoit G, Moukarzel M, Hiesse C, et al: Transplant renal artery stenosis: Experience and comparative results between surgery and angioplasty. Transplant Int 3:137–140, 1990.
2. Halimi JM, Al-Najjar A, Buchler M, et al: Transplant renal artery stenosis: Potential role of ischemia/perfusion injury and long-term outcome following angioplasty. J Urol 161:28–32, 1999.
3. Patel NH, Jindal RM, Wilkin T, et al: Renal arterial stenosis in renal allografts: Retrospective study of predisposing factors and outcomes after percutaneous transluminal angioplasty. Radiology 219:663–667, 2001.
4. Sarkari BR, Geisinger M, Zelch M, et al: Post-transplant renal artery stenosis: Impact of therapy on long-term kidney function and blood pressure control. J Urol 155:1860–1864, 1996.
5. Voiculescu A, Hollerbeck M, Plum J, et al: Iliac artery stenosis proximal to a kidney transplant: Clinical findings, duplex-sonographic criteria, treatment, and outcome. Transplantation 76:332–339, 2003.

30. VASCULAR INTERVENTION IN LIVER AND PANCREAS TRANSPLANTATION

Wael E. A. Saad, MBBCh

1. Name the most common vascular (arterial or venous) complication in liver transplant recipients.

Hepatic artery thrombosis (HAT) occurs in 2–12% of adult transplant recipients (Fig. 1).

2. What age group is most vulnerable to HAT after liver transplant?

Children, especially under 1 year of age, who can have a HAT rate of up to 30%. However, children handle HAT better than adults do.

3. List the predisposing causes and risk factors that are associated with HAT in liver transplant recipients.
- Low donor-to-recipient age ratio
- Children (weight less than 10 kg)
- Poor surgical techniques
- Preservation injury to the graft artery
- Diminutive size of the donor or recipient artery
- Blood group incompatibility
- Coagulation abnormalities, including smoking
- Kinking (long arterial stump)
- Persistent pre-existing recipient inflow disease (e.g., celiac axis stenosis)
- Transplant rejection

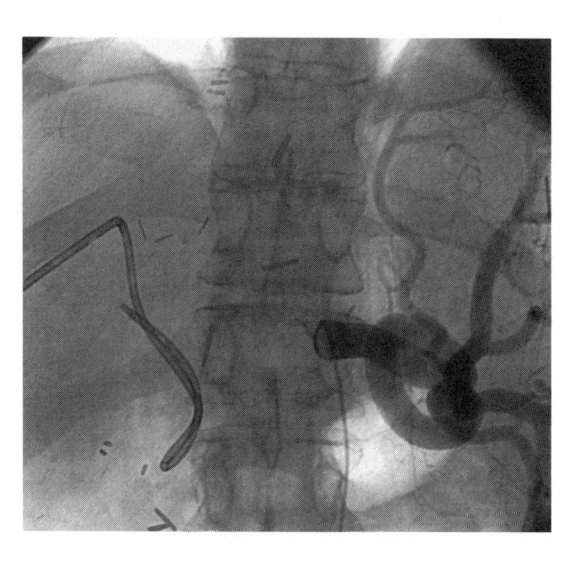

FIGURE 1. After transplant the patient's liver enzymes were noted to be increasingly abnormal. Ultrasound, the first-line modality to evaluate hepatic arterial flow, revealed no arterial flow. An angiogram confirmed the finding. Selected celiac axis injection shows no arterial flow in the hepatic artery. In transplanted livers, the bile ducts are dependent on hepatic artery flow. Occlusion of the hepatic artery may lead to ductal necrosis.

4. How does HAT present in liver transplant recipients? Give the mortality rate associated with each presentation.

HAT presents in three different ways with almost equal frequency:

1. Transient bacteremia that responds to antibiotics and is accompanied by abnormalities in liver function tests (LFTs): 29% mortality rate.
2. Biliary tract complications, which include stenoses, necroses, and delayed biliary leaks from the surgical anastomosis: 57% mortality rate.
3. Hepatic parenchymal infarction and necrosis, which can rapidly lead to septicemia and death: 75% mortality rate.

5. Name the most prevalent complication of HAT in liver transplant recipients.

Up to 80% of liver transplant recipients with HAT have abnormal cholangiograms. These biliary complications range from biliary strictures to necrosis of the bile ducts with biliary leaks or biloma formation (Fig. 2).

6. Why are biliary complications most prevalent after hepatic artery complications (including HAT)?

The intrahepatic biliary epithelium is totally reliant on the hepatic artery and does not receive adequate blood supply from the portal circulation.

7. Can HAT be asymptomatic?

Yes—in up to 20% of cases.

8. How can HAT be diagnosed radiographically?
- Doppler ultrasonography
- Helical computerized tomography
- Digital subtraction angiography (the gold standard for evaluating hepatic artery complications)

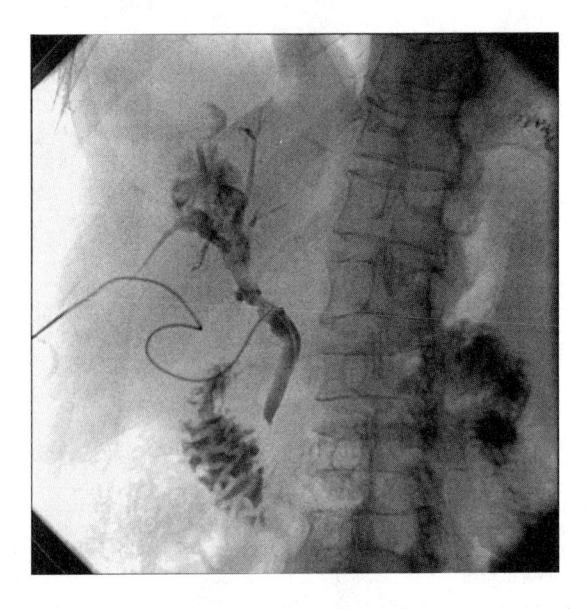

FIGURE 2. Multiple filling defects are seen within the biliary system. This characteristic finding of biliary necrosis commonly begins at the confluence of the bile ducts.

9. **What are the Doppler criteria for diagnosing HAT or hepatic artery stenosis (HAS)?**
   A parvus tardus waveform with a resistive index (RI) of less than 0.50 (parvus component) and a prolonged systolic acceleration time more than 0.08 seconds (tardus component).

10. **How is HAT traditionally treated?**
    Cases of acute, early thrombosis with extensive necrosis and cases of diffuse biliary structuring and multiple intrahepatic abscesses are treated with retransplantation, which still carries high morbidity and mortality rates.

11. **What are the alternative treatments for HAT?**
    Prompt thrombectomy and revision of the arterial anastomosis may salvage as many as 70% of livers without extensive necrosis. The literature related to endoluminal therapy (thrombolysis with or without angioplasty or stenting) is limited. Approximately six technically successful cases have been reported.

12. **What is the prevalence of HAS in liver transplant recipients?**
    HAS is the second most common hepatic artery complication in liver transplant recipients (after HAT). It occurs in 3–11% of transplants.

13. **Name the less common hepatic artery complications in liver transplant recipients.**
    - Hepatic artery rupture
    - Hepatic artery dissection
    - Hepatic artery pseudoaneurysm
    - Hepatic artery-to-portal vein fistulas

14. **What is the most common site of HAS?**
    HAS is most common at the anastomosis (46–77% of cases).

15. **List the more common causes of HAS in liver transplant recipients.**
    - Surgical/technical faults
    - Angulated anastomoses due to size discrepancy between donor and recipient arteries
    - Clamp injury
    - Preservation injury/ischemic injury to the intrahepatic (graft) artery
    - External compression
    - Pre-existing stenoses in the recipient (celiac trunk stenoses)

16. **What is the significance of HAS in liver transplants?**
    Up to 60% of liver transplants with HAS have biliary complications (strictures and/or necrosis), ultimately leading to allograft dysfunction. In addition, it has been postulated that HAS may lead to HAT with its graver consequences.

17. **Name the treatment alternatives for HAS.**
    - Anticoagulation therapy
    - Surgical revision (excision and reanastomosis)
    - Endoluminal therapy by angioplasty or stenting

18. **What is the HAT rate after treatment of HAS with surgery or hepatic artery stenting?**
    - 26% for surgery
    - 8% for stenting (treated after stenting with anticoagulation and antiplatelet agents)

19. **What is the technical success rate of hepatic artery angioplasty for HAS?**
    81% with a complication rate of 9.5% (Fig. 3).

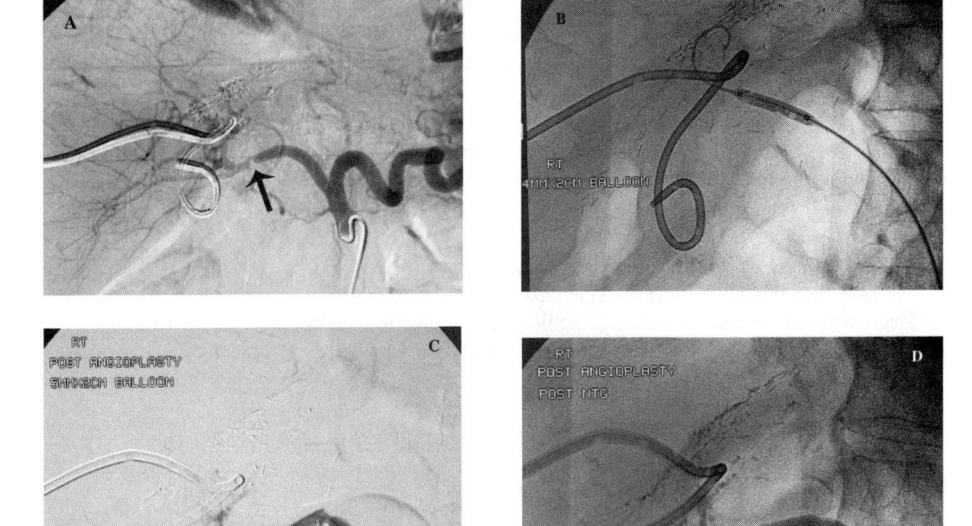

FIGURE 3. A, Selective celiac arteriogram shows a significant stenosis of the hepatic artery at an anastomosis in a patient with liver transplant *(arrow)*. **B,** Angioplasty of the stenosis was performed. **C,** The angiogram after angioplasty demonstrates intense spasm. **D,** Selective arteriogram obtained after injection of vasodilators shows resolution of the spasm and good results of angioplasty. Vascular complications are among the most serious problems encountered with liver transplantation, with hepatic artery stenosis accounting for 30%.

20. What are the primary patency and primary assisted patency rates of hepatic artery stenting at 1 year after stenting?

53% (± 14) and 60% (± 22), respectively. To date, no patency rates are available for hepatic artery angioplasty.

21. What are the restenosis rate and HAT rate of hepatic artery stenting?

31% and 8%, respectively.

22. Identify the indication for splenic artery embolization in liver transplant ischemia.

Splenic arterial steal, which in patients who present with hypersplenism, dilated splenic artery, and hepatic graft dysfunction. Angiographically, the majority of flow goes to the splenic artery and not to the hepatic artery.

23. List the causes of hepatic artery pseudoaneurysms in liver transplant recipients.
- Infection (mycotic pseudoaneurysm)
- Iatrogenic pseudoaneurysm from biopsies and/or biliary drainages

24. Name the treatment options for portal vein thrombosis after liver transplantation.
- Transcatheter thrombolysis (can be administered up to several days after transplantation)
- Transjugular intrahepatic portosystemic shunt (TIPS), which provides better access for

larger sheaths to the thrombosed portal vein and increased outflow after revascularization
- Treatment of the underlying cause of portal vein thrombosis, such as portal vein stenosis and/or hypercoagulable states

25. What are the complications of portal vein stenosis after orthotopic liver transplantation (OLT)?
Portal hypertension and portal vein thrombosis. Both present with variceal bleeding and/or ascites.

26. List the treatment options for portal vein stenosis after OLT.
- Surgical reconstruction of the transplant portal vein (usually difficult due to abundant scar tissue)
- Endoluminal angioplasty with or without stenting through a percutaneous or transjugular approach

27. Summarize the response to portal vein angioplasty in liver transplant recipients.
- One-third of stenoses recoil and require stenting.
- One-third of stenoses restenose (usually within 6 months) after an initially successful angioplasty and require reangioplasty or stenting.
- One-third of stenoses respond well to angioplasty without restenoses.

28. Summarize the response to endoluminal treatment of hepatic vein stenosis in hepatic transplant recipients.
- 100% technical success rate
- 73% clinical success at 1 year

Some authorities believe that recurrence of stenosis (after angioplasty or stenting) is the rule rather than the exception.

29. What kind of hepatic transplant carries a higher risk for hepatic vein stenosis?
Hepatic vein stenosis is more common in segmental transplants.

30. Discuss the causes of stenosis of the inferior vena cava (IFC) after liver transplantation.
Early stenoses (44%) are usually due to technical factors such as kinking or torsion of the graft, a tight suture line, or compression from an over sized transplant.
Late stenoses (56%) are usually due to fibrosis or intimal hyperplasia (Fig. 4).

31. What is the preferred endoluminal treatment for IVC stenoses after liver transplantation?
Early stenoses usually need stenting, whereas late stenoses usually respond well to angioplasty alone.

32. Which stent is preferred for treatment of IVC stenoses in transplant recipients? Why?
Z-stents are preferred over Wallstents for the following reasons:
- They are less likely to slip than Wallstents
- They ave a greater radial force
- They have larger interstices protecting against hepatic vein orificial occlusion in the event of intimal hyperplasia

33. List the advantages of pancreatic islet cell transplants over whole-gland pancreatic transplants.
1. Minimally invasive procedure
2. Unique option for tolerance induction because islet cells can be pretreated in culture before transplantation.

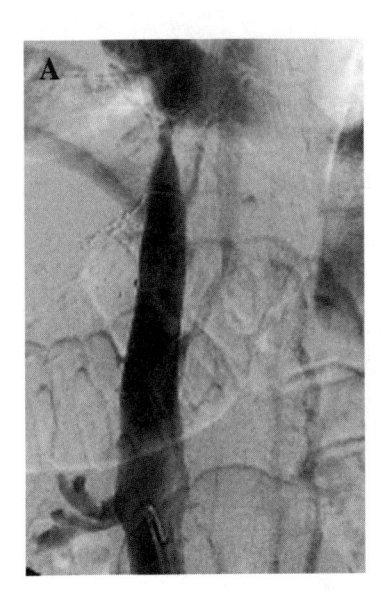

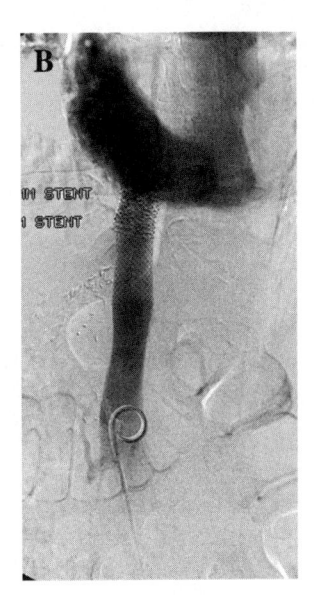

FIGURE 4. A patient presented with recurrent ascites after liver transplantation (**A**). A cavagram showed narrowing of the intrahepatic inferior vena cava. Mulitple balloon dilatations did not improve the pressure gradient across the stenosis. The pressure gradient was only 4 mmHg across this lesion. Stenting of the lesion (**B**) greatly improved the ascites.

  3. Donor tissue availability can become unlimited through the use of xenogeneic islets (in vitro islet expansion)
  4. Potential to circumvent the need for chronic immunosuppressive therapy
  5. Points 1 and 4 potentially reduce the costs for endocrine replacement therapy.

34. Briefly outline the history of pancreatic islet cell transplantation (PIT).
  1972: First successful PIT in animals.
  1974: First PIT in humans.
  1999: Summary of international islet registry data indicates that PIT was performed on 305 patients from 1974 to 1998; 267 procedures were performed between 1990 and 1998. The 1-year rate of insulin independence in the 1990s was 8.2%.
  2000: Canadian investigators establishing the novel immunosuppression regimen (Edmonton Protocol) report 7 consecutive successful cases with insulin independence at a mean follow-up of 1 year.
  2000–2003: Success of Edmonton group continues for 10 additional cases and is reproduced by other institutions.

35. How many PIT sessions are required to achieve insulin independence?
  Before 1999 (according to PIT Registry Report) insulin independence was achieved by one session, two to three sessions, and more than three session in 49%, 30%, and 21% of patients, respectively. The Edmonton group results were achieved with at least 2–3 sessions from islet cells acquired from 2–4 donors per successful PIT.

36. Name the most common site of PIT embolization/deposition.
  The portal vein, which is accessed by a transhepatic approach. However, successful PIT also has been described in islet cell deposition in the spleen, epiploic fat, and peritoneal cavity.

37. What is the main predictor of insulin independence?

The main predictor is the number of islet cells transplanted. Seventy-four percent of patients who received > 300,000 islets were insulin-independent for more than 2 years.

38. Briefly give an example of the islet cell suspension that is infused into diabetic recipients.

Edmonton suspension: 4000 islet equivalents/kg body weight of the recipient in a packed-tissue volume of less than 10 ml are suspended in 120 ml of medium-199 that contains 500 U of heparin and 20% human albumin.

39. Discuss the technical protocols for PIT in the portal vein.

The portal vein is accessed in a transhepatic approach (it has been described in a transjugular approach) by ultrasound and/or fluoroscopic guidance. Usually 1–6 attempts are made until successful access is achieved. Once access is confirmed a Seldinger technique is used to place a 5-French Kumpe catheter (or a 6-French sheath) in the main portal vein. Portal vein pressure is measured at baseline and after the islet infusion is completed. Some authors select either the right or left portal vein for infusion. The pancreatic islet cell suspension is infused over 5 minutes. Some authors infuse 17 U/kg of heparin in the portal vein before withdrawal of the catheter. The transhepatic/parenchymal tract is sometimes embolized with gelfoam, especially if heparin is used.

40. List the known complications associated with PIT along with their incidence.

- Bleeding requiring blood transfusion (0–9%)
- Subcapsular hematomas or peritoneal bleeding not requiring transfusion (0–2%)
- Injury to gallbladder (0–10%)
- Injury to right kidney (0–2%)
- Segmental portal vein thrombosis (0–4%)
- Bacteremia due to contaminated islet cell suspension (rare)

41. What is expected in the early posttransplant period?

Most patients stay in the hospital for 0.5–5 days (median = 2 days). Abdominal pain and nausea with vomiting are seen in 71% and 59% of patients, respectively, and correlate with the volume of islet cells transplanted. Transient, asymptomatic transaminitis peaking within 5–8 days from the PIT is seen in almost all patients.

42. What happens to the portal venous pressure after sequential clinical islet transplantation?

Posttransplant portal vein pressures rise significantly with sequential transplantation. In one study the portal vein pressure rose from a mean of 12.4 mmHg to a mean of 17.3 mmHg. Portal pressure changes correlate significantly with islet cell volume.

43. What is the portal vein pressure cut-off at which PIT is aborted?

Some authors will not transplant if the portal pressure is above 20 mmHg.

BIBLIOGRAPHY

1. Abbasoglu O, Levy MF, Vodapally MS, et al: Hepatic artery stenosis after liver transplantation: Incidence, presentation, treatment, and long term outcome. Transplantation 63:250–255, 1997.
2. Brantcatelli G, Katyal S, Federle MP, Fontes P: Three-dimensional multislice helical computed tomography with the volume rendering technique in the detection of vascular complications after liver transplantation. Transplantation 73:237–242, 2002.
3. Casey JJ, Lakey JRT, Ryan EA, et al: Portal venous pressure changes after sequential clinical islet transplantation. Transplantation 74:913–915, 2002.
4. Cotroneo AR, DiStasi C, Cina A, et al: Stent placement in four patients with hepatic artery stenosis or thrombosis after liver transplantation. J Vasc Intervent Radiol 13:619–623, 2002.

5. Denys AL, Qanadli SD, Durand F, et al: Feasibility and effectiveness of using coronary stents in the treatment of hepatic artery stenoses after orthotopic liver transplantation: preliminary report. Am J Roentgenol 178:1175–1179, 2002.
6. Goss JA, Sultes G, Goodpastor SE, et al: Pancreatic islet transplantation: The radiographic approach. Transplantation 76:199–203, 2003.
7. Haskal ZJ, Naji A: Treatment of portal vein thrombosis after liver transplantation with percutaneous thrombolysis and stent placement. J Vasc Intervent Radiol 4:789–792, 1993.
8. Hering BJ, Ricordi C: Results, research priorities, and reasons for optimism: Islet transplantation for patients with type I diabetes. Graft 2:12–27, 1999.
9. Ko GY, Surg KB, Yoon HK, et al: Endovascular treatment of hepatic venous outflow obstruction after living-donor liver transplantation. J Vasc Intervent Radiol 13:591–599, 2002.
10. Markmann JF, Deng S, Huang X, et al: Insulin independence following isolated islet transplantation and single islet infusions. Ann Surg 237:P741-P750, 2003.
11. McNulty JG, Hickey N, Khosa F, et al: Surgical and radiological significance of variants of Buhler's anastomotic artery: A report of three cases. Surg Radiol Anat 23:277–280, 2001.
12. Orons PD, Zajko AB: Angiography and interventional procedures in liver transplantation. Radiol Clin North Am 33:541–548, 1995.
13. Orons PD, Zajko AB, Bron KM, et al: Hepatic artery angioplasty after liver transplantation: Experience in 21 allografts. J Vasc Intervent Radiol 6:523–529, 1995.
14. Ozaki CF, Katz SM, Monsour HPJ, et al: Surgical complications of liver transplantation. Surg Clin North Am 74:1155–1167, 1994.
15. Settmacher U, Stange B, Haase R, et al: Arterial complications after liver transplantation. Transplant Int 13:372–378, 2000.
16. Shapiro AMJ, Lakey JRT, Ryan EA, et al: Islet transplantation in seven patients with type I diabetes mellitus using a gluco-corticoid-free immunosuppressive regimen. N Engl J Med 343:230–238, 2000.
17. Weeksw SM, Gerber DA, Jaques PF, et al: Primary Gianturco stent placement for inferior vena cava abnormalities following liver transplantation. J Vasc Intervent Radiol 11:177–187, 2000.

III. Nonvascular Intervention

31. TRACHEOESOPHAGEAL AND GASTROINTESTINAL INTERVENTION
Wael E. A. Saad, MBBCh

1. **What are the indications for percutaneous gastrostomy tubes (G-tubes)?**
   - Decompression of gastroenteric contents in gastric outlet and/or proximal small bowel obstruction (in 10% of cases) (Fig. 1).
   - Enteral feeding for nutritional support (in 90% of cases). Enteral feeding is less costly and more nutritious and has fewer long-term complications than parenteral nutrition.
   - As an access for percutaneous interventions at a more distant site; for example, balloon dilation and/or stenting of a distal small bowel stricture/anastomosis.
   - For palliation by partially diverting oral intake in cases of distal enteric fistulas.

2. **List the contraindications of G-tube placement.**
   Relative
   - Correctable coagulopathy
   - Overlying viscera (colon, hepatosplenomegaly)
   - Ascites
   - Prior gastric surgery
   - Ventriculoperitoneal shunt (especially if recent)
   - Gastric outlet obstruction (with the intent to feed via G-tube)

   Absolute
   - Uncorrectable coagulopathy
   - Portal hypertension with gastric varices

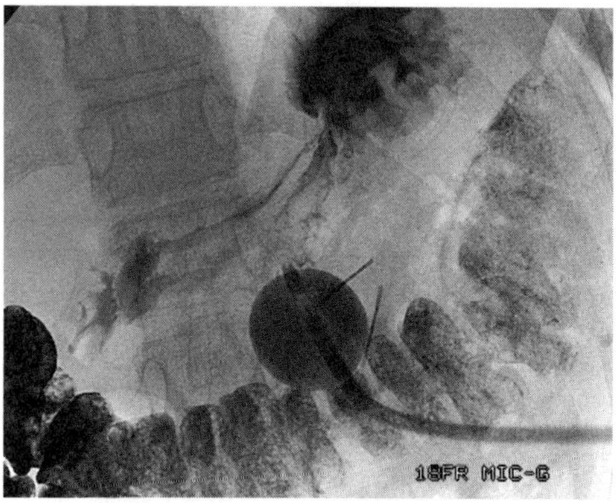

FIGURE 1. Contrast was given 12–24 hours before placement of a gastrostomy tube to outline the colon. In this case, two gastropexy sutures were placed. The use of this method is controversial. In our practice a Tractmaster dilatation system is used before the G-tube is inserted.

- Extensive abdominal burns
- Gastric carcinomatosis
- Total gastrectomy

3. Are gastropexy "T-fasteners" warranted?

The absolute need for gastropexy sutures is controversial. However, gastropexy is almost always needed in patients taking steroids or patients who have ascites.

4. Where is the ideal gastric site for percutaneous G-tube placement?

The puncture site should be between the mid-body of the stomach and the body-central junction. The puncture site should be midway from the greater and lesser curvatures, making the puncture distant from the left gastric artery and the right and left gastroepiploic arteries. (These arteries course along the greater and lesser curvatures). The site should be correlated with the abdominal wall puncture site, which should be at least 1 inch from the costal margin for added comfort of the patient.

5. How should the puncture (in the anterior abdominal wall tract) be angulated?

If the percutaneous G-tube is intended for enteral feeding, it is best directed toward the pylorus in case a jejunal extension is required. This is a major advantage over endoscopic G-tubes, which are usually placed in the direction of the fundus/gastroesophageal junction, as dictated by the endoscopic approach from the esophagus.

6. What are the prerequisites to placing a percutaneous G-tube?

In addition to the routine preinterventional work-up, such as ruling out or correcting coagulopathy and checking for contraindications, the patient should avoid oral ingestion (NPO) for 12–24 hours. Some authors prefer to give diluted barium 24 hours before the procedure so that the colon can easily be visualized and thus avoided. A nasogastric (NG) tube or 5-French catheter should be placed to insufflate air into the stomach. One milligram of glucagons is also given to augment the air insufflation of the stomach.

7. Discuss the advantages of insufflating the stomach.

Insufflating the stomach delineates its anatomy and enlarges the target for the percutaneous puncture, pushing the curvature arteries away from the puncture site. In addition, insufflating the stomach may displace bowel (especially the traverse colon) away from the puncture tract and pushes the anterior gastric wall (entry wall) closer to the anterior abdominal wall. Furthermore, enlarging the stomach can displace the distal half of the body of the stomach (target entry site) below the costal margin, thus making percutaneous G-tube placement more feasible.

8. When should a jejunal extension be considered? When should a gastrostomy portal be maintained?

A jejunal extension (Fig. 2) should be entertained in patients with significant gastroesophageal reflux and aspiration as well as patients with partial gastric outlet/duodenal obstruction. Maintaining a gastrostomy portal is necessary in patients with gastric outlet obstruction requiring decompression and in patients taking an oral medication that must be deposited in the stomach and not in the small bowel.

9. Discuss the post G-tube procedural considerations.

Patients are kept NPO and without tube feeds for 12–24 hours. The G-tube is left to drainage/gravity. Feeding can be started right away through the jejunostomy portal if the jejunostomy tube (J-tube) component is beyond the ligament of Treitz. On postoperative day 1, signs of peritonitis (gastric content spillage) should be ruled out, including fever, high white cell count, and rebound tenderness. In the absence of these signs, G-tube feeding can be started. Gastropexy sutures, if any, can be removed in 7–14 days postoperatively.

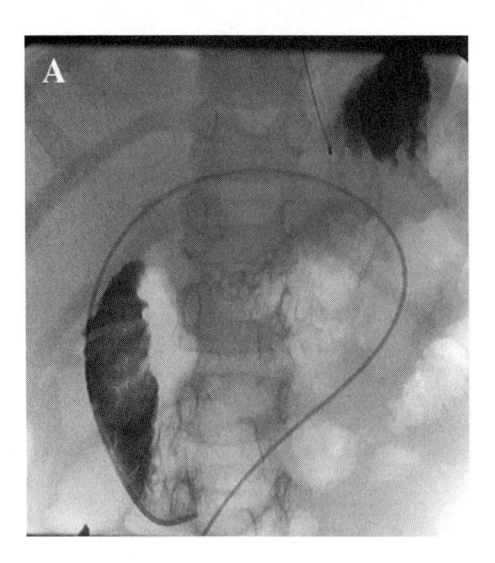

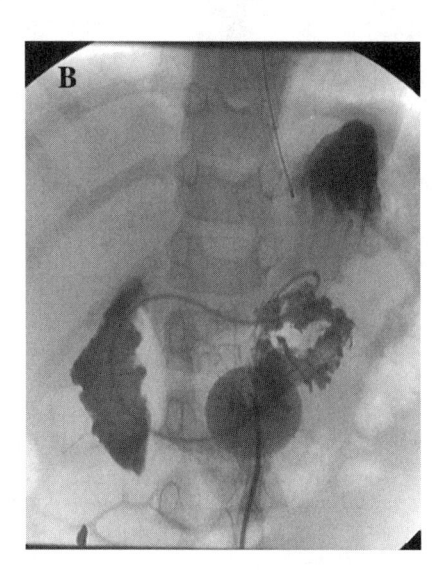

FIGURE 2. Gastrostomy-to-jejunal extension tubes are used when patients have difficulty with gastric reflux or dysmotility. Initially a catheter is manipulated through the stomach into the duodenum under fluoroscopic guidance (**A**). The gastrostomy-to-jejunal tube is then passed over a wire (**B**). The tube has two parts: one exits into the stomach, and the other empties into the jejunum.

10. Of all-comers, how many patients are considered not safely amenable to percutaneous G-tubes or G-J tubes?

Up to 7–8% of patients may be turned down due to overlying viscera, high stomach, and/or massive ascites.

11. Which are more convenient—nasogastric tubes or gastrostomy tubes?

G-tubes are more convenient. In a study by Hoffman et al. of patients with NG tubes or G-tubes placed for decompression after colon surgery, 4% of patients with G-tubes considered them to be the most irritable drainage tube that they had. This percentage was 43% in patients with NG tubes.

12. Briefly describe the two routes of radiologically placed G-tubes.

1. In the **direct percutaneous transabdominal route** the G-tube is placed through the anterior abdominal wall.

2. In the **peroral route (gastric pull-through)** the stomach is accessed from the transabdominal approach, but the tube itself is placed from the inside out by snaring it from the mouth.

13. List the type of retention devices used to anchor the G-tube and prevent dislodgement.
Gastric pull-through: silastic mushroom.
Direct percutaneous G-tube: Malecot anchor, balloon, locking pig-tail.

14. Give the technical success rates and complication rates of radiologically placed G-tubes.
- Technical success rate: 90–100%
- Minor complications: 3–10%
- Major complications: 0–5%
- Procedure-related mortality: 0–1%
- 30-day mortality (not related to procedure): 4–17%

The overall morbidity and mortality rates are approximately 10–20% and less than 2%, respectively. They compare favorably with surgical morbidity and mortality rates, which are 13–23% and 2–6%, respectively.

15. List the complications that may be encountered during G-tube placement.
1. Injury to surrounding organs and/or structures
   - Solid organs: liver and spleen
   - Hollow viscera: small and large bowel
   - Vessels: gastric and gastroepiploic arteries, splenic and hepatic vessels
2. Malposition of the G-tube
   - In the peritoneal cavity
   - Through the posterior wall of the stomach (in the lesser sac)
3. Peritonitis due to gastric content spillage
4. Aspiration
5. Vasovagal reaction and hypotension

16. List the postprocedural complications.
- Wound and stoma infection
- Stoma breakdown (necrosis)
- Tube clogging by inspissated feedings and/or crushed medications
- Dislodgement of the tube
- Tube migration into the pylorus/duodenum with or without gastric outlet obstruction or dumping syndrome
- Peri-tube leakage

17. A patient suffers from abdominal cramping and diarrhea every time bolus feeds are administered. What is the diagnosis? How should the patient be treated?
In this condition, sometimes called "dumping syndrome," the G-tube has migrated through the pylorus and the tube feeds are being "bolused" directly into the duodenum. This condition is treated by pulling back the G-tube so that its tip is back into the stomach.

18. Give the technical success rate and complication rates of pull-through G-tube placement.
- Technical success rate: 97–100%
- Minor complications: 3–12%
- Major complications: 0–5%

19. What type of retention devices has the lowest long-term complication rate?
Mushroom retention devices (placed by the peroral pull-through technique) have the lowest long-term complication rate. The long-term complication rates of balloon-retained catheters, pigtail-retained catheters, and mushroom-retained catheters are 67%, 36%, and 4%, respectively.

20. Name the type of G-tube (retention device) that is ideal for combative, noncooperative patients.
Peroral pull-through G-tubes with mushroom retention devices are the most secure tubes; inadvertent pulling is rarely reported. The dislodgement rates of balloon-retained tubes and pigtail-retained tubes are 60% and 11%, respectively.

21. Months after a peroral pull-through G-tube is placed in a patient with head and neck cancer, a CT exam demonstrates a soft tissue mass encasing the mushroom-retaining device. What diagnosis must be excluded?
Metastatic implantation of the head and neck cancer at the exit site of the G-tube. This complication is rarely reported but should be excluded by biopsy of the soft tissue mass.

22. List the indications for placement of a J-tube.
Major
- Gastric resection
- Gastric pull-up
- Complete gastric outlet obstruction

Minor
- High risk of aspiration
- Gastric dysmotility
- Partial gastric outlet obstruction

The minor indications are minor because they may be managed by a G-J tube.

23. How are direct jejunostomy tubes placed?
Direct jejunostomy tubes are placed in a similar manner to percutaneous G-tubes. However, the nasogastric tube is advanced to the duodenum (if possible), and air is insufflated directly into the distal duodenum/proximal jejunum. T-fasteners are invariably required. The added difficulty lies in the increased motility of the small bowel (reduced by glucagons) and the soft, pliable small bowel wall, which pushes back and is challenging to puncture. In addition, the small bowel loop is likely to "fall-back" leading to leakage and/or extraintestinal J-tube placement.

24. How successful are radiologically placed direct percutaneous jejunostomy tubes?
The initial case reports from small series place the technical success rate at 60–100%. The general experience is more likely to be closer to 60% than 100%

25. How are endotracheal stents introduced through the upper airway?
Stents are passed by placing them through an endotracheal tube with the patient in suspended respiration. They may also be passed through a tracheostomy site.

26. How is the airway visualized for adequate placement of a tracheobronchial stent?
The airway is usually visualized fluoroscopically without further visual aids. If airway stenoses are difficult to see, the tracheobronchial tree can be opacified by a lipid-based contrast such as Lipiodol (Laboratoire Guerbet, Aulnay-sous-Bois, France).

27. List the advantages of metal stents vs. traditional silicone stents.
- Thin delivery system: better tolerated and softer.
- Less bulky and greater expansile properties: create a larger airway.
- Small area of mucosa covered by stent: associated with superior respiratory-mucociliary clearance.

28. Discuss the types of stents used to treat tracheobronchial lesions.
Self-expanding metallic stents
- Gianturco-Z stents: balloon dilation is required only if lesions are highly resistant to stenting. Most lesions gradually resolve over days to weeks under the continuous radial force of these stents.
- Wallstents: usually require post-stent balloon dilation.

Balloon-expandable Palmaz stents: recently described in the treatment of tracheobronchial lesions.

Silicone stents: the traditional stents used in tracheobronchial tree lesions. They have a small internal-to-external diameter ratio with increased likelihood for occlusion by mucous secretion. Due to their large outer diameter, they can be deployed with difficulty, and their deployment may be traumatic. Another disadvantage is that they are more liable to migrate from their original position.

29. When can covered stents be used in tracheobronchial lesions?

In cases of malignant tracheobronchial obstruction. Early failure of noncovered stents (bare stents) in treating these lesions has been attributed to tumor protruding through the interstices of the stents. Covered stents avoid this problem.

30. When are "hinged" covered stents used?

In lesions at or near the carina requiring covered stents, the contralateral main bronchus must remain unobstructed by the stent; thus a "hinge" is located between two stent bodies (the proximal stent in the distal trachea and the distal stent in one of the main bronchi) along the lateral wall of the bronchus. This technique allows an opening in the covered-stent directed toward the contralateral bronchus. An additional stent can be deployed through this opening into the contralateral bronchus if needed.

31. Can balloon dilation of tracheobronchial lesions be used without stent placement?

Some authors believe that balloon dilation has good results in treating benign tracheobronchial strictures (including strictures caused by tuberculosis). It avoids the long-term complications of stents (e.g., stent fractures) in patients who have a prolonged life expectancy.

32. List the complications that may result from tracheobronchial stent placement.
- Strut fractures
- Tracheobronchial ruptures with or without fistula formation
- Stent blockage with secretions or granulation tissue (seen in up to 13% of cases)
- Hemoptysis
- Dislodgement from excessive coughing (seen in up to 20% of cases)

33. Summarize the results of tracheobronchial balloon dilation and/or stent placement.
- Clinical improvement after stent placement in 83–100% of cases
- Up to 41% of patients may require repeat procedures to maintain airway patency
- Up to 33% of patients may experience stent blockage and/or dislodgement
- Major intraprocedural complication rate: 1%
- 30-day mortality rate: up to 17%
- Balloon dilation for benign strictures have a clinical improvement rate of 73% at 6 months and 64% at 3–4 years

34. Discuss the causes of tracheobronchial stenoses after lung transplantation.

Airway stenoses may be due to inherent weakness in the airway walls (tracheobronchiomalacia). In addition, lung transplantation is performed without restoration of the bronchial arterial blood supply, leading to ischemia of the donor tracheobronchial tree with lethal dehiscence or fibrotic stenosis of the bronchial anastomoses. Bronchial stenoses lead to poor lung function, diminished mucociliary clearance, infection, and occlusion with subsequent obstructive lobe collapse.

35. Discuss the results of balloon dilation and/or stent placement in the tracheobronchial tree after lung transplantation.

Clinical improvement (improved respiratory function tests and reduced respiratory infection) is achieved in 92% of cases with a complication rate of 4%. The 6-month primary patency rates of tracheomalacia and anastomotic stenosis are 71% and 29%, respectively. The overall recurrence rate of stenoses is 17%, and the secondary patency rate at 1 year for both tracheomalacia and anastomotic stenoses is 100%.

36. List the indications for esophageal stenting or balloon dilation.

1. Malignant dysphagia to liquids (grade III or IV; grade II dysphagia may also benefit from stents) (Fig. 3)
    - Grade I: dysphagia to solids
    - Grade II: dysphagia to soft solids

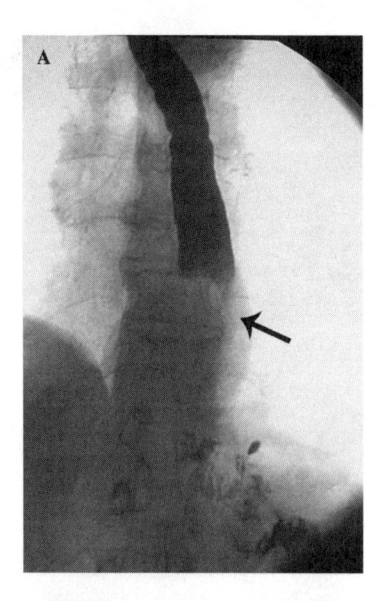

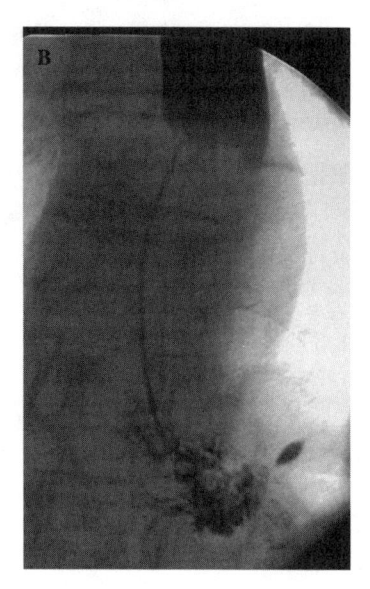

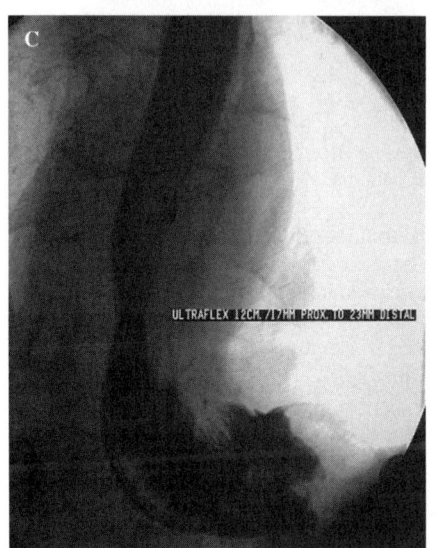

FIGURE 3. A postsurgical patient with a history of gastric cancer extending to the esophagus presented for stent placement because of recurrent disease. Endoscopy failed because of the inability to pass a wire through the lesion. Contrast is injected through a catheter, and the level of complete obstruction is identified in the distal esophagus (**A**). The obstruction was successfully traversed (**B**), and an Ultraflex stent was placed with good results (**C**).

- Grade III: dysphagia to solids and liquids
- Grade IV: dysphagia to saliva

2. Benign postoperative dyshagia (Fig. 4), gastroesophageal disease (GERD), post-radiation strictures causing dysphagia
3. Esophagorespiratory fistula

37. What is the prevalence of esophagorespiratory fistulas in esophageal cancer? How are they treated endoluminally?

Esophagorespiratory fistulas occur in 5–10% of patients with esophageal cancer. They can be treated with covered stents in the esophagus, the trachea, or both (parallel stents). Complete relief of symptoms and improvement of symptoms occur in 20–46% and 58–95% of patients, re-

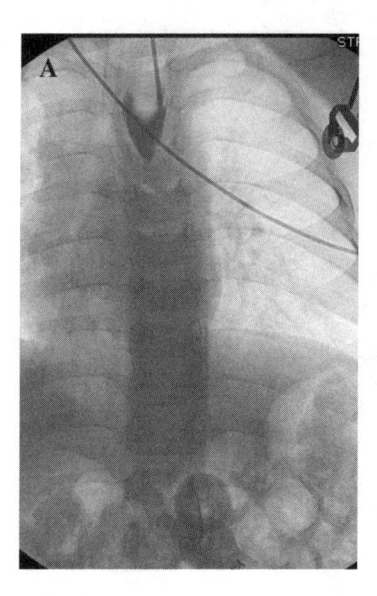

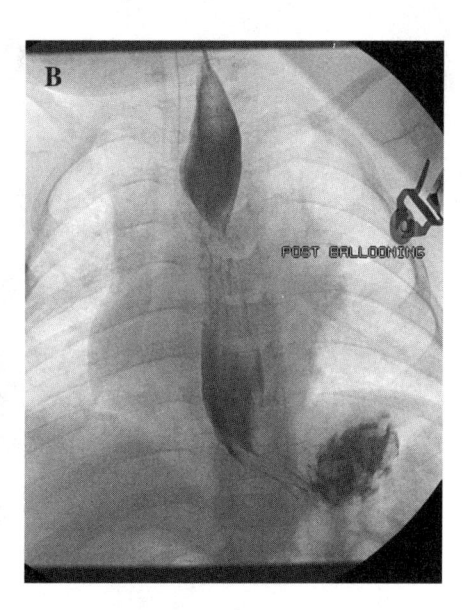

FIGURE 4. A patient born with esophageal atresia underwent surgery and developed a severe narrowing at the anastomosis (**A**). Management consisted of continual serial dilatation (**B**). He is now 2 years old and eating solid foods. We continue to see him every 2–3 months for repeat dilatations.

spectively. Fistulas may recur in 8–20% of patients. Dyspnea from airway compression secondary to esophageal stent placement occurs in up to 20% of patients.

38. Discuss the problems encountered in high (proximal) esophageal stenting.

High lesions must be approached with caution because patients may experience a foreign body sensation and/or upper airway compromise, which can be so severe as to require stent removal. Some authors believe that lesions 3 cm from the cricopharyngeus muscle should not be stented. Other authors have shown that cervical esophageal stenting is feasible, with only 18% of patients experiencing a foreign body sensation after stenting.

39. What problems may be encountered in stenting gastroesophageal lesions? How are they managed?

The problems encountered are stent migration (50%) into the stomach and unimpeded gastroesophageal reflux. Both of these problems are pretreated with placement of specially designed stents: conical covered stents to reduce migration or antireflux stents and proton pump inhibitors for post-stenting GERD. Antireflux stents have three polyurethane leaflets (configured like aortic valve cusps) that reduce GERD in 59% of cases and completely alleviate GERD in the remaining patients (41%).

40. Which is better for malignant esophageal lesions—covered or uncovered stents?

The short answer is covered stents. Uncovered stents are prone to tumor ingrowth (20–30%), which occurs in only 2% of patients treated with covered stents. Uncovered stents had fewer migration problems compared with first-generation covered stents, which had a migration incidence of 10–30%. New covered stents (such as the Ultraflex endoprosthesis and the conically shaped Flamingo Wallstent) have virtually eliminated the problem of distal migration.

41. How effective are esophageal stents compared with laser therapy?

The short answer is that covered stents are better for palliation than laser therapy. Reduction in dysphagia is seen in 83–100% of stented patients compared with 80% of laser-treated patients.

Complications, particularly esophageal perforation, are higher in laser therapy (5–9%) than in esophageal stents (0–5%). The main drawback of laser therapy is the requirement for multiple treatments (mean of 3.3 laser sessions per patient).

42. Describe the morphologic types of esophageal cancer in which esophageal stents are best avoided.
- Highly exophytic (fungating) tumors
- Cases with significant proximal esophageal dilation

43. What is the treatment regimen for esophageal perforation during stenting or laser therapy?
- H_2 blockers
- Antibiotics
- NPO status and total parenteral nutrition
- Mortality rate: $\geq 13\%$

44. Ideally, how is a stent positioned in cases of malignant esophageal narrowing?
The stent should extend $\geq$ 2 cm proximally and distal to the malignant lesion to avoid "shouldering" and malignant ingrowth.

45. How are benign esophageal strictures best treated?
Benign esophageal strictures are treated with balloon dilation. Results are successful in 86–90% of cases. Repeat dilation is required in approximately one-third of patients, with a median time to repeat dilation of 4–5 months. Stents should be reserved for lesions that are refractory to balloon dilation in patients who are poor surgical candidates. When stents are used, noncovered stents are preferred over covered stents due to decreased risk of migration.

46. How effective is fluoroscopically guided balloon dilation in the treatment of achalasia?
Balloon dilation under endoscopic guidance alone achieves only modest success because positioning is often inaccurate. Fluoroscopically guided balloon dilation is more effective, with immediate and a 1-year improvement rates in dysphagia of 98% and 78%, respectively. Only 5–6% of patients are refractory to fluoroscopically guided dilation and require surgical myotomy.

47. How are benign esophageal strictures (including achalasia) treated with balloon dilation?
The patients must be heavily sedated because esophageal dilation is very painful. Balloon dilation is performed with sequentially larger balloons increased at 5-mm increments and usually starting with a 15- to 20-mm balloon. The procedure is terminated if blood is seen on the balloon.

48. Describe the alternative approach to a patient who has a significant proximal esophageal stricture that cannot be "crossed" with a balloon from above (peroral route).
Such patients are not eating or drinking and need nutritional support. A percutaneous G-tube should be placed for enteral feeding and after 6 or more weeks (to allow time for the gastrostomy tract to mature) a retrograde attempt (up the gastroesophageal junction) at balloon dilation of the esophageal stricture can be attempted from the G-tube tract.

49. Discuss the management of esophageal stent migration.
If a stent migrates completely into the stomach and is asymptomatic, it can be left within the stomach. If the stent migration is symptomatic, the stent can be removed via a minor gastrostomy. Partial migration is treated with a proximal overlapping, noncovered stent in an attempt to anchor the migrated stent.

50. Discuss the delayed complications related to esophageal stent placement for malignant esophageal lesions.
Delayed complications can be devastating and may occur in up to 65% of patients with multiple and life-threatening complications (21% and 23% of patients, respectively). The delayed

stent-related mortality rate may be as high as 16%. These complications include hemorrhage (hemoptysis, 2%; hematemesis, 7%), fistula formation (5%), dyspnea (6%), migration (6%), and recurrent dysphagia due to tumor ingrowth (13%).

The prevalence of life-threatening complications decreases with stenting of distal lesions. The prevalence of life-threatening complications in proximal, mid, and distal lesions is 46%, 18%, and 0%, respectively.

51. Describe the "funnel phenomenon" seen after stent placement for malignant esophageal lesions.

The funnel phenomenon is defined as development of a space between the esophageal wall and the proximal part of the stent, caused by progressive dilation of the upper esophagus after stent placement and resulting in loss of apposition of the stent against the esophageal wall. The funnel phenomenon occurs in up to 8.5% of patients and may be the cause of esophagotracheal fistula recurrence. The etiology of this phenomenon is unknown, but possibilities include neural plexus injury from tumor invasion and/or stent compression.

52. Can stent design affect delayed complications of stents in the setting of malignant esophageal lesions?

The delayed complication rates for Ultra-Flex stents, Wallstents, and Z-stents are 44%, 68%, and 75%, respectively. Funnel-shaped stents, such as the Flamingo-Wallstent, may reduce the occurrence of the funnel phenomenon. Retrievable covered Nitinol stents can be retrieved successfully in cases of patient intolerance and/or delayed complications.

53. List the routes and approaches taken to place gastroduodenal stents.
- Peroral route: least invasive and most desired
- Percutaneous gastrostomy or even jejunostomy
- Through an enterocutaneous fistula
- Transhepatic (transbiliary) approach

54. What are the indications for gastroduodenal stent placement?
- Malignant antropyloric obstruction (including cases of linitis plastica)
- Malignant duodenal obstruction
- Malignant external compression on the duodenum by pancreatic cancer or malignant pancreaticoduodenal lymph nodes
- Recurrent malignancy leading to stenoses of surgical anastomoses

55. What kind of stents are used for malignant gastroduodenal obstruction?

Self-expanding, uncovered stents are used. Balloon-expandable stents are too rigid, and covered stents do not anchor well. Until recently radiologists used Wallstents or esophageal stents. However, Wallstents are usually insufficiently wide (maximum diameter = 16 mm), and esophageal stents are relatively inflexible. Recently the Schneider enteral stent (Boston Scientific/Medi-tech) has become available. It is self-expanding and both flexible and wide (18–22 mm in diameter). This stent is also now used for colonic stenting. The Song stent is a centrally covered stent with bare ends and is specifically designed for the gastroduodenal region.

56. Describe placement techniques for stenting malignant gastroduodenal lesions.

The stent(s) should be placed 1–2 cm beyond the malignant stenosis, both proximally and distally. If multiple stents are needed, they should be placed from distal to proximal with an overlap of 1–2 cm. Post-stent dilation is not necessary because most stents will self-expand over time.

57. Summarize the results of stenting malignant gastroduodenal lesions.
- Technical success rate: 75–100%
- Short-term clinical success rate: 67–100%

- Reobstruction rate: 12–25%
- 6-month patency rate of stents: 39%

In a meta-analysis by Mauro et al of 11 case series (total of 91 patients), the clinical success rate was 89%. Fifty percent of the clinical failures were attributed to synchronous small bowel lesions that were not detected at the time of stent placement. Therefore, it is imperative to rule out distal small bowel lesions/obstruction before embarking on gastroduodenal stent placement.

58. What are the indications for colonic stenting?
   1. Temporary colonic decompression in cases of acute colonic obstruction in cases of:
      - Left hemicolon cancer (main indication) (Fig. 5)
      - Crohn's disease
      - Diverticulitis
      - Ischemic strictures
      - Postsurgical strictures

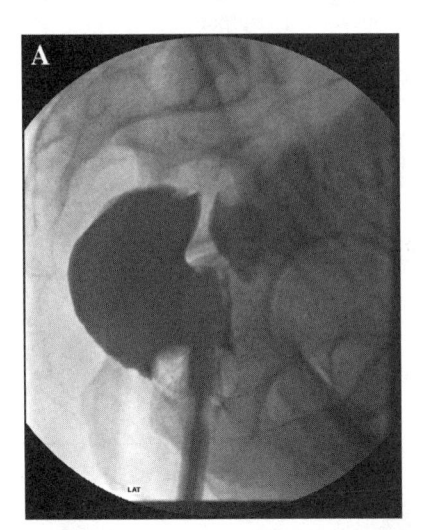

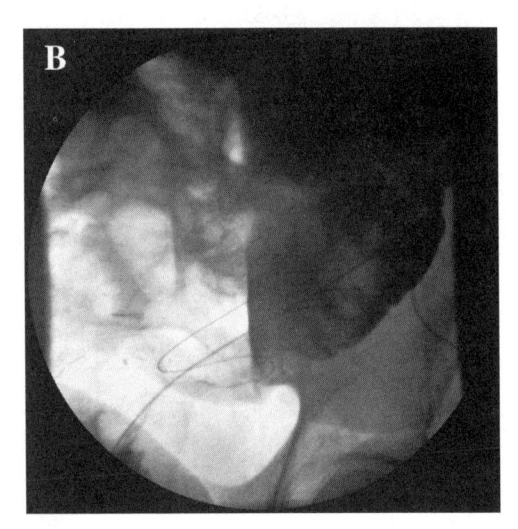

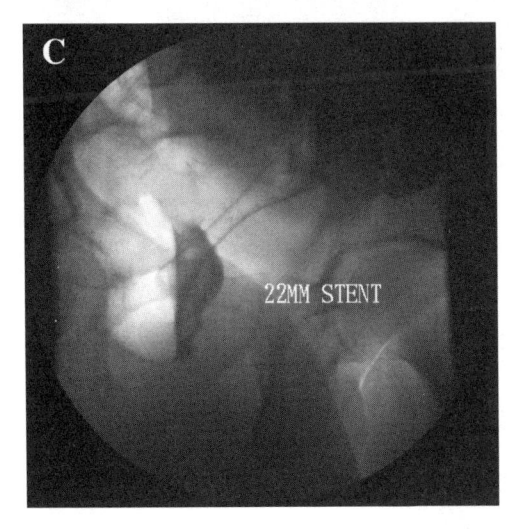

FIGURE 5. A patient with colon cancer developed acute colonic obstruction. Contrast enema demonstrates obstruction at the rectal sigmoid junction (**A**). A colonic 22-mm Wallstent was placed (**B**) under fluoroscopic guidance. Over the next 24 hours the patient experiences significant relief. He was then prepared for safer surgery. Colonic stents (**C**) may be placed using either standard fluoroscopic techniques or colonoscopy.

2. Palliative colonic decompression in cases of nonresectable primary vs. recurrent colonic cancer

59. What is the main contraindication to colonic stenting?
Colonic perforation.

60. List the advantages of colonic stenting over surgical decompression.
- No major patient preparation is required.
- Colonic decompression can be achieved with a minimally invasive procedure with reduced morbidity and mortality compared with emergent surgery, which has morbidity and mortality rates of 50% and 15–27%, respectively.
- Colostomy is avoided in most patients.
- Stenting allows time for tumor staging with better planning for definitive therapy/surgery.
- Stenting allows time for optimal medical management of the patient (rehydration, electrolyte correction, antibiotics) and colonic cleansing/preparation. Thus a precarious emergent surgical procedure is converted into a well-planned elective procedure.

61. At what distance from the anus are colonic lesions generally stentable? What is the length of stentable lesions?
In a study by Mainar, et al (who had a clinical success rate of 96%) the mean distance of the lesion from the anus was 20 cm (range = 4–75 cm) and the mean lesion length was 46 mm (range = 34–65 mm).

62. How successful is colonic stenting with the intent for a subsequent definitive surgery?
The technical success rate is 78–100% (mean = 89%) with 85% and 92% of stented patients having relief of bowel obstruction at 24 and 96 hours, respectively.

63. Compare colonic stenting with primary surgery for acute colonic obstruction in patients with resectable colon cancer.

	COLONIC STENTS	PRIMARY SURGERY
Percentage of patients in whom primary anastomosis is possible	85%	41%
Percentage of patients in whom colostomy is required	15%	59%
Major complications	12%	42%
Hospital stay	Significantly lower (p = 0.015)	Significantly higher (p = 0.04)
Cost-effectiveness	28% cheaper	

64. Summarize the results of colonic stenting with the intent of palliation in unresectable malignant colonic obstruction.
An average of 64–91% of stents remain patent until the patient's demise. Stent obstruction occurs in 15–29% of cases. The mean survival time is 5 months after stent placement with reported survival rates at 3, 6, and 9 months of 55%, 44% and 25%, respectively.

65. List the complications encountered after colonic stenting.
The procedure-related mortality rate is 1.3–1.4%. The complication rate is 15–42%. Complications may include the following:
- Rectal bleeding (usually mild)
- Anorectal pain
- Tenesmus
- Stent malposition/migration (mean = 6.5%)
- Stent obstruction (mean = 15–27%)

- Perforation with or without sepsis

66. **Summarize the causes and management of colonic perforation during colonic stenting.**
    Microperforation
    - Can exist subclinically before stenting as a result of the initial pathology.
    - May be caused by catheter and wire manipulation.
    - May result from erosion of colon by stent ends (barbs).
    - Usually treated conservatively (if diagnosed in the first place).

    Macroperforation
    - Can be due balloon dilation before and/or after stent deployment. Such maneuvers should be avoided.
    - Treatment is surgical.

67. **List the factors that increase the risk of colonic stent migration.**
    - Placement of covered stents
    - Placement of multiple stents to cover a long lesion
    - Stenting obstructions due to extrinsic compression

68. **What are the indications for percutaneous cecostomy?**
    - Distal colonic obstruction not amenable to being crossed endoscopically and/or fluoroscopically in unstable, poor surgical candidates
    - Cases of colonic pseudo-obstruction

69. **Discuss the technical aspects of percutaneous cecostomy.**
    Patients are given prophylactic antibiotics. CT images are reviewed to rule out cecal wall pathology. The cecum is accessed under fluoroscopy or CT guidance as if it were an abscess. Locking pigtail cathetes (8–14 French) can be placed after 2–3 pexy, T-fasteners are placed.

70. **How can sigmoid volvulus be managed radiographically?**
    1. Decompress the sigmoid colon by placing a transrectal tube as a prelude for elective surgery.
    2. Perform a water-soluble contrast enema both to diagnose the volvulus and to identify its site.
    3. Using a 5-French Cobra catheter and a glidewire, the twist is crossed and the glidewire is exchanged for an Amplatz wire.
    4. A 14-French nasogastric tube with an endhole and sideholes is advanced over the Amplatz wire to decompress the obstruction. Alternatively a silastic stent can be deployed for decompression.

BIBLIOGRAPHY

1. Aviv RI, Shyamorlan G, Khan FH, et al: Use of stents in the palliative treatment of malignant gastric outlet and duodenal obstruction. Clin Radiol 57:587–592, 2002.
2. Bell SD, Carmody EA, Yeung EY, et al: Percutaneous gastrostomy and gastrojejunostomy: Additional experience in 519 procedures. Radiology 194:817–820, 1995.
3. Block RD, Peterson B, Saxon RR, et al: Tracheal and esophageal stent placement. SCVIR Syllabus 1997: Thoracic and visceral nonvascular interventions: Part I, Chapter 17. 1997, pp 197–216.
4. Burns KE, Orons PD, Dauber JH, et al: Endobronchial metallic stent placement for airway complications after lung transplantation: longitudinal results. Ann Thorac Surg 74:1934–1941, 2002.
5. Chait PG, Weinberg J, Connolly BL, et al: Retrograde percutaneous gastrostomy and gastrojejunostomy in 505 children: A 4 1/2-year experience. Radiology 201:691–695, 1996.
6. Clark JA, Pugash RA, Pantalone RR: Radiologic peroral gastrostomy. J Vasc Intervent Radiol 10:927–932, 1999.
7. Currier AA Jr, Hallisey MJ: Direct percutaneous jejunostomy. SCVIR Syllabus 1997; Thoracic and visceral nonvascular interventions: Part I, Chapter 12. 1997, pp 155–158.

8. Do YS, Choo SW, Suh SW, et al: Malignant esophagogastric junction obstruction: Palliative treatment with an antireflux valve stent. J Vasc Intervent Radiol 12:647–651, 2001.
9. Ferral H: Colonic stents: clinical perspective, devices and outcomes. SIR 2003 Proceedings; Categorical Course (GI Stenting), 2003, pp 272–276.
10. Funaki B, Peirce R, Lorenz J, et al: Comparison of balloon and mushroom retained large-bore gastrostomy catheters. Am J Roentgenol 177:359–362, 2001.
11. Funaki B, Zeleski GX, Lorenz J, et al: Radiologic gastrostomy placement: Pigtail versus mushroom retained catheters. Am J Roentgenol 175:375–379, 2000.
12. Gaissert HA, Grillo HC, Wright CD, et al: Complications of benign tracheobronchial strictures by self-expanding metal stents. J Thorac Cardiovasc Surg 126:744–747, 2003.
13. George PJ, Irving JD, Khaghani A, Dick R: Role of the Gianturco expandable metal stent in the management of tracheobronchial obstruction. Cardiovasc Intervent Radiol 15:375–381, 1992.
14. Giuliano AW, Youn HC, Lomis NN, Miller FJ: Fluoroscopically guided percutaneous placement of large-bore gastrostomy and gastrojejunostomy tubes: review of 109 cases. J Vasc Intervent Radiol 11:239–246, 2000.
15. Hoffman S, Koller M, Plaul U, et al: Nasogastric tube versus gastrostomy tube for gastric decompression in abdominal surgery: A prospective, randomized trial comparing patients' tube-related inconvenience. Langenbecks Arch Surg 386:402–409, 2001.
16. Jung GS, Song HY, Seo TS, et al: Malignant gastric outlet obstructions: Treatment by means of coaxial placement of uncovered and covered expandable nitinol stents. J Vasc Intervent Radiol 13:275–283, 2002.
17. Kishi K, Kobayashi H, Suruda T, et al: Treatment of malignant tracheobronchial stenosis by Dacron mesh-covered Z-stents. Cardiovasc Intervent Radiol 17:33–35, 1994.
18. Lee KW, Im JG, Han JK, et al: Tuberculous stenosis of the left main bronchus: Results of treatment with balloons and metallic stents. J Vasc Intervent Radiol 10:352–358, 1999.
19. Lewis CA: Radiographically guided percutaneous gastrostomy and gastrojejunostomy. SCVIR Syllabus 1997: Thoracic and Visceral Nonvascular Interventions.
20. Lopera JE, Alvarez O, Castro R, Castaneda-Zuniga W: Initial experience with Song's covered duodenal stent in the treatment of malignant gastroduodenal obstruction. J Vasc Intervent Radiol 12:1297–1303, 2001.
21. Macdonald S, Edwards RD, Moss JG.; Patient tolerance of cervical esophageal metallic stents. J Vasc Intervent Radiol 11:891–898, 2000.
22. Mainar A, DeGregorio MA, Tejero E, et al: Acute colorectal obstruction: treatment with self-expandable metallic stents before scheduled surgery: results of a multicenter study. Radiology 210:65–69, 1999.
23. Marx MV, Williams DM, Perkins AJ, et al: Percutaneous feeding tube placement in pediatric patients: Immediate and 30-day results. J Vasc Intervent Radiol 7:107–115, 1996.
24. Mauro MA, Koehler RE, Baron TH, et al: Advances in gastrointestinal intervention: the treatment of gastroduodenal and colorectal obstructions with metallic stents. Radiology 215:659–669, 2000.
25. Morgan R, Adam A:Review article: Use of metallic stents and balloons in the esophagus and gastrointestinal tract. J Vasc Intervent Radiol 12:283–297, 2001.
26. Orons PD, Amesur NB, Dauber JH, et al: Balloon dilation and endobronchial stent placement for bronchial strictures after lung transplantation. J Vasc Intervent Radiol 11:89–99, 2000.
27. Park KB, Do YS, Kang WK, et al: Malignant obstruction of gastric outlet and duodenum: palliation with flexible covered metallic stents. Radiology 219:679–683, 2001.
28. Petersen BD, Uchida BT, Barton RE, et al: Gianturco-Rosch Z stents in tracheobronchial stenoses. J Vasc Intervent Radiol 6:925–931, 1995.
29. Prego CX, Munton FA, Cimadevila XE, et al: Volvulus of the sigmoid colon: Treatment by transrectal fluoroscopic catheterization and stenting. In Castaneda-Zuniga WR (ed): Interventional Radiology, 3rd ed. Baltimore,Williams and Wilkins, 1997.
30. Rofanan AL, Mehta AC: Stenting of the tracheobronchial tree. Radiol Clin North Am 38:395–408, 2000.
31. Ryan JM, Hahn PF, Boland GW, et al: Percutaneous gastrostomy with T-fastener gastropexy: results of 316 consecutive procedures. Radiology 203:496–500, 1997.
32. Saad CP, Ghamande SA, Minai OA, et al: The role of self-expandable metallic stents for the treatment of airway complications after lung transplantation. Transplantation 75:1532–1538, 2003.
33. Slonim SM, Razavi M, Lee S, et al: Transbronchial Palmaz stent placement for tracheo-bronchial stenosis. J Vasc Intervent Radiol 9:153–160, 1998.
34. Song HY, Lee DH, Seo TS, et al: Retrievable covered Nitinol stents: Experience in 108 patients with malignant esophageal strictures. J Vasc Intervent Radiol 13:285–292, 2002.
35. Szymski GX, Albazzaz AN, Funaki B, et al: Radiologically guided placement of pull-type gastrostomy tubes. Radiology 205:669–673, 1997.
36. Tan HM, Song HY, Lee JM, et al: Esophagorespiratory fistulae due to esophageal carcinoma: palliation with a covered Gianturco stent. Radiology 199:65–70, 1996.

37. van den Bongard HJ, Boot H, Baas P, Taal BG: The role of parallel stent insertion in patients with esophagorespiratory fistulas. Gastrointest Endosc 55:110–115, 2002.
38. vanSonnenberg E, Casola G, D'Agostino H, Mueller PR.: Percutaneous cecostomy for Ogilvie's syndrome: Laboratory observations and clinical experience. In Castaneda-Zuniga WR (ed): Interventional Radiology, Vol. 2, 3rd ed. Baltimore, Williams & Wilkins, 1997.
39. Wong MQ, Sze DY, Wang ZP, et al: Delayed complications after esophageal stent placement for treatment of malignant esophageal obstruction and esophagorespiratory fistulas. J Vasc Intervent Radiol 12:465–474, 2001.
40. Wood DE, Liu YH, Vallieres E, et al: Airway stenting for malignant and benign tracheobronchial stenosis. Ann Thorac Surg 76:167–174, 2003.

32. HEPATOBILIARY INTERVENTION

Wael E.A. Saad, MBBCh

1. **Who first described transhepatic cholangiography via a right intercostal approach?**
   Seldinger in 1966.

2. **Who first used flexible, long, thin needles in percutaneous transhepatic cholangiography (PTC)?**
   Okuda in 1974. This technique reduced the morbidity and mortality associated with large-bore needle cholangiography and thus popularized the procedure.

3. **List the contraindications for PTC.**
   - Bleeding disorders
   - Life-threatening reaction to contrast medium
   - Known hepatic vascular tumors
   - Ascites (relative)
   - Polycystic liver disease
   - Parasitic cysts (e.g., *Echinococcus* species)

4. **List the indications for PTC.**
   1. Diagnostic evaluation for cause and level of obstruction (Fig. 1A)
   2. Relief of biliary obstruction
   3. Diversion of bile flow in cases of bile leak (Fig. 1B)
   4. Provide a landmark for surgical biliary diversion (Fig. 2)
   5. Provide access for intracorporeal radiation
   6. Provide access for biliary manipulations such as:
      - Brush biopsy
      - Balloon dilation for strictures

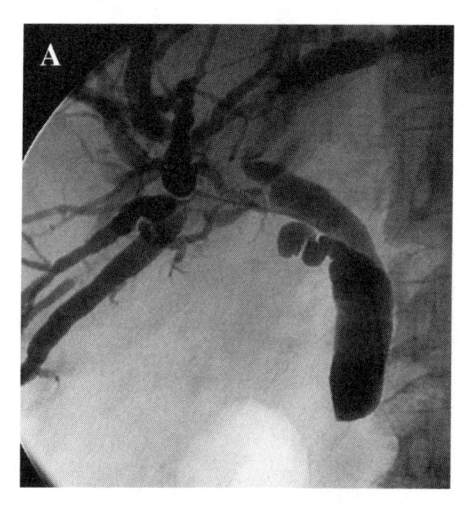

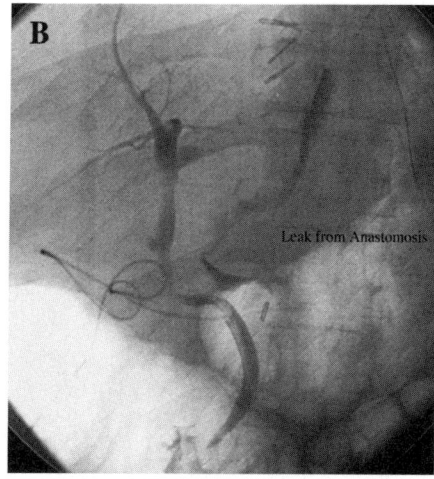

FIGURE 1. A, PTC depicting level of obstruction in a patient with ampullary cancer. **B.** PTC demonstrating bile leak from surgical anastomosis at common bile duct.

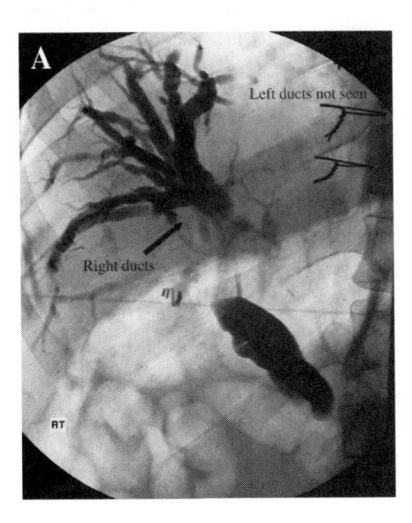

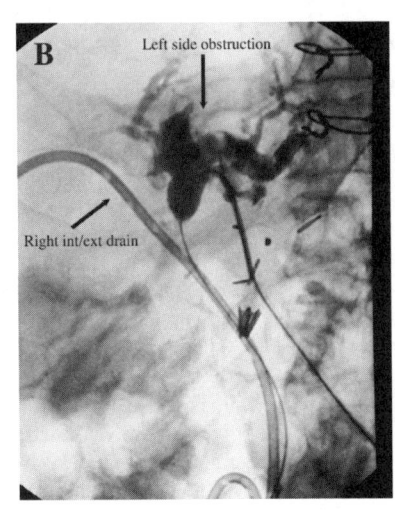

FIGURE 2. A, PTC via right biliary duct shows no filling of left duct in a patient with Klatskin tumor. Hence separate access to drain left duct is required. **B,** PTC via left duct demonstrates obstruction to left duct (same patient as in A).

- Bile stent placement
- Stone therapy and extraction

5. **What is the incidence of infected bile in the setting of biliary obstruction?**
   - 25–36% with malignant biliary obstruction
   - 71–90% with choledocholithiasis
   - Up to 100% in liver transplant recipients

6. **What is the incidence of bacteremia or septicemia following PTC?**
   In a study by Clark et al, 5% (7/148) of patients had culture-proven bacteremia following PTC despite prophylactic antibiotics (cefotetan). Clinical septicemia has an incidence of less than 3% after PTC.

7. **List the complications of PTC along with their incidence.**
   - Death ($< 1\%$)
   - Bleeding ($\leq 3\%$)
   - Sepsis ($\leq 3\%$)
   - Pancreatitis ($< 1\%$)
   - Peritonitis ($\leq 2\%$)
   - Pleural injury ($< 1\%$)
   - Catheter-related complications such as obstruction or dislodgement or wound infection
   - Overall major complication rate: $\leq 8\%$

8. **What kind of imaging guidance is used to perform PTC?**
   - Strictly fluoroscopy.
   - Combined ultrasound guidance access followed by fluoroscopy

9. What approaches are available in performing PTC?
- Left lobe approach from a subxiphoid puncture site
- Right lobe, midaxillary line approach

10. When should both approaches be used?
When both the left and the right intrahepatic biliary systems are obstructed by a central lesion at their confluence (right and left intrahepatic ducts). Draining one side will not result in an overall reduction in the bilirubin or in the risk of biliary source septicemia (see Fig 2).

11. What eponymous term is used to describe a cholangiocarcinoma involving the confluence of left and right intrahepatic biliary systems?
Klatskin tumor (see Fig 2).

12. Cholangiocarcinomas cause segmental atrophy of the liver parenchyma, including, in some cases, entire left lobe atrophy. Which vessel obstruction leads to this atrophy—the hepatic artery, portal vein, or hepatic vein?
None of the above. The primary cause of parenchymal atrophy is obstruction of the biliary ducts.

13. Briefly describe the two classes of cholangiocarcinomas.
Intrahepatic cholangiocarcinoma
- 10% of cholangiocarcinomas
- Prominent desmoplastic (fibrotic) reaction (delayed enhancement on contrast-enhanced computed tomography [DECT])
- Second most common primary hepatic tumor after hepatoma
- Includes Klatskin tumors

Extrahepatic cholangiocarcinoma
- 90% of cholangiocarcinomas

14. List the top four factors that predispose to cholangiocarcinoma.
1. Inflammatory bowel disease (10-fold increase in risk)
2. Sclerosing cholangitis
3. Caroli disease
4. Clonorchis sinensis infestation (most common cause worldwide)

15. List a short differential diagnosis for the following findings by cholangiography: multifocal strictures, especially at bifurcations, that give a "beaded" appearance to bile ducts and a "pruned tree" appearance to the biliary tree.
1. Primary sclerosing cholangitis (Fig. 3)
2. Secondary sclerosing cholangitis, which includes:
    - Chronic bacterial cholangitis
    - AIDS cholangitis
    - Bile duct ischemia
    - Floxuridine therapy

16. Name the organisms causing sclerosing cholangitic changes related to AIDS.
- Cytomegalovirus
- *Cryptosporidium* species

17. To which disorders is primary sclerosing cholangitis related?
- Inflammatory bowel disease, especially ulcerative colitis
- Retroperitoneal fibrosis
- Cholangiocarcinoma

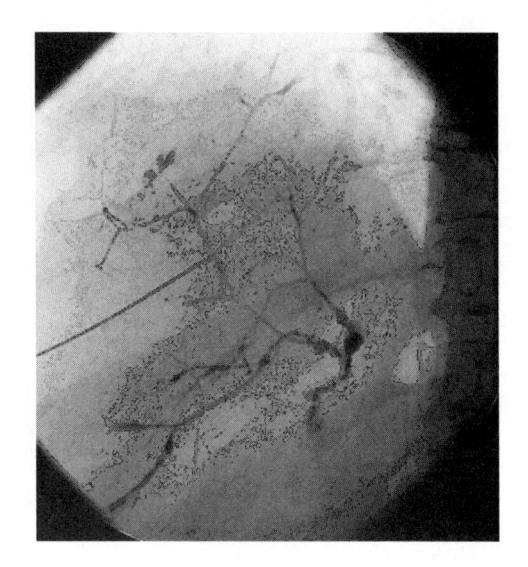

FIGURE 3. Patient with primary sclerosing cholangitis.

18. Why should the skinny needle (Chiba needle) be passed over the superior aspects of the ribs in the midaxillary line and not under them?

Immediately under the ribs run the intercostals arteries and nerves. Avoiding them reduces the risks of bleeding and pain during and after the procedure.

19. What should be done before performing a left-side, subxyphoid approach?

All abdominal imaging should be reviewed to determine whether or not major organs (e.g., transverse colon) are interposed between the subxyphoid skin entry site and the left lobe of the liver.

20. Should antibiotics be given before PTC?

Yes—and they should be continued for 24 hours. Biliary interventions are considered "dirty procedures" during which potential pathogens colonizing the biliary tract may escape into the blood stream and cause bacteremia/septicemia. The antibiotic of choice at the author's institution is Zosyn (piperacillin and tazobactam). Later single-dose antibiotics are used for asymptomatic patients requiring routine tube changes.

21. What is the next step after a diagnostic PTC reveals an anatomic defect, such as a bile stone (Fig. 4) or stricture, that can be treated percutaneously?

The next step is to place a percutaneous biliary drain. You should not approach the anatomic problem at this point in time in order to reduce the risk of septicemia. The stricture or stone should be dealt with in at least 1–3 days. The biliary drain is placed to maintain access and to decompress (drain) the biliary system.

22. In attempting balloon dilation of a benign biliary stricture, with what balloon size should you begin?

The answer, of course, depends on the size of the duct and whether the stricture is in a smaller peripheral branch or a larger more central branch. In general, in the case of a common bile duct stricture, you should begin with an 8- to 10-mm diameter balloon. If no waist is seen during balloon dilation at the site of biliary stricture, a larger balloon is used.

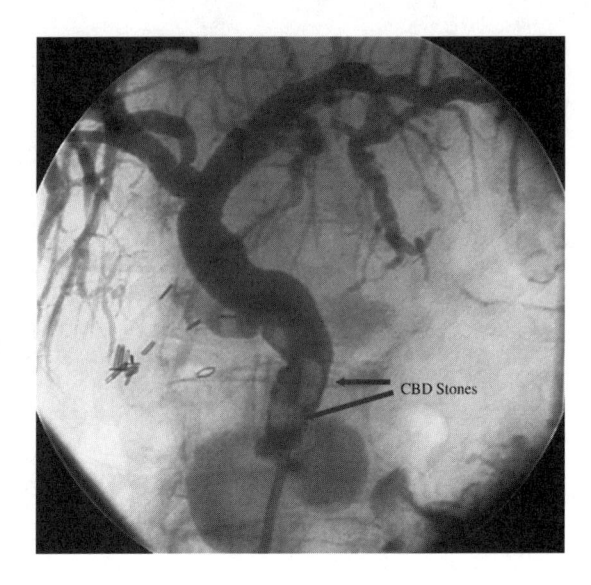

FIGURE 4. Two filling defects in the distal common bile duct that represent common bile duct stones.

23. Should the biliary drain be removed after a technically successful biliary stricture dilatation?

No. The drain should stay in place. The duration of drain placement is controversial. Some authors like to keep the drain in place for a minimum of 3 months after balloon dilation. The final decision is based on clinical and laboratory parameters and biliary flow dynamics.

24. If biliary stones coexist with strictures, which take priority?

The patient must undergo endoscopic and/or percutaneous removal of stones before balloon dilation of the stricture(s). Patients with extensive stone burden with multiple biliary strictures should receive surgical biliary reconstruction with creation of a Roux-en-Y hepaticojejunostomy after a preoperative PTC/PBD followed by combined transhepatic percutaneous cholangioscopy with stone fragmentation and cholangioplasty.

25. Name another percutaneous option in treating biliary calculi if percutaneous extraction fails.

Percutaneous intracorporeal electrohydraulic lithotripsy.

26. How amendable are postlaparoscopic cholecystectomy strictures to percutaneous management?

Unlike primary noniatrogenic biliary strictures and postcholecystectomy biliary strictures, postlaparoscopic strictures are markedly resistant to percutaneous management. Surgical repair is the treatment of choice; however, interventional procedures before and after surgery are important in the management of such patients.

27. Discuss the steps involved in removing an indwelling biliary drain.

Before losing transhepatic access, an over-the-wire cholangiogram is performed by exchanging the drain over a wire for a sheath (7-French) that is not introduced all the way but only as far as the peripheral bile ducts. If the stricture appears patent by this cholangiogram, a decision is made to initiate a clinical trial. For this purpose, a shortened biliary drainage catheter is reintroduced. The tip of this catheter is placed above (proximal) to the biliary stricture site. This catheter is capped for 1–2 weeks (up to 4 weeks by some authors). If the patient remains asymptomatic during this clinical trial, the drain is removed.

28. Are there any predictors of patency before removal of the biliary drain?
Yes. Successful balloon dilation, an asymptomatic clinical trial, and normal pressures (< 20 cmH$_2$O) during biliary manometric perfusion test have a positive predictive value of 85–90% for biliary duct patency at 1 year.

29. What is the overall patency rate of balloon dilation of benign strictures?
76% at 3 years and 55% at 5 years.

30. How is primary sclerosing cholangitis (PSC) treated?
Combined percutaneous (for intrahepatic) and endoscopic (for the common bile duct) balloon dilation and surgical resection for strictures refractory to balloon dilation. Ultimately PSC is treated with liver transplantation.

31. Name the applications of fiber optics (transhepatic endoscopy) as an adjunct to biliary interventions.
1. Treating calculi with lithotripsy under direct vision
2. Biopsy of suspicious lesions

32. What size needle is used in percutaneous transhepatic cholangiography? How are the bile ducts identified?
Usually a 21–22 Chiba needle is used. There are two ways to identify the bile ducts:
1. A common way is to "puff-inject" contrast by using a syringe and tubing while the needle is slowly withdrawing. Try to avoid staining of the hepatic parenchyma, which obscures further interventions.
2. A less common way, which is not ideal for mildly dilated bile ducts, is to aspirate while the needle is withdrawn. This method avoids staining.

33. Define the features of a needle-bile duct entry site that is most amenable to percutaneous bile duct placement.
The entered bile duct should be a peripheral—not a central—bile duct. The trajectory angle between the needle and the bile duct should be smooth and obtuse (a duct with a horizontal course is selected to facilitate subsequent manipulations). Some authors prefer, but do not mandate, a bile duct bifurcation site.

34. What should be done if the initial access needle, which is used to opacify the biliary tree, does not meet the criteria above?
The access needle should be left in place to further opacify the biliary tract using contrast. Another 22-gauge Chiba needle is used to access a more favorable bile duct, which is now delineated by the cholangiogram (Fig. 5).

35. How do you access an already opacified bile duct using a Chiba needle?
Visualize the intended bile duct, and choose an access site that gives a direct trajectory to the bile duct with an obtuse angle between the intended trajectory and the targeted bile duct. The needle is passed to a depth that the needle tip projects over the intended bile ducts.

36. How do you know that the needle tip is in the desired bile duct on an anteroposterior fluoroscopic projection?
If the bile duct moves or kinks on passage of the needle tip; you know that you are close to, if not in, the bile ducts. Then get a left anterior oblique (LAO) projection. If the needle tip moves "**p**ast" the bile duct on the LAO projection, the needle is **p**osterior to the duct. If the needle tip moves "**a**way" from the bile duct on the LAO projection, the needle is **a**nterior to the duct (Fig. 6).

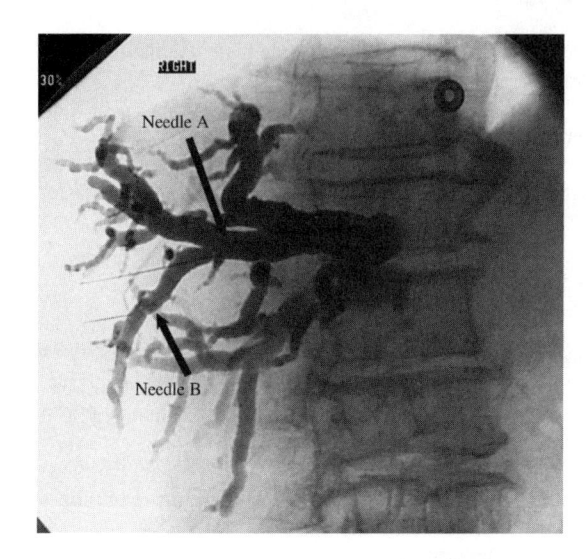

FIGURE 5. A, PTC needle is not in an ideal location for catheter placement. **B,** Needle shows good access site for catheter placement.

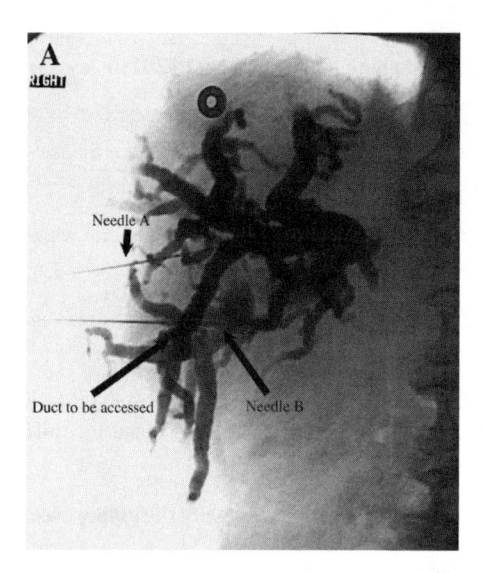

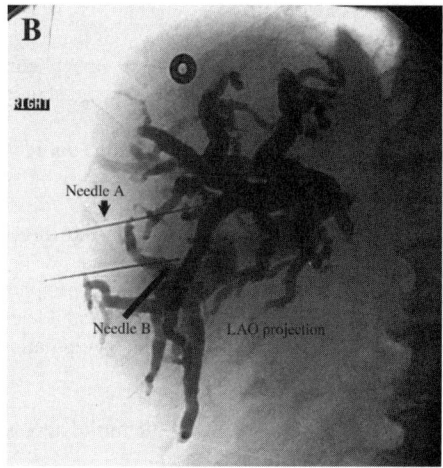

FIGURE 6. A, LAO projection demonstrates needle tip "past" the duct, indicating that the needle is posterior. **B,** LAO projection demonstrates needle tip "away" from the duct, indicating that the needle is anterior.

37. Why is biliary drain placement beyond (distal) a stricture/lesion preferred over a placement above (proximal) a stricture/lesion?

External drains (not crossing a stricture) are more likely to fall out than internal-external drains that cross a lesion and end in the bowel. In addition, external drains result in loss of fluids and electrolytes, which must be replaced to prevent renal impairment.

38. List the indications of a left hepatic PTC approach.
1. Operator preference
2. Obstruction of the main left hepatic duct with patent right-sided ducts

3. As part of combined drainage of both the right and left lobes in cases of hilar obstruction
4. With extensive neoplastic involvement of the right lobe by primary or secondary tumor

39. When should metallic endoprostheses (stents) be used in biliary strictures?

They should be reserved for malignant strictures and should not be used for benign strictures. Metallic endoprostheses have a poor long-term patency and should be reserved for patients who have a life expectancy (generally < 6–9 months) less than the expected patency of the biliary stent (Fig. 7).

40. What type of stents (metallic endoprostheses) are preferred for placement in the biliary tract?

Most interventionalists use self-expanding metallic stents for the percutaneous relief of biliary obstruction, mainly because of their increased flexibility compared with balloon-expandable stents. The Wallstent is the most popular self-expanding stent used by biliary interventionalists.

41. Name two techniques of percutaneous endobiliary biopsy procedures.

1. Passing a brush biopsy catheter back and forth across a potentially malignant stricture.
2. Procuring a piece of tissue with a percutaneous transhepatic biopsy forceps.

42. What finding in the setting of malignant biliary strictures favors plastic endoprosthesis placement over metallic stent placement?

Evidence of extensive involvement of the duodenum at or distal to the ampulla, a metallic stent is contraindicated.

43. In malignant hilar disease, which side (right or left) of the intrahepatic biliary tree should be decompressed to attempt to achieve clinical improvement?

Advanced hilar disease (including Klatskin tumors) usually causes dilation of the right and left intrahepatic biliary tree. Both the left and the right systems should be decompressed if clini-

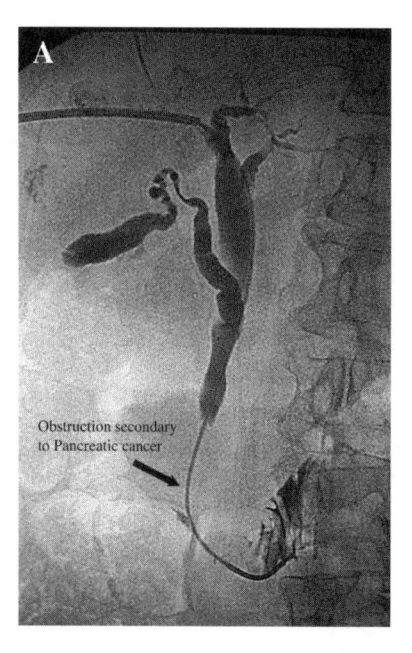

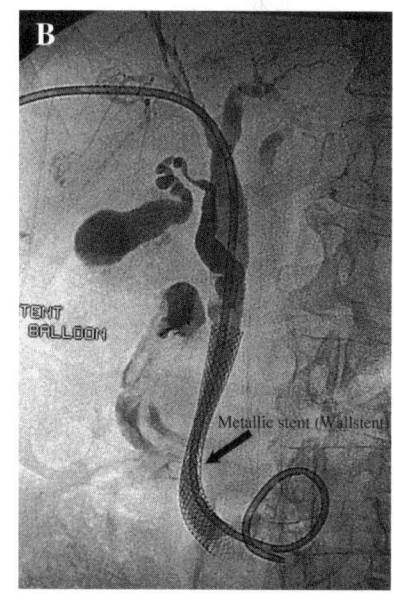

FIGURE 7. A, Distal common bile duct obstruction secondary to pancreatic cancer. **B,** Metallic stent demonstrates good response.

cal improvement is to be achieved. Rarely, clinical improvement is achieved by decompressing the right intrahepatic biliary system only.

44. Discuss the two methods of deploying metallic stents in both the right and left bile ducts.

1. Single transhepatic tract technique. Two stents are placed. One passes from right to left and the second from the right lobe to the ampulla, forming a T configuration.

2. Bilateral stenting using two transhepatic tracts, one through a right hepatic approach and the other through a left hepatic approach. Both stents go down the common bile duct in a Y configuration (Fig. 8).

45. What is the incidence of hemorrhage after PTC?
- Mild hemobilia is common and is seen in up to 16% of cases.
- Severe hemorrhage is seen in up to 3% of cases.

46. In the setting of severe hemobilia, should the PBD be upsized or downsized?

It should be upsized in an attempt to tamponade the hemorrhagic tract. The PBD should be flushed regularly to clear any thrombus.

47. If upsizing the PBD fails, list in order the sequential steps at attempting to stop the hemorrhage.

1. Placing a wire in the transhepatic tract to maintain access. Over this wire an end-hole catheter is placed, and contrast is injected to visualize the vascular site of hemorrhage by gradually withdrawing the catheter. If a vessel is identified, it is embolized by a sterile sponge or coils.

2. If no vessel is identified, a hepatic arteriogram is performed with the PBD removed over a wire (detamponading the tract). If a hepatic artery branch is visualized, that branch should be embolized (Fig. 9).

3. If no hepatic artery branch is seen bleeding and the hemorrhage is life-threatening, the hepatic artery is embolized in an attempt to reduce the hepatic perfusion pressure.

48. What are the advantages and disadvantages of a left hepatic lobe approach for a PTC?

Advantages
- Fewer pleural complications
- Less painful for patient

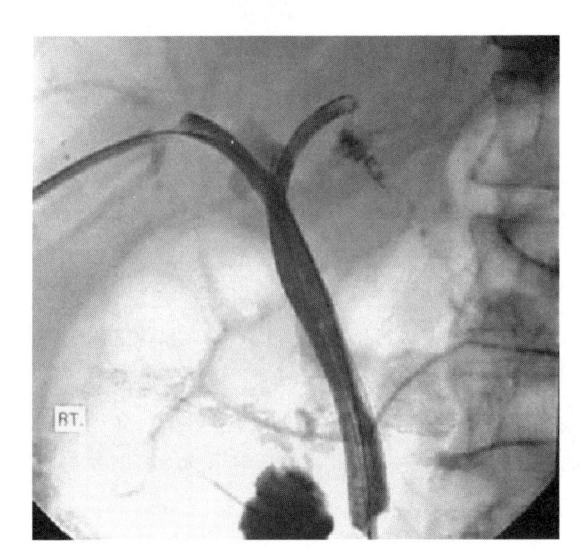

FIGURE 8. Bilateral stenting using two separate accesses with Y configuration.

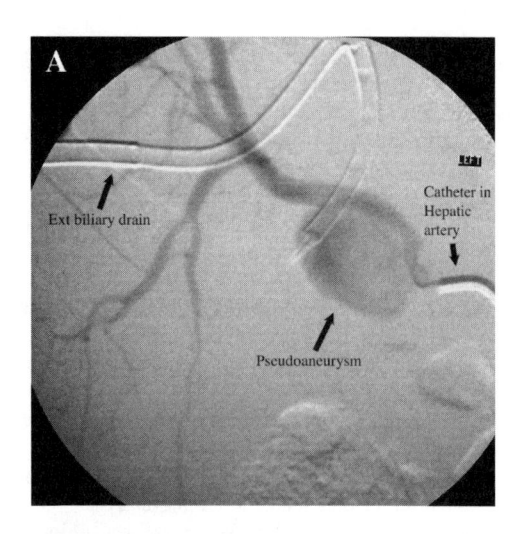

FIGURE 9. A, Hepatic artery pseudoaneurysm secondary to PTC. **B,** Pseudoaneurysm successfully embolized with coils.

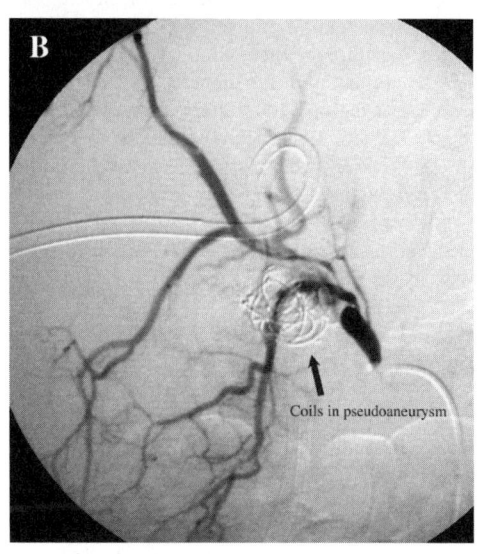

- Decreased respiratory motion during the procedure
- Because it is an anterior approach, it is be easier for the patient to take care of the tube.

Disadvantage
- More radiation to operator's hands

49. What is the next step if the biliary tract cannot be opacified by a transhepatic approach in an attempt to perform a PTC?

If the patient has a distended gallbladder; a cholecystostomy can be performed and the intrahepatic biliary tree can be opacified in a retrograde manner.

50. What are the causes of metallic endoprosthesis occlusion?
1. Tumor overgrowth (most common).
2. Occlusion by food debris

3. Bile inspissation/encrustations
4. All of the above

51. How are the occluded metal endoprosthesis managed if the percutaneous transhepatic drain has been removed?

Most are treated with another stent placement from an endoscopic approach. If this approach is not successful, a direct anterior needle puncture into the stent is used to opacify the biliary tree, and another stent is placed through an opacified bile duct.

52. List the indications for percutaneous transhepatic biliary endoscopy.
- History of recurrent biliary stones
- Retained intrahepatic or extrahepatic stones in the setting of a complex biliary-enteric surgical anastomosis
- Failure to remove stones when using conventional, fluoroscopically guided percutaneous methods
- Failure to remove stones when using standard endoscopic procedures (e.g., endoscopic retrograde pancreatocholangiography).
- Evaluation of filling defects on cholangiography in which stones, polyps, tumors, and clots must be differentiated
- Need for adjunctive biliary procedures such as lithotripsy
- Evaluation of functional surgical anastomoses
- Evaluation of the biliary drainage catheter tract
- Debulking of ductal tumors and theoretical application of local radiation
- Assistance in crossing eccentric high-grade strictures, which may have otherwise failed treatment by fluoroscopic means

53. What size must the transhepatic biliary tract be to accommodate a choledochoscope?

15–16 French and perhaps up to 18 French, depending on the type of choledochoscope.

54. How quickly can a transhepatic biliary tract be upsized to 16–18 French?

The routine biliary drain tract (at the time of establishing the tract) is 8–10 French. If the tract has just been established ("fresh tract"), it can be upsized by 2 French increments per day. If the biliary drainage catheter has been in place 1 week or longer, the tube may be directly upsized to 16–18 French.

55. Can a choledochoscope be used once a 16–18 French tract is established?

No. A choledochoscope can be used 48 hours after a freshly established tract is upsized to 16–18 French or 24 hours after a week-old tract is upsized to 16–18 French.

56. How early can choledochoscopy be performed through a surgically placed T tube?

Traditionally 6 weeks are required for tract maturation, although some authors have used T tube tracts that are 3 weeks old without serious consequences.

57. Describe the fluid requirements needed to reduce bile loss in cases of external percutaneous biliary drainage.

Normal bile output is 400–800 ml per day. This amount should be replaced ml for ml by IV Ringer's lactate.

58. What are the functional types of biliary drains?

1. External biliary drains: do not cross the area of bile pathology (stenosis, obstruction, or leak) (Fig. 10A)
2. Internal biliary drains: biliary endoprosthesis stents
3. Internal-external biliary drains: placed across the bile pathology (obstruction). They have two sets of side holes and drain internally as well as externally in a bag. (Fig. 10B)

Hepatobiliary Intervention 279

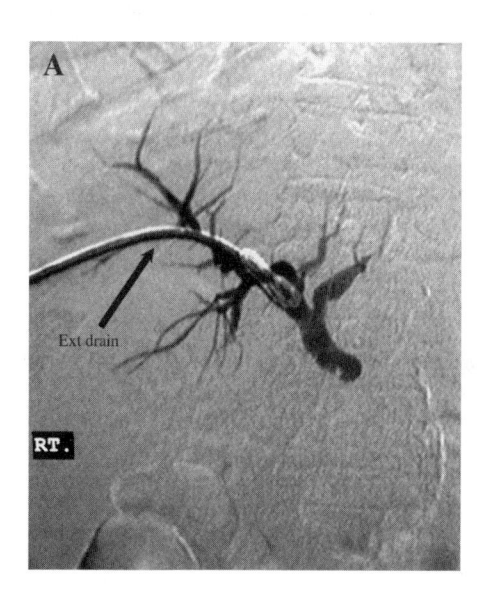

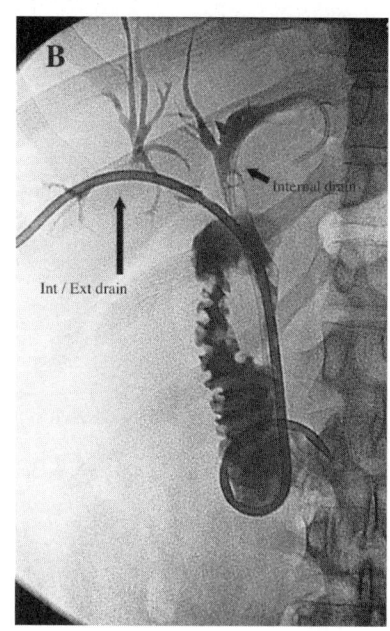

FIGURE 10. A, External drain placed since it could not get past the obstruction. **B,** Internal stent placed by endoscopic retrograde cholangiopancretography in the left duct and internal-external biliary drain placed by interventional radiologist in the right duct.

59. What is the rate of migration of biliary endoprostheses (internalized stents)?

Migration of plastic endoprostheses has been observed in up to 5.5% of such stents. Metallic endoprostheses migrate less frequently.

BIBLIOGRAPHY

1. Clark CD, Picus D, Dunagan WC: Bloodstream infections after interventional procedures in the biliary tree. Radiology 191:495–499, 1994.
2. Keighley MRB: Microorganisms in the bile: A preventable cause of sepsis after biliary surgery. Ann R Coll Surg Engl 59:328, 1977.
3. Lillemoe KD, Pitt HA, Cameron JL: Current management of benign bile duct strictures. Adv Surg 25:119–174, 1992.
4. McCormick CD, Cameron JL, Lillemoe KD, et al: Choledochoscopy as adjuvant therapy in the percutaneous management of patients with intrahepatic cholelithiasis. J Vasc Intervent Radiol 12:594–595, 2001.
5. Picus D, Weyman PJ, Marx MV: Role of percutaneous intracorporeal electrohydrolytic lithotripsy in the treatment of biliary tract calculi. Radiology 170:989–993, 1989.
6. Savader SJ, Cameron JL, Pitt HA, et al: Biliary manometry versus clinical trial: Value as predictors of success after treatment of biliary tract strictures. J Vasc Intervent Radiol 5:757–763, 1994.
7. Trerotola SO, Savader SJ, Lund GB, et al: Biliary tract complications following laparoscopic cholecystectomy. 184:195–200, 1992.
8. Venbrux AC, Osterman FA: Percutaneous management of benign biliary strictures. Techn Vasc Intervent Radiol 4(3):141–146, 2001.
9. Venbrux AC, Osterman FA: Percutaneous biliary endoscopy. In Laberge JM, Venbrux AC (eds): Biliary Interventions. SCVIR Syllabus. Reston, VA, SCVIR, 1995, pp 246–258.
10. Venbrux AC, Robbins KV, Savader SJ, et al: Endoscopy as an adjuvant to biliary radiology intervention. Radiology 180:355–361, 1991.

33. NONVASCULAR INTERVENTION IN SOLID ORGAN TRANSPLANTATION

Wael E. A. Saad, MBBCh

1. List the vascular complications that may result from percutaneous biopsy of renal transplant allografts.
- Arteriovenous fistulas (AVFs)
- Arteriocalyceal fistulas
- Pseudoaneurysms
- Extravasation and perinephric hematomas

2. What is the incidence of vascular complications of renal transplants after percutaneous biopsy?
0.2–2.0%. These complications coexist (particularly AVFs and pseudoaneurysms) in up to 30% of cases.

3. Summarize the success rates of AVF embolization in renal transplants.
- Technical success rate: 71–100%
- Clinical success rate: 57–88%

4. Summarize the complication rates of AVF embolization in renal transplants.
- Significant complications rate: 0–29%
- Minor renal infarcts (< 30% of renal parenchyma) have been reported in 100% of coil embolizations of AVFs and/or pseudoaneuryms.
- Major renal infarcts (> 30–50% of allograft parenchyma) have been reported in up to 29% of coil embolization combined with polyvinyl alcohol (PVA) and/or gelfoam. These infarcts lead to allograft loss.

5. With what factors is biliary cast syndrome associated?
- Posttransplant graft ischemia (70%) (Fig. 1)
- Biliary strictures (50%)
- Prolonged ischemia time

6. What is the incidence of biliary cast syndrome?
In recent years the incidence has been 4–18%. In the early transplant years the incidence was 26–34%.

7. List the biliary complications and their prevalence after liver transplantation.
- Biliary leak (4%)
- Strictures (8–12%) (Fig. 2)
- Biliary casts (4–18%)
- Ductopenia (3–4%)

8. What factors are associated with posttransplant biliary strictures?
- Hepatic artery thrombosis (HAT)
- Hepatic artery stenosis (HAS)
- Primary sclerosing cholangitis (PSC)
- Choledochojejunostomies
- Certain graft preservatives

FIGURE 1. Cholangiogram in a patient with liver transplant demonstrates filling defect in almost all of the ducts — a finding that is also seen in repeat cholangiograms. A hepatic angiogram demonstrated hepatic artery thrombosis, which is consistent with biliary cast syndrome.

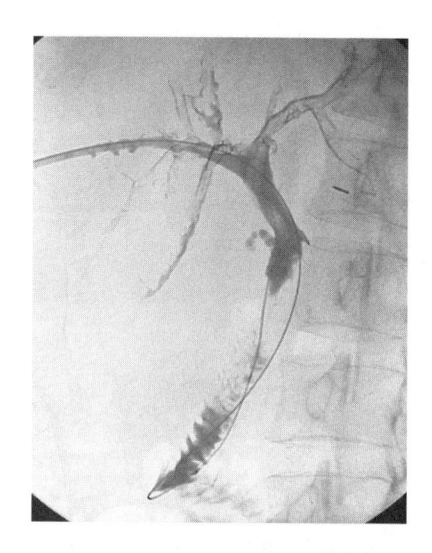

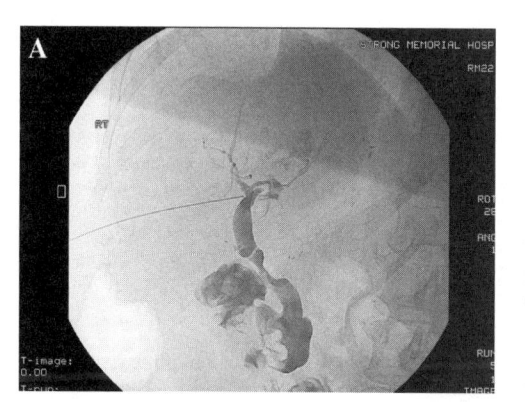

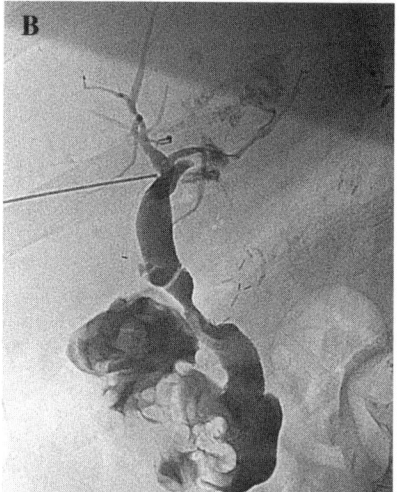

FIGURE 2. A and **B,** Narrowing at the duct-to-duct anastomosis after liver transplant, which was treated with consecutive balloon dilatation. The patient showed a slight elevation in liver enzymes and bilirubin. Hepartic artery thrombosis must be excluded.

9. **What is the recurrence rate of PSC after orthotopic liver transplantation?**
    5–20%. However recurrence does not affect patient survival.

10. **Compare the prevalence of multiple vs. solitary biliary strictures.**
    Multiple strictures (76%) are more common than solitary biliary strictures (24%).

11. **Compare the prevalence of central vs. peripheral biliary structures.**
    Central strictures (at bifurcation) are seen in 35% of cases. Peripheral strictures are seen in 34% of cases. Combined central and peripheral strictures are seen in 31% of cases (Fig. 3).

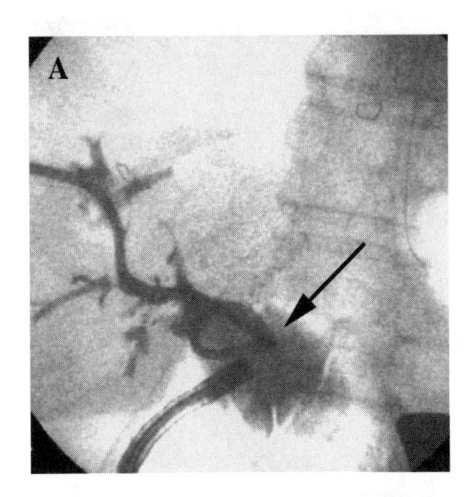

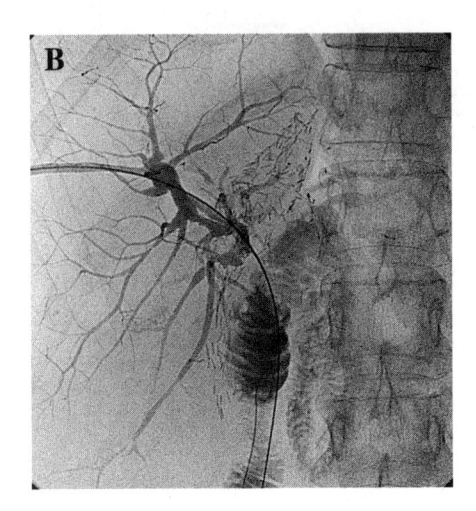

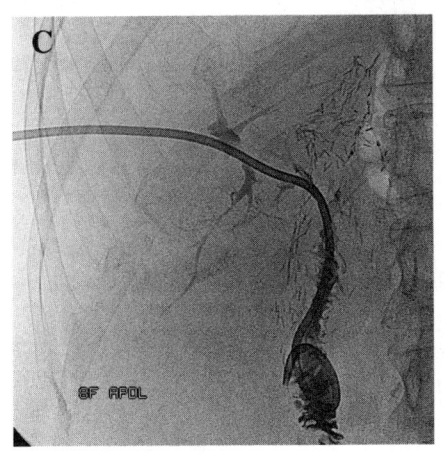

FIGURE 3. Complete occlusion of the biliary duct anastomosis in a patient who underwent living related liver transplantation. **A,** A scope was inserted into the bowel from a laparoscopic incision and placed at the anastomosis *(arrow)*. **B,** From above a wire was passed through the liver into the bowel, creating a neoanastomosis. **C,** The patient is maintained on chronic internal-external biliary drainage.

12. How successful is transhepatic balloon dilation of biliary strictures in liver transplant recipients?

The technical success rate is 89% with an 81% patency rate at 6 months. Nonanastomotic strictures have a better 6-month patency rate (94%) than anastomotic stenoses (77%) (Fig. 4).

13. Discuss the technical success rate and complication rates of percutaneous biliary drain placement in adult transplant recipients.

Placement of percutaneous biliary drains in transplanted livers is considered technically challenging. In adults, the technical success rate is 89–90% with minor and major complication rates of 5–11% and 2–4%, respectively.

14. What is the technical success rate of percutaneous biliary drain placement in children?

The technical success rate drops to 76% in nondilated biliary tracts in pediatric recipients, who are considered the most challenging patients.

15. Define ductopenia. How common is it?

Ductopenia or vanishing duct syndrome is pathologically defined as the absence of bile ducts in more than 50% of the portal triads. It occurs in 3–4% of transplant recipients, mostly in the first year after transplant.

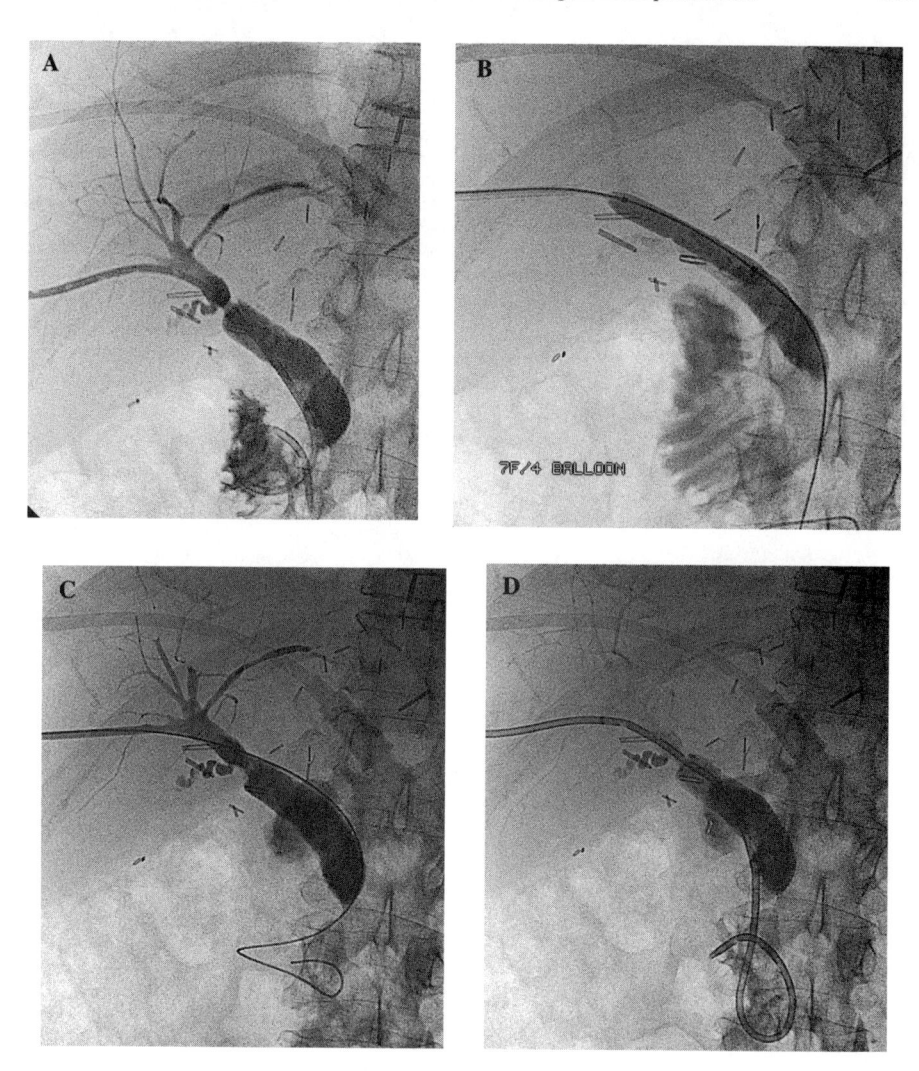

FIGURE 4. A, Stenosis at the bile duct anastomosis in a liver transplant recipient. **B,** The stenosis was dilated with a balloon. **C,** Moderate improvement is seen after dilatation. **D,** a drainage catheter is placed back within the duct.

16. With what phenomenon is ductopenia associated?

It is associated with chronic rejection due to bile duct cytotoxicity (reversible component) and ischemia (irreversible component).

BIBLIOGRAPHY

1. Benoit G, Moukarzel M, Hiesse C, et al: Transplant renal artery stenosis: Experience and comparative results between surgery and angioplasty. Transplant Int 3:137–140, 1990.
2. Campbell WL, Sheng R, Zajko PB, et al: Intrahepatic biliary strictures after liver transplantation. Radiology 19:735–740, 1994.
3. Funaki B, Zaleski GX, Straus CA, et al: Percutaneous biliary drainage in patients with nondilated intrahepatic bile ducts. Am J Roentgenol 173:1541–1544, 1999.

4. Graziadei TW: Recurrence of primary sclerosing cholangitis after liver transplantation. Liver Transplant 8:575–581, 2002.
5. Inomata Y, Tanaka K: Pathogenesis and treatment of bile duct loss after liver transplantation. J Hepatobil Pancr Surg 8:316–322, 2001.
6. Lorenz JM, Funaki B, Leek JA, et al: Percutaneous transhepatic cholangiography and biliary drainage in pediatric liver transplant patients. Am J Roentgenol 176:761–765, 2001.
7. Shah JN, Haigh WG, Lee SP, et al: Biliary casts after orthotopic liver transplantation: Clinical factors, treatment, and biochemical analysis. Am J Gastroent 98:1861–1867, 2003.
8. Zajko AB, Sheng R, ZeHi GM, et al: Transhepatic balloon dilation of biliary strictures in liver transplant patients: A 10-year experience. J Vasc Intervent Radiol 6:79–83, 1995.

34. GENITOURINARY INTERVENTION
Ryan K. Lee, MD

1. Define percutaneous nephrostomy.
It is an interventional procedure whereby access into the renal collecting system is obtained through the skin.

2. What are the indications to percutaneous nephrostomy?
One of the main indications is for external drainage of the collecting system because of a pyeloureteral obstructive process. External drainage may also be necessary to drain a fluid collection within the kidney, such as an abscess. Other reasons to perform a percutaneous nephrostomy include dilatation and/or stenting of a stricture within the collecting system. The nephrostomy can also be used for direct access into the collecting system to administer antibiotics, chemotherapeutic drugs, or agents for dissolving stones.

3. Discuss contraindications to percutaneous nephrostomy.
There are no absolute contraindications. Untreated infections and any potentially complicating anatomic problems, such as severe splenomegaly or scoliosis, are relative contraindications. Other relative contraindications that apply to any procedure (e.g., clotting diathesis) should also be evaluated on a case-by-case basis. The risks and benefits to the patient should be weighed carefully.

4. What should be done before percutaneous nephrostomy is performed?
Informed consent, preprocedural laboratory data (complete blood count, electrolytes, blood urea nitrogen/creatinine), IV access, and avoidance of oral ingestion (NPO status) for 6–8 hours before the procedure are standard preparations at most institutions. Routine antibiotics for all patients can be also be given, although this practice varies from institution to institution. Many institutions reserve antibiotics for patients with complicating factors (e.g., urinary tract infections, kidney stones).

5. What modalities can be used for guidance?
Access can obtained with guidance by one of two modalities: fluoroscopy or ultrasound. Fluoroscopy can often visualize the kidneys well, and opacification of the collecting system can be obtained by using iodinated contrast. Alternatively, ultrasound can be used to identify the collecting system (Fig. 1).

FIGURE 1. Ultrasound demonstrates hydronephrosis in a 32-year-old woman with left pelvic transplant kidney. The patient presented with increased levels of blood urea nitrogen and creatinine.

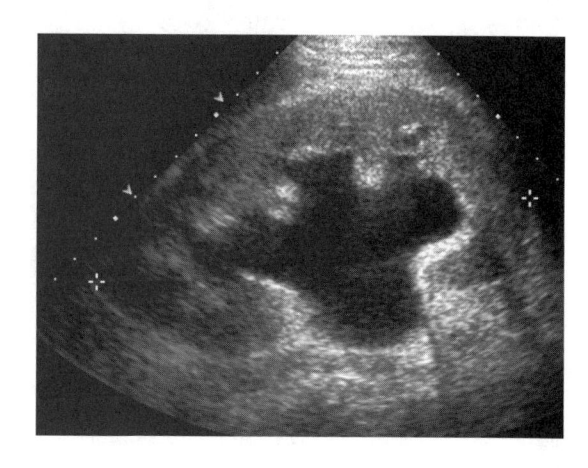

6. In what position should the patient be placed to obtain access into the collecting system?

The patient should be placed in the prone or oblique prone position, with the affected side elevated up to 45°.

7. Discuss the best approach to obtain access.

The best approach to access the collecting system is low enough to avoid the thoracic cavity and lateral enough to avoid the major lumber muscle groups. A useful anatomic landmark for the inferior extent of the parietal pleura is the eighth rib anteriorly, tenth rib along the midaxillary line, and twelfth rib posterioly. A posterolateral approach with the introducing needle toward the mid-to-lower calyx (unless a calyx bearing a stone needs to be accessed) is preferable. This approach approximates Brodel's avascular line, which avoids large vascular structures.

8. What size should the introducing needle be?

A 21- or 22-gauge needle, such as a Chiba needle, can be used.

9. Outline the steps for placement of a nephrostomy.

1. Confirm that the collecting system has been entered. Reflux of urine from the needle is a good indicator.

2. After some urine has been aspirated, inject a small amount of contrast through the needle to opacify the collecting system. This step is useful to confirm that the needle is well placed and also for preliminary assessment of the status of the collecting system.

3. After dilating the tract, a nephrostomy tube, such as a self-retaining Cope loop nephrostomy tube, can be placed over the guidewire.

4. After placement is confirmed, the distal loop is formed in the renal pelvis by pulling on the string of the locking loop (for the Cope loop) (Fig. 2).

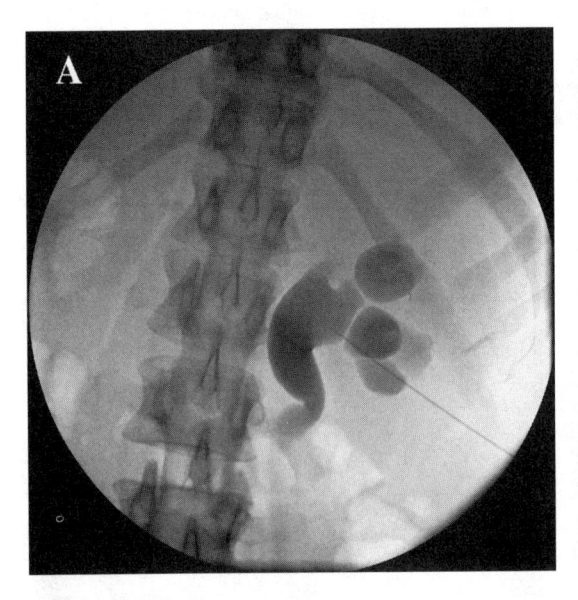

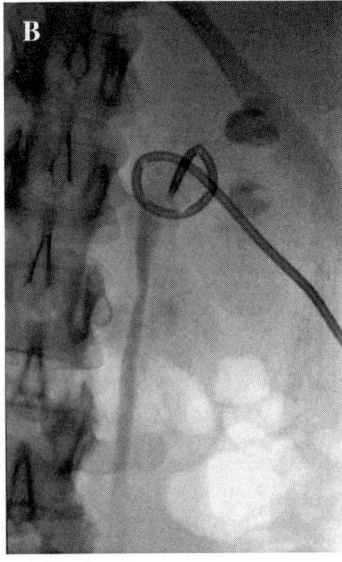

FIGURE 2. Classic nephrostomy tube placement. Under fluoroscopic guidance a 21-gauge Chiba needle was placed through a calyx into the renal pelvis (**A**). The optimal place for the puncture is through the calyx because of the decreased vascular supply within this area. Today the puncture would have been made under ultrasound guidance. After dilatation of the tract, a nephrostomy tube was placed and pigtail formed within the renal pelvis (**B**).

10. Discuss the complications of percutaneous nephrostomy.

As with any procedure, bleeding is a possible complication. The percentage of cases requiring transfusion has been reported to be as high as 3.6%, and the percentage of cases requiring surgery has been reported to be as high as 2%. Bleeding is more likely if punctures are made too medially due to injury to major vessels. Other complications include hydrothorax or pneumothorax (1%) and life-threatening sepsis (1–2%). Minor complications include microscopic hematuria, pain, and urine extravasation.

11. What size nephrostomy tubes are typically used?

Typically, an 8- to 10-French Cope nephrostomy tube is used. Larger nephrostomy tubes (e.g., 12 or 14 French) may be necessary for draining thick proteinacious fluid such as pus.

12. How should the nephrostomy tube be maintained?

For long-term drainage, catheters should be changed every 2–3 months on a fixed schedule. If a problem develops or the patient has an infection, the nephostomy tube should be changed sooner. Many institutions send the patient home with a 7-day supply of oral antibiotics initially after the procedure.

The patient should be instructed to keep the nephrostomy site dry and to change the dressing daily. A physician should be contacted for fever > 101°F, drainage at the tube site, foul-smelling urine, pain and redness at the site, or dislodgement of the tube.

13. How successful is percutaneous nephrostomy?

Generally speaking, percutaneous nephrostomy is an effective, safe, and minimally invasive procedure that is successful in 98% of patients.

14. What are the indications for ureteral stenting?

One of the main indications for placing ureteral stents is to relieve an obstruction, on either a temporary or permanent basis. Ureteral stenting is also used as part of the management of stone therapy, either before or after extracorporeal shock wave lithotripsy. It is often helpful in diverting urine leaks due to fistulas in the kidney or ureter. Finally, it can be used preoperatively to localize the ureter.

15. What causes ureteral obstruction?

Intrinsic factors: tumor (Fig. 3), calculi (Fig. 4), blood clots, sloughed papilla, infectious process (tuberculosis, schistosomiasis), strictures.

Extrinsic factors: infection (pelvic abscess, pelvic inflammatory disease), adenopathy, retroperitoneal fibrosis, metastatic disease, endometriosis.

16. Discuss the contraindications for ureteral stenting.

Untreated urinary tract infections are a contraindication to stenting, and drainage with a nephrostomy tube as well as antibiotics should be administered first. Any bladder problems should also be resolved first, such as bladder outlet obstruction, fistula/leak, or cystitis. Of course, general contraindications for any procedure apply, such as bleeding diathesis.

17. How can ureteral stents be placed?

Stents can be placed in antegrade fashion using the percutaneous nephrostomy as the access site. Alternatively, a stent can be placed in retrograde fashion, using a cystoscope. A newer technique is use of an angiographic catheter to access the ureter through the urethra and into the bladder.

18. Define internal stent.

An internal stent is completely within the body, with the proximal tip in the renal pelvis and the distal tip within the bladder.

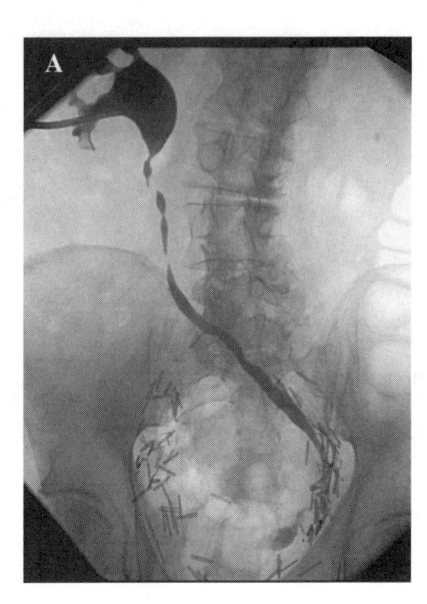

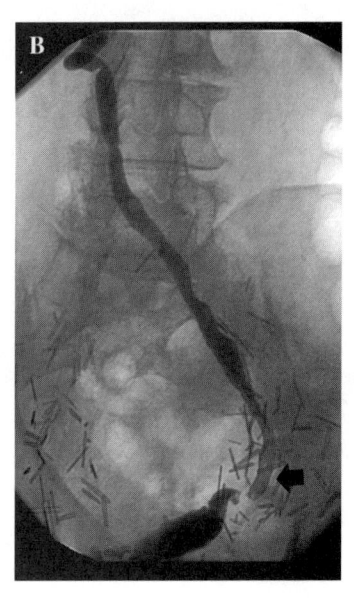

FIGURE 3. A 62-year-old man with a history of transitional cell cancer of the bladder underwent bladder surgery and now has an ilial-loop conduit. He developed hydronephrosis, and a percutaneous nephrostomy tube was placed (**A**). A persistent distal ureteral filling defect (**B**) was seen at 3-month follow-up. A brush biopsy confirmed transitional cell cancer.

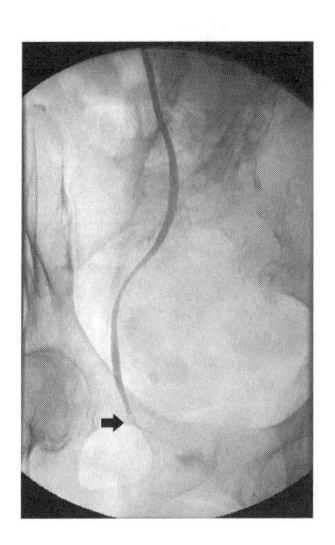

FIGURE 4. A patient with a history of nephrolithiasis presented with hydronephrosis. An antegrade nephrostogram was performed, and a nephrostomy tube was placed. A small filling defect in the distal ureter *(arrow)* represented a distal ureteral stone.

19. Define internal-external stent.

An internal-external stent has an external component that may exit either through a nephrostomy tube (Fig. 5) or through the urethra. Alternatively, the external component may exit via a stoma, as might be the case with an ileo-loop conduit.

20. Discuss the advantages and disadvantages of the internal stent vs. the internal-external stent.

The **internal stent** has the advantage of being less unwieldy compared with the internal-external variety, because it requires no external bags or tubes. Since it does not have a break through

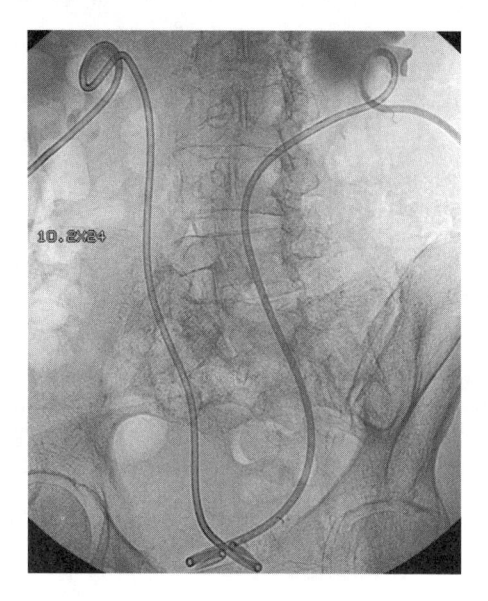

FIGURE 5. A patient with cervical cancer and extension of the cancer into the pelvis underwent radiation therapy and later developed bilateral distal ureteral obstruction. Bilateral internal-external nephroureteral stents were placed.

the skin site like the external types, infection is also less of a problem. In addition, an internally placed stent has the advantage of a percutaneously placed nephrostomy in place before the stent is placed; thus, the patient can have urinary drainage while any preexisting infection or other problems are corrected.

An **internal-external stent** has the advantage of convenient exchanges over guidewire. The procedure is considerably more involved for internal stents, in which the distal end must be snared through the bladder. Because of their less invasive nature, internal-external stents are excellent for short-term use.

21. Discuss the complications of stent placement.

Complications immediately after the procedure include perforation of the collecting system. Bladder irritability resulting in frequent urination and discomfort also may occur but usually resolves within several days. Stents, of course, have the possibility of occlusion. In the acute setting, occlusion is often caused by blood clots, although more recently transient obstruction from mucosal edema has also been described. In the chronic setting, stents can also obstruct by inciting an inflammatory reaction within the ureters that causes stricture. Other delayed complications include infection and stent migration. Stent fractures are much less common today with newer materials. Ureters can also undergo necrotic changes, especially from stents that are too wide and cause constant pressure on the ureteral walls.

22. How about dilatation of ureteral strictures?

Some success with stricture dilatation has been reported, although the high patency rates appear to be only on a short-term basis. The study by Shapiro et al. reports an 8% patency rate by 2 years.

23. Explain selective salpingography.

Selective salpingography can be thought of as an extension of hysterosalpingography (HSG). Both procedures involve injection of contrast into the female reproductive tract and visualization of relevant structures under fluoroscopy. Whereas HSG involves the nonselective catheterization of the cervix to identify the uterus and secondarily the fallopian tubes by retrograde filling, selective salpingography selectively catheterizes the fallopian tube in question for visualization.

24. What is the most common cause of female infertility?

Most cases of female infertility are caused by blockage of the fallopian tube. Normally after ovulation, an egg is released by the ovary into the fallopian tube and ultimately arrives to the uterus. If the fallopian tube is blocked or narrowed, pregnancy can be prevented.

25. Explain tubal recanalization.

Fallopian tube recanalization involves passing some type of guidewire past an obstruction in the fallopian tube identified on selective salpingography. Sometimes however, the force of contrast injection from selective catheterization of a fallopian tube actually restores patency, and passing a guidewire may be unnecessary.

26. Define infertility.

Infertility is defined as the inability to achieve pregnancy after 1 year of unprotected sex or after 6 months, if the patient is over 35 years of age. Because selective salpingography and tubal recanalization are often performed as part of the work-up for infertility, the diagnosis should be considered only after this time frame.

27. What are the indications for selective salpingography?

Further evaluation of a potential obstruction from a previous HSG is a typical reason to perform selective salpingography. An abnormal HSG may be due to tubal spasm or a true tubal disorder. Alternatively, the HSG may be inconclusive due to technical difficulties. Selective salpingography is indicated to further evaluate these findings (or nonfindings). Another indication for selective salpingography is to resolve discordance between HSG findings and the clinical diagnosis or laparoscopy. Finally, selective salpingography is performed for reevaluation if the patient has not achieved pregnancy either after tubal recanalization or after surgical tubocornual anastomosis.

28. What are the indications for tubal recanalization?

The main indication for tubal recannulization is infertility secondary to proximal fallopian tube occlusion. Recanalization can also be performed for persistent occlusion after reversal of a tubal ligation.

29. Discuss the contraindications for performing selective salpingography and tubal recanalization.

An active pelvic infection, such as pelvic inflammatory disease, is a common contraindication. Although occlusion of the distal portions of the fallopian tubes is not a true contraindication, studies have failed to substantiate the role of tubal recanalization in such cases. Severe intrauterine adhesions and any tubal pathology that may be amenable to surgical repair are other contraindications.

30. When should selective salpingography be scheduled?

Ideally, selective salpingography and tubal recanalization should be performed within the first 5 days after menstrual bleeding has ended.

31. How should the patient be prepared for selective salpingography?

Before the procedure, an infertility specialist should evaluate the patient, and sometimes a pelvic ultrasound or laparoscopic procedure is performed.

Antibiotics (e.g., doxycycline, 100 mg 2 times/day orally) should be administered on the evening before and continued for several days after the procedure. Conscious sedation should be administered according to institutional protocol.

32. Describe the proper positioning of the patient.

The patient should be placed in the lithotimy position, with the legs elevated by stirrups. Drapes should be carefully positioned to cover the legs, and the entire area, including the perineum, should be prepared in sterile fashion.

33. How is selective salpingography performed?
  1. The cervix should first be cannulated with an HSG catheter and an HSG performed. If the HSG demonstrates tubal occlusion, selective salpingography should be performed.
  2. The HSG catheter is then removed, and an introducing catheter is used to cannulate the cervix.
  3. A 5-French catheter is then inserted coaxially through the introducing catheter to selectively cannulate the ostium of the occluded tube.
  4. Contrast is then injected.
  5. If the selective salpingogram confirms a proximal occlusion, it is appropriate to proceed with fallopian tube recanalization.
  6. A 3-French catheter is then inserted coaxially through the already placed 5-French catheter, and an 0.0018 guidewire is used to attempt to pass the obstruction.
  7. When the obstruction is successfully passed, the 3-French catheter is slowly advanced past the obstruction.
  8. The guidewire is removed, and contrast is injected to determine distal tubal patency (Fig. 6).
  9. The procedure can be repeated for the opposite side, and a final HSG may be performed to document tubal patency.

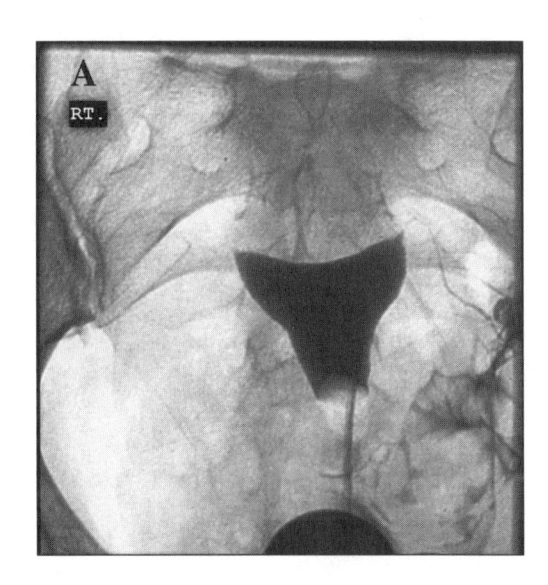

FIGURE 6. A, Initial image of the uterus and fallopian tubes demonstrates occlusion of the right tube. **B,** Placement of a 3-French catheter on an 0.018-inch guidewire into the tube allows free flow of contrast.

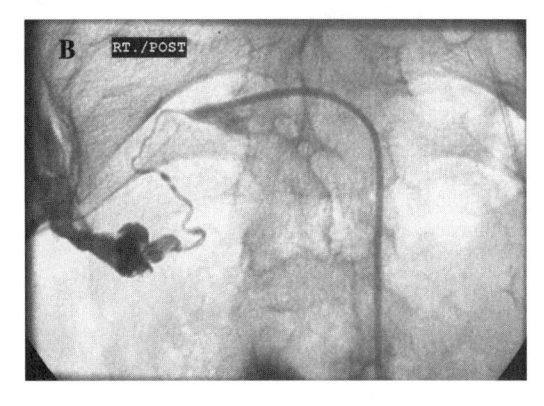

34. Discuss complications of selective salpingography.
Because of direct manipulation of the fallopian tubes, tubal perforation is a possible complication. Other complications include ectopic pregnancy and pelvic infections. Mild cramping and spotting are not unusual during the first week after the procedure.

35. How should the patient be managed after the procedure?
The patient should be observed for a short period of time (1–2 hours). If stable, she can be discharged with another adult who can drive her home. She should be reminded that mild spotting and cramping are not unusual. Some also recommend that pads instead of tampons be used until the next menstrual cycle and that intercourse be avoided for the next day or so.

36. How often is infertility due to tubal occlusion from any cause?
Depending on the sources, anywhere from 20–40% of female infertility is due to proximal tubal occlusion.

37. What is the success rate of restoring tubal patency in proximal occlusion?
The technical success rate depends on the cause of the occlusion. Idiopathic occlusion has success rates ranging from 71% to 100%, and occlusion secondary to salpingitis isthmica nodosa (SIN) has a success rate as high as 82%.

38. What is the success rate for achieving pregnancy after tubal recanalization?
Depending on the study, anywhere from 9% to 44% of patients ultimately achieve pregnancy after recanalization. The majority of these pregnancies occur within the first 6 months after the procedure. These results compare favorably with those of surgery, and selective salpingography may have complementary role to in vitro fertilization.

BIBLIOGRAPHY

1. Kandarpa K, Aruny JE: Handbook of Interventional Radiologic Procedures. Philadelphia, Lippincott Williams & Wilkins, 2002.
2. Laberge JM, et al: Interventional Radiology Essentials. Philadelphia, Lippincott Williams & Wilkins, 2000.

35. PERCUTANEOUS MANAGEMENT OF ABNORMAL FLUID COLLECTION
Wael E. A. Saad, MBBCh

1. What is the preferred method of managing intra-abdominal abscesses?

In the past surgery was required to treat intraabdominal abscesses by exploratory laparotomies, abscess evacuation, and peritoneal irrigation. Surgery was associated with high rates of morbidity and abscess recurrence. Advances in imaging technology and percutaneous techniques over the past two decades have enabled intra-abdominal collections to be drained percutaneously by interventionalists, with open surgical drainage reserved only for the most complex cases.

2. Describe the role of percutaneous drainage of abdominal abscesses.

Percutaneous drainage brings about complete resolution of the abscess in most cases with reduced morbidity and mortality compared with surgery. In the remaining cases it allows simpler, safer definitive surgery once the acute process has resolved.

3. Describe the characteristics of intra-abdominal collections that are most amenable to percutaneous drainage.

Simple, unilocular, superficial collections are the most amenable to percutaneous drainage. However, deeper and certain multilocular collections can also be drained if a safe route exists. Inter-bowel-loop abscesses, organized nonliquified hematomas, phlegmonous collections, and collections with extensive loculations are generally difficult to treat successfully with percutaneous techniques.

4. Which is better for percutaneous drainage—ultrasound guidance or computed tomography (CT) guidance?

The answer is highly dependent on operator preference. Ultrasound has the advantage of real-time needle visualization, speed, and simplicity and is best for superficial collections with direct, short-passage, safe routes. CT is preferred for deep collections because CT more precisely delineates adjacent bowel loops, organs, and vascular structures.

5. Describe the two-drain placement techniques.

Seldinger technique: A needle is placed in the collection, and a wire is advanced into the collection through the needle. The percutaneous tract is dilated, and the drainage catheter is then advanced over the wire into the collection.

Tandem trocar technique: The drainage catheter with a sharp inner stylet is advanced in one step (in tandem) into the collection.

6. What are the respective advantages of the trocar technique and Seldinger technique?

The trocar technique is a one-step procedure, whereas the Seldinger technique involves 3–5 steps, depending on whether a micropuncture needle is used initially or an 18-gauge needle. The Seldinger technique allows some margin of error in the initial needle passage into the collection, particularly if a micropuncture needle is used initially.

7. What should be done if a suspected collection is not infected?

Some interventionalists initially aspirate the collection and send a sample for culture and sensitivity and do not leave an indwelling drain. This approach is an attempt to avoid seeding a potentially sterile collection by placing an indwelling drain and thus converting a sterile collection to an abscess. If the aspirate is infected, drainage can then be performed.

8. When should percutaneous abscess drains be flushed?
Percutaneous abscess drains are flushed when the output is viscous and thick at the offset of the drainage or when the abscess drainage rate drops.

9. When should a percutaneous abscess drain be checked with a sinogram?
When sepsis has improved, patients routinely return for a catheter sinogram 2–3 days after initial catheter placement or when the drainage rate has decreased to 10 ml/day for 2–3 consecutive days and drainage removal is contemplated. In both situations the sinogram is performed to check tube position and to evaluate for possible fistulous tracts between the collection and bowel, biliary tract, or pancreatic duct.

10. When should a repeat/follow-up CT scan be obtained?
If the patient's clinical status does not improve within 2–3 days after the initial drainage, a repeat CT scan should be obtained to evaluate for residual undrained collections and for tube positioning. Additional drainage tube placement may be required for complex fluid collections.

11. When should an abscess drain be considered for removal?
When the following criteria are fulfilled:
- The patient is clinically well (afebrile, normal white blood count).
- No residual fluid collection is seen on a follow-up CT.
- Tube output is < 10 ml/day for 2–3 days.
- No residual cavity or fistula is seen on tube check.

12. What should be done if on a tube check/sinogram the collection has become considerably smaller and now is the same size as the pigtail (Cope) loop of the drainage catheter?
The drainage tube should be changed for a tube with a smaller pigtail loop to allow further shrinkage of the collection/cavity.

13. When should you suspect an enteric to collection fistula?
The search for a fistulous tract should be prompted by persistent unexpected output (out of proportion to initial collection size)—particularly in collections associated with any of the following:
- Postoperative collections involving bowel surgery and bowel anastomoses
- Crohn's disease
- Pancreatitis
- Bowel obstruction

14. What must be ruled out before attempting to treat an enterocutaneous/collection fistula?
Distal bowel obstruction must be ruled out. In the presence of distal bowel obstruction the prospects of an enterocutaneous fistula healing are dismal.

15. How can enterocutaneous fistulas be managed?
- Resolve distal bowel obstruction if present.
- Treat underlying condition (e.g., Crohn's disease).
- Ensure adequate nutrition (total parenteral nutrition)
- Ensure bowel rest.
- Place a straight drain adjacent to the fistulous tract and gradually withdraw the catheter over long intervals. A tube check/sinogram should be performed before an interval catheter withdrawal.

16. Do any local remedies promote fistulous tract healing?
A stoma/wound care consultation is recommended to reduce cutaneous breakdown and promote healing at the cutaneous end of the fistula. In addition, fibrin glue can be instilled in the fistulous tract as the catheter is gradually withdrawn.

17. **List the complications associated with percutaneous abscess drainage and the methods used to minimize them.**
    Complications occur in < 10% of cases and may include the following:
    1. **Septicemia,** which is managed with:
       - Broad-spectrum antibiotics
       - Avoiding overdistention of the cavity
       - Adhering to sterile technique
       - Avoiding aggressive tube flushing
    2. **Injury to surrounding organs and/or structures,** which is managed with:
       - Careful procedure planning
       - Appropriate image guidance. If the patient needs to be drained under CT guidance, then do it under CT guidance.

18. **Summarize the success rates of percutaneous management of intra-abdominal collections and enterocutaneous fistulas.**
    - 70–100% success rate for abdominal collections
    - 57–84% success rate for enterocutaneous fistulas

19. **List the types of hepatic abscesses.**
    - Amoebic abscess (most common worldwide)
    - Pyogenic abscess (most common in the United States) (Fig. 1)
    - Fungal abscess (in immunocompromised patients)
    - Echinococcal cyst/abscess

20. **List the causes of pyogenic abscesses.**
    - Ascending pyogenic cholangitis
    - Portal vein seeding from appendicitis, diverticulitis, and inflammatory bowel disease
    - Hepatic arterial seeding from systemic bacteremia
    - Infected penetrating trauma
    - Postoperative abscess formation
    - Infected hepatic infarcts, particularly in liver transplant recipients

21. **Can the organism isolated from a hepatic abscess suggest the cause of the abscess?**
    Yes, but this is not a hard-and-fast-rule. Gram-negative rods are *suggestive* of a pancreaticobiliary source. Mixed flora or anaerobic isolates are *suggestive* of an enteric source (especially colonic).

22. **List the radiographic differential diagnosis of an intrahepatic abscess.**
    - Hepatic abscess
    - Hepatic hematoma
    - Necrotic hepatic tumor
    - Intrahepatic biloma, especially in liver transplant recipients
    - Intrahepatic cysts

23. **How are pyogenic hepatic abscesses treated?**
    Generally they are treated with percutaneous catheter drainage and antibiotics. Small (< 3 cm), unilocular abscesses, however, may resolve with antibiotic treatment alone. In addition, unilocular abscesses under 5 cm have been treated with needle aspiration and antibiotic therapy (without indwelling catheter drain) with success rates of over 90–95%. These success rates compare favorably with the success rates of catheter drainage.

24. **Describe how pyogenic hepatic abscess aspiration is performed.**
    The catheter is placed under image guidance. Then the collection is completely aspirated and the cavity irrigated with a volume of normal saline or an antiseptic solution that is approximately

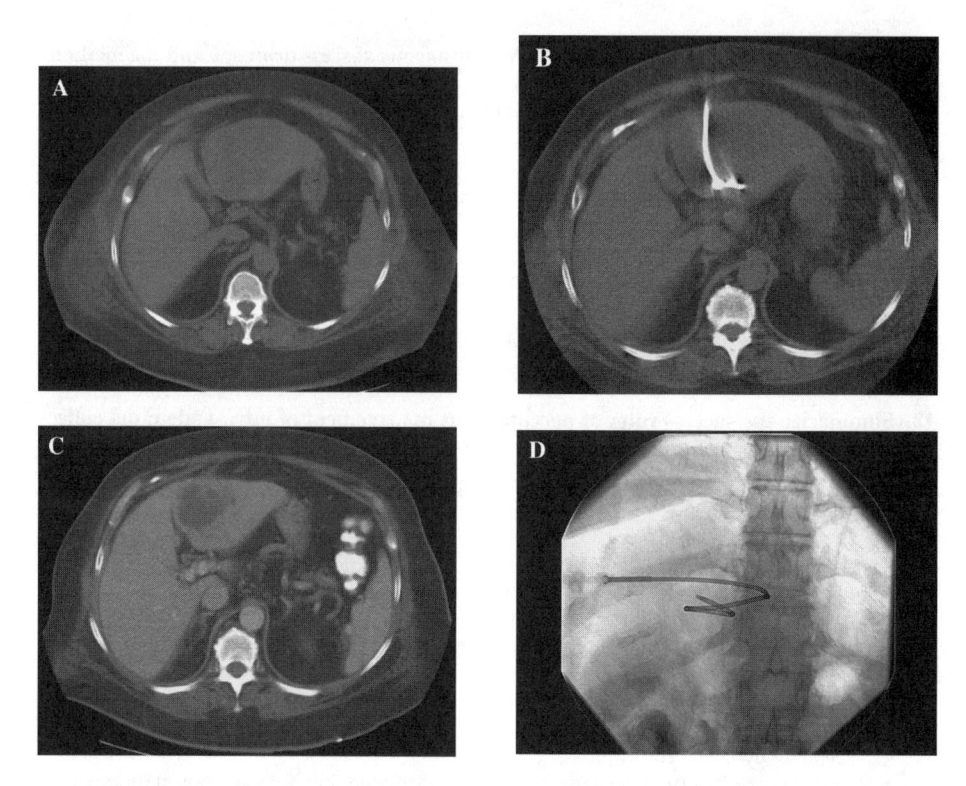

FIGURE 1. Initial CT scan (**A**) in a patient with fever, chills, and right upper quadrant pain showed low attenuation in the left lobe of the liver. No contrast was given because of elevated levels of blood urea nitrogen and creatinine. The initial drainage tube was placed under CT guidance (**B**). Over the next several weeks the patient improved, and the catheter drainage dropped below 20 ml/day. The catheter was removed. Over the next several weeks the patient developed intermittent low-grade fevers. The patient was re-imaged with contrast CT (**C**), which showed a smaller abscess. This abscess was drained under ultrasound guidance (**D**). The patient has done very well, and the catheter was removed over 6 months ago. Most likely, the abscess was initially a septated collection in which a pocket of moderate size was left undrained.

two-thirds the volume of the initial aspiration. Irrigation is repeated until the return fluid is clear. A sinogram is then obtained to assess for any communication with the biliary system. If no communication is found, the catheter is removed.

25. How do pyogenic hepatic abscesses with biliary communication differ from those without biliary communication?

The cure rates are similar. However, abscesses with biliary communications run a longer course. Abscesses communicating with an obstructed biliary tract require that the obstruction be addressed.

26. List the complications associated with percutaneous hepatic abscess drainage.
Early complications: sepsis (10% of patients), hemorrhage, pneumothorax, bowel injury.
Delayed complications: empyema, peritonitis, arterioportal fistulas.

27. How successful is percutaneous hepatic abscess drainage?
- Curative drainage: 80–85%
- Partial success: 5–10%

28. Describe how hepatic echinococcal cysts are treated percutaneously.

Conventional treatment of echinococcal cysts is surgical resection. The fear of managing this condition percutaneously is the potential for anaphylaxis and/or peritoneal dissemination. When they are treated percutaneously, the following steps are recommended:
  1. For superficial/subcapsular lesions, care should be taken to traverse a segment of liver parenchyma rather than to make a direct transperitoneal/transcapsular puncture.
  2. A small-caliber drain should be used (5–8 French).
  3. The cavity is aspirated dry.
  4. The cyst is then sclerosed with alcohol or hydrogen peroxide.

29. Discuss the prevalence and causes of pelvic abscesses.

Approximately 25% of intra-abdominal abscesses are pelvic. Seventy-one percent of pelvic abscesses are secondary to surgeries (e.g., bowel, gynecologic, urologic). Spontaneous or primary pelvic abscesses (29%) result from appendicitis (Fig. 2), diverticulitis, and inflammatory bowel disease.

30. Describe the technical challenge involved with a percutaneous transgluteal approach to draining deep pelvic abscesses.

Catheter placement in a transgluteal approach traverses the greater sciatic foramen and has the potential to injure the sciatic neurovascular bundle, which includes the superior and inferior gluteal vessels, internal pudendal artery, and sciatic nerve.

31. Describe the ideal trajectory of a transgluteal catheter to avoid the sciatic neurovascular bundle.

On predrainage CT it is important to identify the piriformis muscle. Most of the neurovascular structures are located superior and lateral to this muscle. Every attempt should be made to stay inferior to the piriformis muscle and as adjacent to the sacrum as possible. In cases of a cephalad-located collection, the piriformis muscle can be traversed; however, traversing this muscle may be associated with postprocedural gluteal pain (Fig. 3).

32. Discuss the results associated with transgluteal pelvic abscess drainage.

- Technical success rate: 100%
- Cure rate: 80%
- Postprocedural pain: 20%

Gluteal contraction may kink the catheter, leading to suboptimal drainage. Some authors consider the transgluteal approach as the last resort and prefer the transvaginal, transrectal, or transperoneal approach.

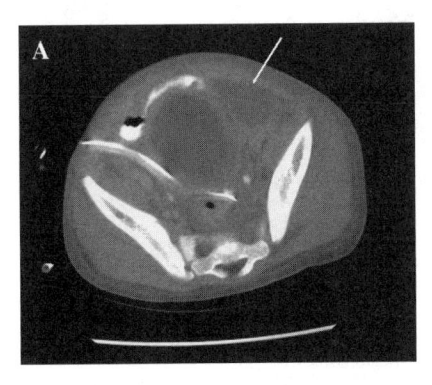

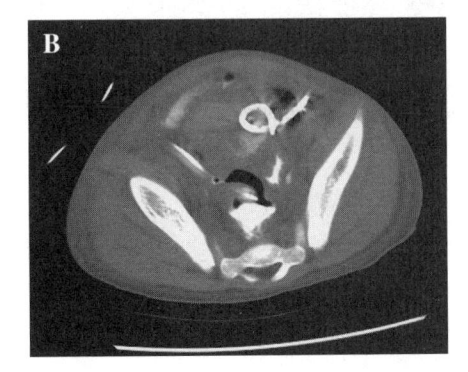

FIGURE 2. A, CT scan revealed multiple abscesses in a 5-year-old child after a perforation of the appendix. The largest was located in the anterior pelvis *(arrow)*. A total of four drainage tubes were placed under CT guidance. **B,** CT scan after placement of the first tube.

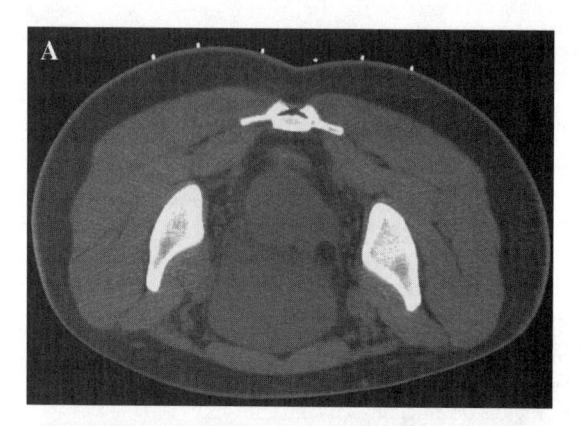

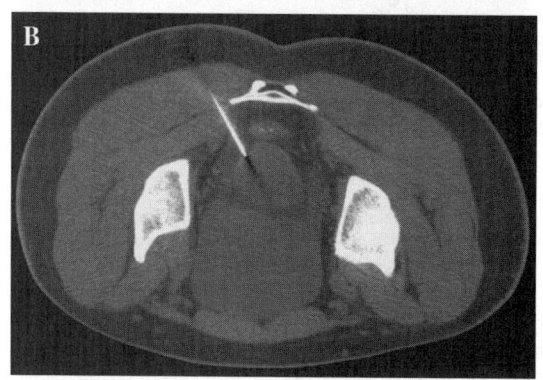

FIGURE 3. **A,** CT scan revealed an abnormal fluid collection immediately anterior to the rectum. **B,** A transgluteal approach was used. **C,** A drainage catheter was placed. The patient was followed clinically. When the drainage drops below 20 ml/day, the tube may be removed if the patient shows clinical improvement. During this type of drainage effort should be made to avoid the sciatic nerve.

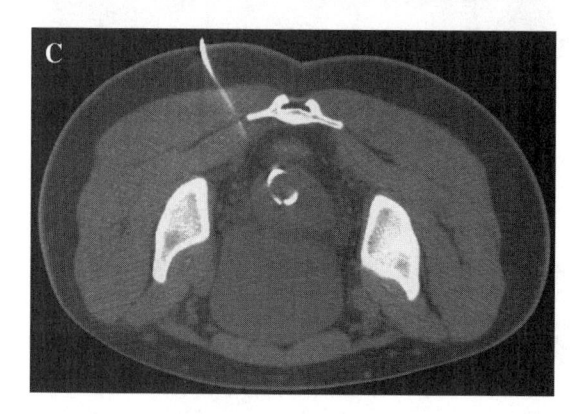

33. When should a transvaginal approach be preferred over a transrectal approach and vice versa?

Transvaginal	**Transrectal**
Obviously in women only	Men or women
Collection anterior to vagina	Presacral collection
	Premenarchal and virgin females

All other factors being equal, a transrectal approach is preferred over a transvaginal approach because it is technically less challenging. However, many women find transvaginal drains more bearable.

34. Describe the patient's position for transvaginal and transrectal pelvic drainage, respectively.
Transrectal: left lateral decubitus position.
Transvaginal: lithotomy position.

35. What are the success rates for endocavitary drainage of pelvic abscesses? What may cause drainage failure?
The success rate of endocavitary drainage is 80–100%. Causes of drainage failure include:
- Drainage of necrotic tumors
- Drainage of organized hematomas
- Drainage of complex collections

36. List the indications for percutaneous drainage of pancreatic fluid collections.
- Infected necrosis (controversial and difficult to drain)
- Postoperative pancreatic abscess
- Pseudocysts larger than 5–6 cm (pseudocysts < 5 cm may resolve spontaneously) (Fig. 4)

37. Describe the management of pancreatic necrosis.
Pancreatic necrosis, although it may appear as an area of low attenuation on CT (fluid attenuation), is difficult to drain percutaneously due to compromising solid debris and fat and nondrainable fluid. Extensive pancreatic necrosis should be treated by surgical debridement.

38. List and describe routes for percutaneous drainage of pancreatic collections.
Left posterolateral transperitoneal approach: a common drainage route because peripancreatic fluid often dissects along the left anterior pararenal space, displacing the descending colon anteriorly.
Posterior transperitoneal approach: through mesocolon or gastrocolic or gastrosplenic ligaments.
Transhepatic approach: through the left hepatic lobe for anterior collections.
Transgastric approach: for lesser sac collections located immediately posterior to the stomach. This drain can be internalized.

39. Why should interventionalists be vigilant and critical of preprocedure images of proposed pancreatic CT images?
Interventional radiologists need to synthesize clinical and radiographic information before embarking on pancreatic drainage because many cases of necrotic pancreatitis appear as liquified collections but are found to be too thick for conventional drainage. In addition, pancreatitis can be associated with vascular complications, and drainage of collections associated with potentially hemorrhagic lesions (e.g., pseudoaneurysms) can be catastrophic.

40. How do complication rates of percutaneous treatment of pancreatic collection compare with complication rates of surgical drainage?
The morbidity and mortality rates associated with percutaneous drainage of **pseudocysts** are 16% and 1%, respectively, compared with 28% and 5% for surgical drainage.
The morbidity and mortality rates associated with percutaneous drainage of **pancreatic abscesses or necrotic collections** are 29% and 11%, respectively, compared with 60% and 27% for surgical drainage.

41. What is the rate of infection in percutaneously drained pseudocysts?
Pancreatic pseudocysts are by definition sterile. Percutaneous drainage carries an 8% risk of making them infected, essentially converting them into pancreatic abscesses. However, the rate of spontaneous pseudocyst infection is similar to that of percutaneously drained pseudocysts.

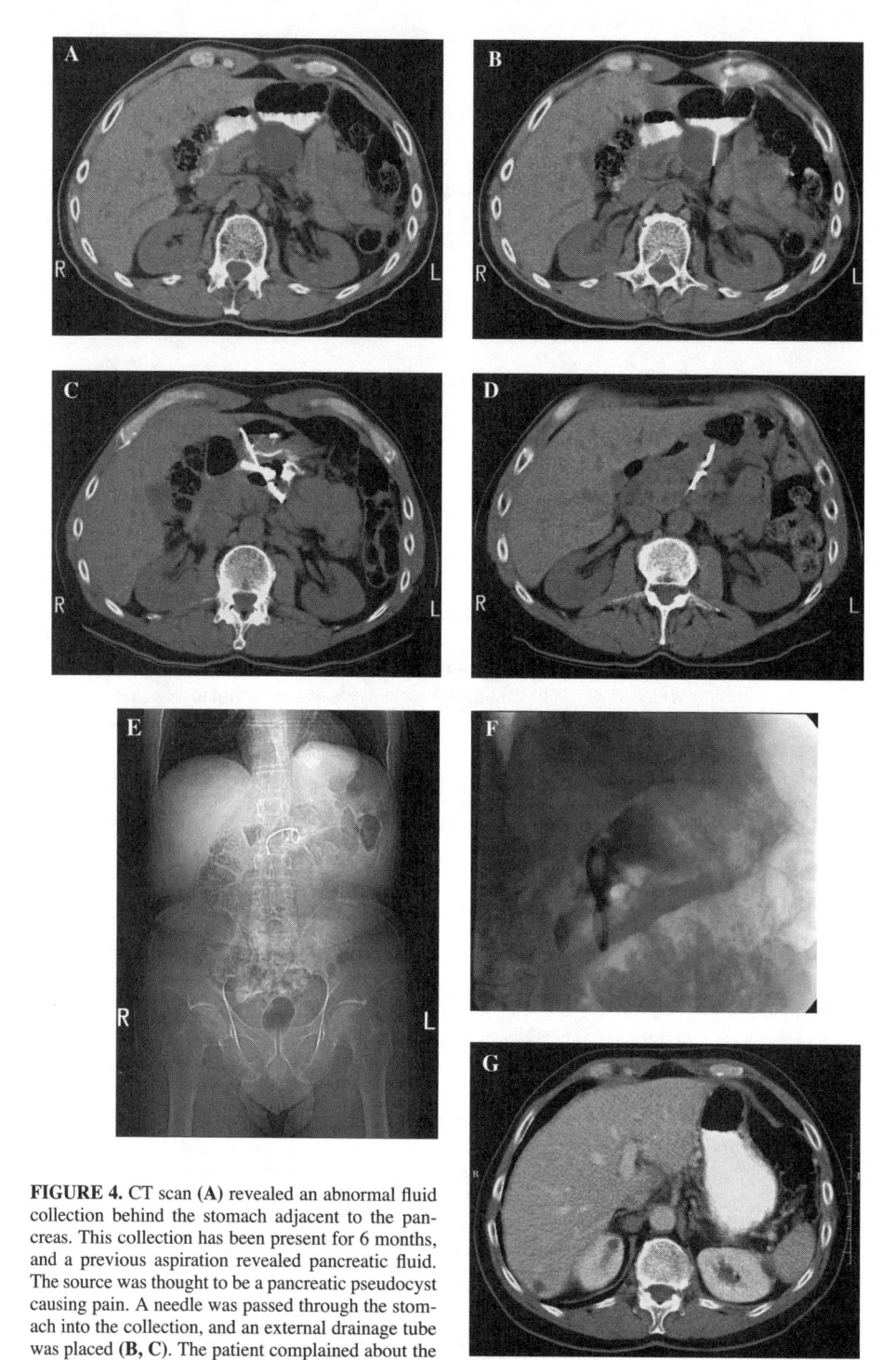

FIGURE 4. CT scan (**A**) revealed an abnormal fluid collection behind the stomach adjacent to the pancreas. This collection has been present for 6 months, and a previous aspiration revealed pancreatic fluid. The source was thought to be a pancreatic pseudocyst causing pain. A needle was passed through the stomach into the collection, and an external drainage tube was placed (**B, C**). The patient complained about the external tube, which was exchanged for a short biliary double J stent. This stent allowed the fluid to be drained via the stomach (**D, E, F**). The stent was removed endoscopically in 6 months. CT at 1-year follow-up (**G**) shows complete resolution of the pseudocyst.

42. List factors that delay healing of pancreatic duct fistulas.
- Distal pancreatic duct disease/obstruction
- Active infection
- Steroids

43. Summarize the success rates of percutaneous pancreatic drainage.
The overall success rate for all pancreatic collections is 70–80% with a recurrence rate of 15–20%.

44. What are the indications for chest tube placement in treatment of pneumothoraces?
- Pneumothoraces greater than 25–35%
- Pneumothoraces with progressive dyspnea
- Increasing size of a pneumothorax on serial chest radiographs
- Tension pneumothorax

45. List the approaches in placing chest tubes for pneumothorax.
- Anterior midclavicular line in the second or third anterior intercostal spaces
- Anterior or midaxillary line in women to avoid traversing breast tissue
- A low anterior approach may be desirable in recumbent patients because it involves the least dependent part of the thoracic cavity

46. Describe the technique in placing chest tubes for pneumothoraces.
The needle or chest tube and trocar are advanced over the superior margin of the rib (to avoid the subcostal vessels) and pointed toward the apex of the lung.

Entrance into the pleural space is confirmed by drawing back air. The chest tube is then placed either by trocar method or Seldinger method to enable wall suction.

47. What are indications for using CT guidance for pleural collection drainage instead of fluoroscopic or ultrasound guidance?
- The access route is difficult.
- Multiple catheters are required for complex collections.
- Need to distinguish underlying lung consolidation for complex, thick pleural collections.

48. List the methods used to improve drainage of a pleural collection that is refractory to drainage.
- Mechanical breakage of septation, using catheter and wire manipulation
- Placement of additional catheters in undrained loculus
- Administration of fibrinolytic agents (such as urokinase or tissue plasminogen activator) in the indwelling chest tube

49. How can an undrained locule in a complex pleural collection be identified?
Diluted contrast is instilled into the indwelling chest tube, and a repeat CT scan is obtained. Loculus without contrast enhancement is easily evident for additional drainage/interventions.

50. Describe a candidate for pleurodesis (sclerosis) of a malignant effusion.
- Life expectancy exceeding 1–2 months
- Chest tube in the most dependent portion of the pleural effusion with a daily output of < 100 ml (to prevent dilution of sclerosant) or chest tube ≥ 16 French
- Adequate coaptation of the visceral and parietal pleura

51. List the sclerosing agents used to pleurodese malignant pleural effusion.
Doxycycline, bleomycin, and talc slurry.

52. What can be offered to a patient with malignant pleural effusion who is not a candidate for pleurodesis (chest tube output > 100 ml/day)?

Tunneled, flexible chest tubes can be placed. These chest tubes can be connected to valve connectors, and patients can be taught to drain the pleural effusion 3–4 times/week. The tunneled chest tubes reduce the infection rate. The "pop-in" valves allow the patient to ambulate without being connected to water-seal containers or wall suction.

53. List the treatment alternatives for managing hepatic hydrothorax.
- Diuretics and protein repletion
- Peritoneojugular (LeVeen) shunt
- Surgical peritoneal-to-pleural fenestration
- Indwelling percutaneous chest tube
- Percutaneous drainage and sclerotherapy
- Transjugular intrahepatic portosystemic shunt (TIPS)
- Liver transplantation

The TIPS procedure should be considered initially because it has been shown to be effective in treating hepatic hydrothorax.

54. Discuss the treatment alternatives in managing lung abscess.

The first-line choice is conservative treatment, which includes postural drainage and antibiotics. This method is successful in 80–90% of patients. Traditionally, if conservative treatment failed, surgical evacuation was warranted. However, percutaneous abscess drainage results in rapid clinical improvement, and surgery can be avoided in 85% of cases (Fig. 5).

55. How common are pelvic lymphoceles after pelvic lymphadenectomy?

Lymphoceles have been reported in up to 30% of cases after pelvic lymph node dissection. This procedure is associated with common surgical procedures, such as prostatectomy or vulvectomy.

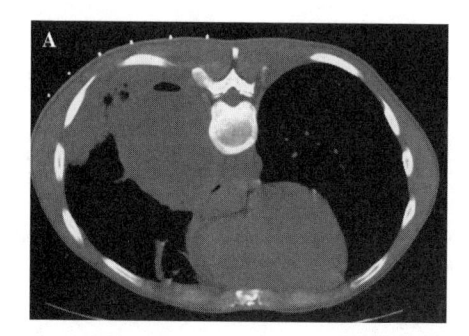

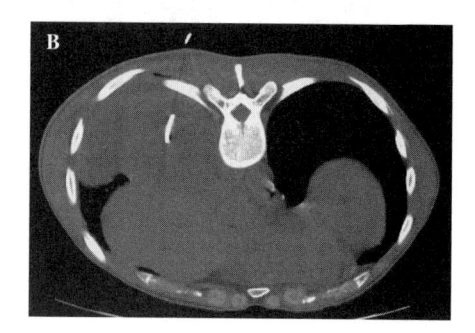

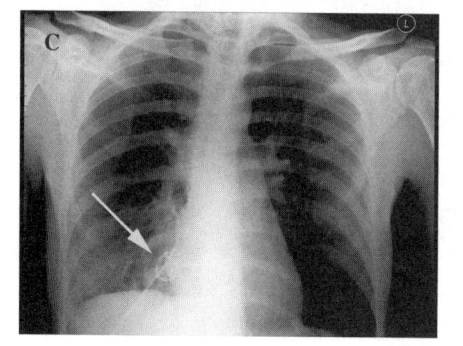

FIGURE 5. CT scan (**A**) shows lung abscess in the right lower lung. Markers were placed on the skin to help guide the drainage. The drainage tube is seen on CT (**B**) and chest x-ray (**C,** *arrow*). When the drainage decreases to less than 20 ml/day, the tube may be removed if the patient shows clinical improvement. Percutaneous drainage is also gaining in popularity. Air within the collection usually indicates a bronchopulmonary fistula.

56. Discuss the treatment options and their success rates for ostoperative lymphoceles.
- Simple surgical drainage: 50–70% successful + surgical complications.
- Surgical marsupialization: 90% successful + surgical complications.
- Percutaneous, indwelling catheter drainage: 50–100% successful + up to 13% recurrence.
- Percutaneous drainage and alcohol sclerosis or doxycycline sclerosis: 79–95% successful.

BIBLIOGRAPHY

1. Abbitt PL, Goldwag S, Urbanski S: Endovaginal sonography for guidance in draining pelvic fluid collections. Am J Roentgenol 154:849–850, 1990.
2. Butch RJ, Mueller PR, Ferrucci JT, et al: Drainage of pelvic abscesses through the greater sciatic foramen. Radiology 158:487–491, 1986.
3. Caliendo MV, Lee DE, Queiroz R, Waldman DL: Sclerotherapy with use of doxycycline after percutaneous drainage of postoperative lymphoceles. J Vasc Intervent Radiol 12:73–77, 2001
4. Clark RA, Towbin R: Abscess drainage with CT and ultrasound guidance. Radiol Clin North Am 21:445–459, 1983.
5. D'Agostino HB, Futoohi M, Aspron DM, et al: Percutaneous drainage of pancreatic fluid collections. Semin Intervent Radiol 13:101–136, 1996.
6. Giorgio A, Tarantino L, Mariniello N, et al: Pyogenic liver abscesses: 13 years of experience in percutaneous needle aspiration with US guidance. Radiology 195:122–124, 1995.
7. Jacques P, Mauro M, Safsit H, et al: CT features of intraabdominal abscesses: Prediction of successful percutaneous drainage. Am J Roentgenol 146:1041–1045, 1986.
8. Kuligowska E, Keller E, Ferrucci JT: Treatment of pelvic abscesses: Value of one-step sonographically guided transrectal needle aspiration and lavage. Am J Roentgenol 165:201–206, 1995.
9. LaBerge JM, Kerlan RK, Gordon RL, Ring EJ: Nonoperative treatment of enteric fistulas: Results in 53 patients. J Vasc Intervent Radiol 3:353–357, 1992.
10. Lambiase RE, Cornan JJ, Dorfman GS, et al: Postoperative abscesses with enteric communication: Percutaneous treatment. Radiology 171:497–500, 1989.
11. Lee MJ, Saini S, Geller SC, et al: Pancreatitis with pseudoaneurysm formation: a pitfall for the interventional radiologist. Am J Ronetgenol 156:97–98, 1991.
12. Moulton JS, Moore PT, Mercini RA: Treatment of loculated pleural effusions with transcatheter intracavity urokinase. AmJ Roentgenol 153:941–945, 1989.
13. Nemcek AA Jr, Vogelzang RL: Managing complications of acute pancreatitis. In Thoracic and Visceral Non-vascular Interventions, Genitourinary Interventions, SCVIR Syllabus, 1997.
14. Robinson LA, Moulton AL, Fleming WH, et al: Intrapleural fibrinolytic treatment of multiloculated thoracic empyemas. Ann Thorac Surg 57:803–814, 1994.
15. Silverman SG, Mueller PR, Sairi S, et al: Thoracic empyema: Management with image-guided catheter drainage. Radiology 169:5–9, 1998.
16. Souza S: Hepatic abscesses: Percutaneous drainage. In Thoracic and Visceral Nonvascular Interventions, Genitourinary Interventions, SCVIR Syllabus, 1997.
17. Van Sonnenberg E, Mueller PR, Ferrucci JT: Percutaneous drainage of 250 abdominal abscesses and fluid collections. Part I: Results, failures, and complications. Radiology 151:337–341, 1984.

36. CATHETER AND TUBE MANAGEMENT

Wael E. A. Saad, MBBCh

1. When should percutaneous abscess drains be flushed?
Percutaneous abscess drains (Fig. 1) are flushed when the output is viscous/thick at the offset of the drainage or when the abscess drainage rate drops.

2. When should a percutaneous abscess drain be checked with a sinogram?
When the sepsis has improved, patients routinely return for a catheter sinogram 2–3 days after initial catheter placement or when the drainage rate has dercreased to 10 ml/day for 2–3 consecutive days and drainage removal is contemplated. In both situations the sinogram is performed to check tube position and to evaluate for possible fistulous tracts between the collection and bowel, biliary tract or the pancreatic duct.

3. How do you flush a drainage catheter?
A drainage catheter or any other drain, such as a biliary drain or nephrostomy tube, can be flushed slowly and steadily with sterile normal saline. Forceful drainage can induce pain and/or bacteremia, and flushing should not be performed forcefully. The saline flush should not be drawn back into the syringe, because it will block the catheter with debris again.

4. If a drainage catheter output suddenly decreases or stops, what are the possible causes? What should be done?
Causes include the following:
- Tube is dislodged or malpositioned
- Tube occluded by debris
- Tube is kinked
- Tube has drained the part of the collection it is in and needs to be repositioned

A tube check (sinogram) with appropriate tube alterations should be performed. If the tube is not being flushed, a saline flush may be attempted to see if it will alter the drainage rate prior to a tube check (sinogram) procedure.

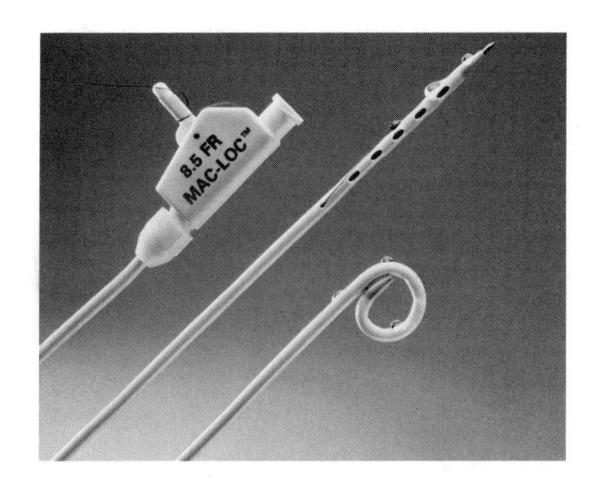

FIGURE 1. Percutaneous drain with a Cope loop at the end. String traveling through the catheter is used to lock the tube. (Courtesy of Cook Inc., Bloomington, IN.)

5. What should be suspected if the drainage catheter output is unexpectedly and persistently high?
A fistulous tract, such as an enterocutaneous fistula.

6. When should a percutaneous abscess drain be removed?
When the following criteria are met:
- Patient is clinically well (afebrile, normal white blood cell count)
- No residual fluid collections by follow-up imaging
- Tube output is persistently < 10 ml/day
- No residual cavity or fistula is seen on tube check

7. During a routine drainage catheter exchange, frank arterial hemorrhage is seen coming out of the tract around the exchange wire. How do you manage this situation?
The drainage tube should be promptly reinserted to tamponade the bleed. A baseline hematocrit and blood type and cross-match should be obtained. The appropriate surgical service should be notified and mobilized.

An urgent angiogram should be performed to interrogate the arterial supply in the vicinity of the drainage tube and fluid collection. The angiogram should be performed with the drainage tube in place and, when the drainage tube is removed, *over a wire*. The tube is removed during the investigative angiogram to detamponade the bleeding and expose the bleeding artery, which is then embolized. The wire allows prompt reinsertion of the tube to control the bleeding.

8. Which drainage route in percutaneous pelvic abscess drainage is associated with the greatest postprocedural pain? How is it managed?
The transgluteal approach is more painful after the procedure than the transvaginal, transrectal, or transabdominal routes. Approximately 20% of the patients who have undergone pelvic drainage by this route experience pain. Patients should be informed of this problem before the procedure and should receive adequate procedural and postprocedural pain management. The pain resolves once the drainage catheter is removed.

9. How are drainage catheters draining pancreatitis related collections managed?
Because of the thick, viscous nature of many pancreatic collections, drains are usually large and are flushed and irrigated copiously and vigorously. Volumes used for flushing/irrigation should not overdistend the cavity. Unlike other drain flushes, the amount of flush injected into the tube should be irrigated.

10. Describe the management of chest tubes placed for pneumothoraces.
Chest tubes are usually small-bore. The catheter is attached to a Pleur-Evac (Deknatel, Inc., Fall River, MA) for drainage on wall suction. The mean duration of drainage is 2–3 days, and once the pneumothorax is obliterated, the catheter is placed under water seal (no suction) for 12–24 hours. A follow-up chest x-ray is obtained, and if no pneumothorax is seen, the chest tube is removed. After chest tube placement, a repeat chest x-ray is obtained.

11. A large loculated, organized (fibrinopurulent) chest empyema is not draining despite an attempted breakage of loculations with a wire and placement of a large chest tube (> 20 French). What is the next step in the management of this patient?
Three doses of thrombolytics every 12–24 hours can be instilled through the chest tube in an attempt to liquefy the collections and its fibrin septa. Thrombolytic agents include urokinase (50,000 μ) or tissue plasminogen activator (2 mg diluted in sterile saline). This method can be used for collections in the abdomen and pelvis that are also refractory to drainage by large-bore catheters/tubes and saline flushes.

12. **What is the difference between percutaneous gastric tube (G-tube) feeding and jejunal tube (J-tube) feeding?**
G-tube feeding is by bolus administration. J-tube or G-J tube feeding through the J-port is by continuous administration.

13. **List the criteria by which tube feeding can be started after a recent percutaneous G-tube placement.**
    - 24 hours after the percutaneous G-tube procedure
    - Afebrile patient
    - No rise in the white blood cell count
    - Soft abdomen with no abdominal tenderness

Fever, an elevated white blood cell count, and a hard abdomen with tenderness are signs of peritonitis due to a leak from the gastrostomy.

14. **A patient with a percutaneous G-tube complains of nausea and diarrhea after bolus feeding. What is the problem? How can it be solved?**
The tip of the G-tube is probably in the duodenum, and the bolus tube feeds are being administered directly into the duodenum, causing nausea and diarrhea (known as "dumping syndrome"). This problem is treated by pulling the G-tube back into the stomach.

15. **If a G-tube (or any other tube) is blocked, how can it be unblocked at bedside?**
First you should address where the blockage is located. Is it in the connector tubing or in the tube itself? If the blockage is in the connector tubing, then change the connector tubing. If the blockage is in the tube itself, a forceful flush attempt can be made. (Soda may also be used to clean out a clogged G-tube). Flushing is performed by using a 1-ml syringe to force saline through the tube. A wire at bedside may also be used to attempt to declog the tube.

16. **Summarize the management of G-tube leaks.**

PROBLEM	MANAGEMENT
Leak from connector tubing	Change connector tubing at bedside.
Leak from a defect in the G-tube itself	Change the G-tube in the IR suite.
Anchoring balloon deflated	Re-inflate G-tube balloon anchor.
Gastric outlet obstruction due to distal migration of G-tube balloon	Pull back balloon/G-tube to be snug against the gastrostomy site.
Gastric outlet obstruction due to pathology (e.g., tumor growth).	Attempt to convert the G-tube to a G-J tube with the J-port tip placed beyond the obstruction and the G-tube port placed proximal to the obstruction and used for decompression drainage.

17. **If a gastrostomy site leak persists without gastric outlet obstruction and without structural and positional problems with the G-tube, what is the cause? How can it be resolved?**
The cause is most likely related to widening of the gastrostomy tract or, worse, tissue breakdown at the gastrostomy site. This situation presents a management dilemma. Some interventionalists "upsize" the tube to coapt the widening tract and thus minimize the leak. However, this strategy usually only temporizes the situation. The patient returns weeks or months later with the same problem but with a bigger tube and even wider tract. A more comprehensive approach is required, including re-evaluating the patient's nutritional status and a formal stoma/wound consultation to evaluate the G-tube site.

18. **Discuss the catheter therapy/management of pelvic lymphoceles.**
Indwelling catheter drainage of lymphoceles is successful in 50–80% of cases (described to be successful in up to 100% of cases) with a lymphocele recurrence of up to 13% of patients.

Sclerosants (ethanol or doxycycline) can be instilled at the end of the drainage to prevent recurrence. The success rate for sclerotherapy is 80–95% with a recurrence of 5% after two doxycycline sclerotherapy sessions.

19. If a percutaneous G-tube falls completely out of the patient, what should be done?
1. If the G-tube has been in place for 4–6 weeks (at least), the tract is most likely mature. A Foley catheter can be placed to maintain the percutaneous gastrostomy tract. Later a definitive G-tube can be placed.
2. If the G-tube has been in for less than 4–6 weeks, the tract should be explored and re-established as soon as possible.

20. How do you explore and re-establish a percutaneous tract of a fallen catheter, drain, or tube?
The cutaneous entry site of the tube or catheter is identified, and a Kumpe catheter tip is inserted into it. A sinogram is then performed under fluoroscopy to identify the tract. The tract is then negotiated/traversed using a Kumpe catheter and a glidewire (0.035 inch) all the way to the target organ or collection. Once the Kumpe catheter is in the target region (as confirmed by contrast injection under fluoroscopy), a definitive catheter or tube can then be replaced.

The above method can be used to re-establish percutaneous nephrostomy tubes, percutaneous biliary drains, abscess drains, and even tunneled central venous catheters.

21. How often are indwelling percutaneous biliary drains, nephrostomy tubes, and double-J ureteric stents changed?
Most indwelling tubes are changed every 2–3 months. Some patients require more frequent changes (Figs. 2 and 3).

22. What is the difference between an external biliary drain, and an internal-external biliary drain?
An **external biliary drain** has one set of side holes positioned along the biliary tract and drains to a bag on the outside. The inner end of the drain is usually looped and is placed in the central biliary tract.

An **internal-external biliary drain** has two sets of side holes. The upper set is positioned in the biliary tract, and the lower, more distal set of side holes at the looped end is positioned in the small bowel. This set drains out to a bag and down into the bowel (anatomically). Capping this drain causes bile to drain anatomically (Fig. 4).

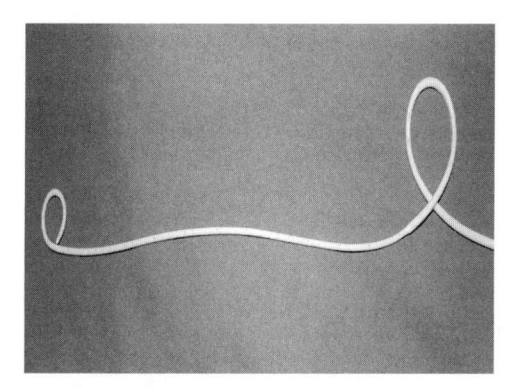

FIGURE 2. Nephroureteral stent. One loop is formed within the renal pelvis. A second loop is formed within the bladder. Holes are present all along the catheter in this example. In other catheters, holes are found only within the loop in the renal pelvis or the loop in the bladder. These catheters need to be changed every 8–12 weeks. Failure to change the catheters may lead to obstruction. (Courtesy of Cook Inc., Bloomington, IN.)

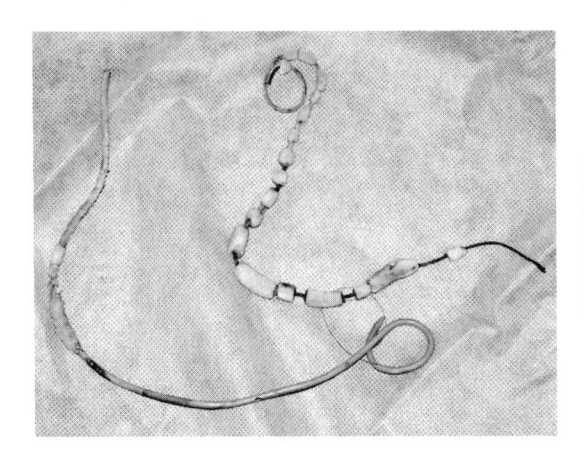

FIGURE 3. Double J-stent from the kidney into an ileo-loop. In one patient the stent had been in place for 3 years and was completely encrusted with stones. It broke upon removal. Extracorporeal shock wave lithotripsy (ESWL) was done to free the remainder of the stent.

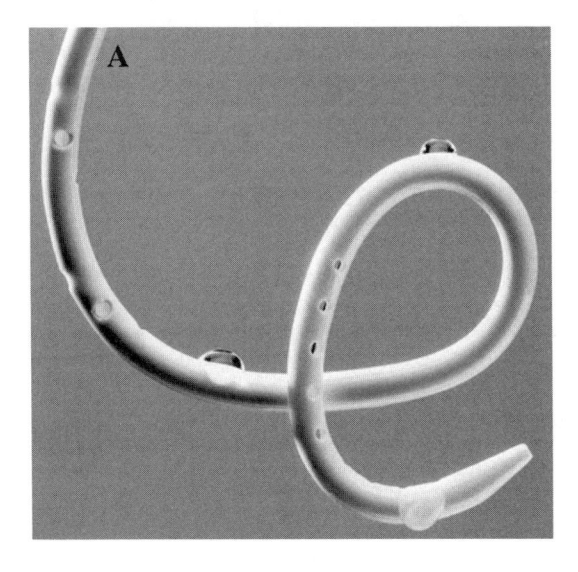

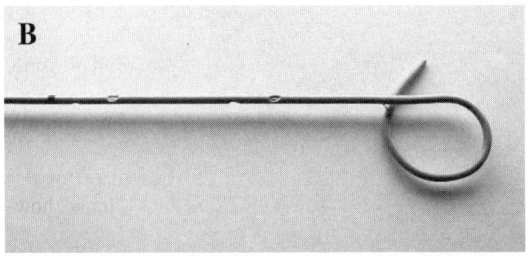

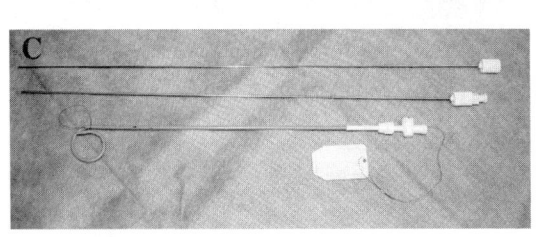

FIGURE 4. A, Loop of a biliary drainage catheter. (Courtesy of Cook, Inc., Bloomington, IN.) **B,** Full view of an internal-external biliary drainage catheter. (Courtesy of Boston Scientific, Watertown, MA.) The loop is placed in the bowel while the side holes are within the ducts. **C,** Modified version is used within the living related liver transplant ducts when there is a short distance between the bile ducts and bowel.

23. Describe the U-shaped biliary drain. When is it used?

A U-shaped biliary drain is a drain that enters through the right biliary system and exits the body through the left biliary system. It has one long set of side holes positioned centrally. The fluid drains out through both the left end and the right end (if both sides are opened).

The U-shaped drain is placed when both the right and left biliary tracts need to be drained and there is no central biliary dilation to accommodate a pigtail loop. A typical scenario is a central bile duct transection with a biliary leak and nondilated bile ducts. The biliary U-tube is a more secure drain than most biliary drains.

24. A capped internal-external biliary drain is leaking around the percutaneous entry site. The patient, as instructed, uncaps the external end and connects it to a bag. The leak diminishes but does not stop. What is the problem?

The internal component may be obstructed, probably by encrusted bile, or it may have been dislodged or kinked. This percutaneous biliary drain needs to be checked and changed.

25. How is a percutaneous biliary drain removed after a metal bile stent or balloon dilation is performed?

1. The percutaneous biliary tract has to be 4–6 weeks old (i.e., mature) to avoid bile backtracking and spilling into the peritoneum. If this prerequisite is fulfilled, a clinical trial is performed (see step 2).
2. A shortened biliary drain of the same caliber is reintroduced, but the tip is placed above the biliary stricture/stent. This technique maintains percutaneous access and allows bile to flow across the dilated stricture/stented lesion.
3. The short tube is capped for 1–2 weeks. If the patient remains asymptomatic and the stent is patent on follow-up cholangiography, the drain is removed.

26. Describe in sequence what should be done in case of severe hemobilia after placement of a percutaneous biliary drain.

1. Type and cross-match blood, order serial complete blood counts, and transfuse as necessary.
2. Upsize catheter diameter to tamponade bleeds.

If the above steps fail:

3. Perform a sinogram over the wire to identify the vascular communication with the tract.
4. If the communication is identified, embolize with gelfoam.

If the above steps fail:

5. Get a hepatic angiogram with the percutaneous drain removed over a wire to expose the bleed.
6. If a hepatic branch is identified to be bleeding, it is embolized (gelfoam and/or coils).

If the above steps fail:

7. Perform an empirical hepatic artery embolization to reduce the hepatic perfusion pressure.

27. Why should there be an oral intake assessment for patients with external biliary drainage?

Normal bile flow is 400–800 ml/day and contains a large quantity of essential electrolytes, which are normally recirculated through bowel absorption. After external biliary drainage, however, this volume of fluid and the electrolytes are lost and should be replaced. If the patient's oral intake is inadequate, the bile output should be replaced milliliter for milliliter with Ringer's lactate solution.

28. Describe the general care and positioning of all percutaneous catheters, drains, and tubes.

Catheters and drains should be sewed to the skin before the patient leaves the interventional suite. This process should include "finger-trap" sutures and sterile dressing. The dressing serves as a sterile barrier and, even more importantly, prevents undue catching on the patient's clothes or bed.

Catheters and drains should not be secured to bed rails. This approach increases the chances of malpositioning or dislodgement. Bags should be safely pinned to the patient's hospital gown and should not be allowed to fill completely before they are emptied. This strategy prevents the weight of bags from pulling or dislodging the tubes.

29. How often should catheters and drains be cleansed and redressed?
They should be dressed daily, and the site should also be cleansed daily with peroxide (or its equivalent).

30. What is the best way to ensure adequate catheter and drain care on discharge?
Patient education and/or education of the patient's family/care provider. Oral and written instructions for the care of tubes/drains should be included. The patient's/care provider's ability to care for the tube should be assessed. The time spent educating the patient will result in a decreased number of follow-up complications and improved quality of life.

31. A patient, initially diagnosed with bile duct obstruction, continues to have fever and pain within the week after successful placement of a percutaneous biliary drain (PBD). What should be done?
- Abdomen and pelvis CECT: to evaluate for perihepatic abscess, biloma, or tube malposition
- Negative CECT: perform a cholangiogram through the existing PBD to look for an isolated biliary segment—that is, an intrahepatic biliary tree segment that is not drained. The posterior biliary segment is a common segment to be isolated, and an RAO projection is the most revealing projection to look for lack of bile duct opacification of the posterior biliary segment.

BIBLIOGRAPHY

1. Butch RJ, Mueller PR, Ferrucci JT, et al: Drainage of pelvic abscesses through the greater sciatic foramen. Radiology 158:487–491, 1986.
2. Caliendo MV, Lee DE, Queiroz R, Waldman DL: Sclerotherapy with use of doxycycline after percutaneous drainage of postoperative lymphoceles. J Cardiovasc Intervent Radiol 12:73–77, 2001.
3. Ho CS, Yee AC, McPherson R: Complications of surgical and percutaneous nonendoscopic gastrostomy: review of 233 patients. Gastroenterology 95:1206–1210, 1988.
4. Kanterman RY, Darcy MD: Complications of the fluoroscopically guided percutaneous gastrostomy. Semin Intervent Radiol 13:317–327, 1996.
5. LaBerge JM, Kerlan RK, Gordon RL, Ring EJ: Nonoperative treatment of enteric fistulas: Results in 53 patients. J Vasc Intervent Radiol 3:353–357, 1992.
6. Lambiase RE, Cornan JJ, Dorfman GS, et al: Postoperative abscesses with enteric communications: percutaneous treatment. Radiology 171:497–500, 1989.
7. Morgan RA, Adam AN: Malignant biliary disease: percutaneous interventions. Tech Vasc Intervent Radiol 4:147–152, 2001.
8. Nemcek AA Jr, Vogelzang RL: Managing complications of acute pancreatitis. In Thoracic and Visceral Non-vascular Interventions, Genitourinary Interventions. SCVIR Syllabus, 1997.
9. Sandhu J: Drainage of deep pelvic abscesses including transgluteal, transrectal and transvaginal approaches. In Thoracic and Visceral Non-vascular Interventions, Genitourinary Interventions. SCVIR Syllabus, 1997.
10. Savader SJ: Management of biliary drainage catheters. In Biliary Interventions, SCVIR Syllabus, 1995.
11. Venbrux AC, Osterman FA Jr: Percutaneous management of benign biliary strictures. Tech Vasc Intervent Radiol 4:141–146, 2001.

37. MUSCULOSKELETAL INTERVENTION

Wael E. A. Saad, MBBCh

1. List the indications for performing percutaneous vertebroplasty.

Primary indication: local pain relief for vertebrogenic pain in cases of compression fractures and bone marrow infiltration.

Secondary/relative indications: prevention of further vertebral body collapse, prophylaxis against collapse of vertebral bodies adjacent to primary vertebroplasty, and prevention of kyphosis in osteoporosis. These indications are controversial and subject to ongoing research and debate.

2. Describe the ideal patient who responds well to vertebroplasty.

Patients with well-defined focal levels (preferably one) (Fig. 1) of pain and tenderness that correspond well to vertebral compression fractures by plain radiographs and/or magnetic resonance imaging (MRI).

Patients with acute fractures and acute on top of chronic fractures respond better than patients with chronic, sclerotic vertebral fractures

3. Before a percutaneous vertebroplasty is performed, what kind of imaging evaluation is required? For what conditions should the patient be evaluated?

Other causes of back pain should be ruled out, such as disc herniation, spinal stenosis, or facet or sacroiliac disease. These conditions can be best evaluated using spine MRI. In addition, MR

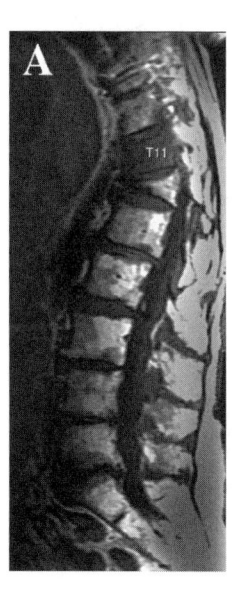

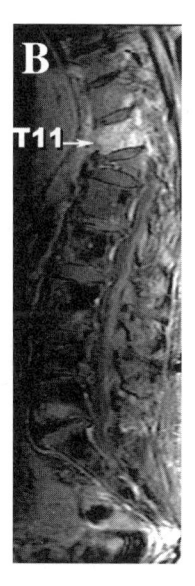

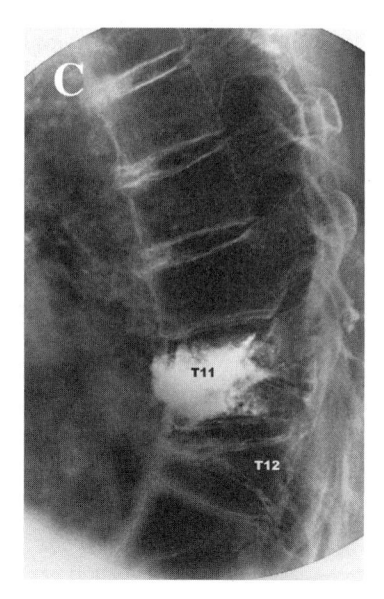

FIGURE 1. Patient with acute back pain. T1-weighted MRI (**A**) demonstrates low signal in the T11 vertebral body that represents edema. There is a compression fracture of T12, although no signal variation is consistent with an acute injury. This fracture represents an old injury and is probably not the cause of acute pain. T1 fat-saturated image after gadolinum injection (**B**) demonstrates abnormally high signal in the same vertebral body, verifying the diagnosis. Vertebroplasty was done at the T11 level (**C**) with excellent pain relief.

evaluation is sensitive for evaluating the chronicity of vertebral compression. Edema (STIR sequences) is a sign of an acute process that responds best to vertebroplasty.

4. Is concomitant disc disease or vertebral disease a contraindication to performing percutaneous vertebroplasty?
Concomitant disc disease and vertebral disease do not contraindicate percutaneous vertebroplasty; however, they may confound the results and temper the perceived success of the procedure.

5. List the infiltrative processes for which percutaneous vertebroplasty has been reported to be successful in treating associated spinal pain.
- Hemangiomas
- Myeloma
- Lymphoma
- Leukemia
- Giant-cell tumor
- Aneurysmal bone cyst
- Metastasis

Percutaneous vertebroplasty is effective in these conditions even though the risk of minor complications may be somewhat higher in these patients.

6. Explain the value of computerized tomography (CT) in the prevertebroplasty evaluation of patients with infiltrative processes.
CT is valuable in evaluating the integrity of the vertebral body cortex, particularly in its posterior aspect, which, if not intact, may cause spinal compression during or after vertebroplasty.

7. Discuss the value of percutaneous vertebroplasty in cases of vertebral hemangiomas.
Percutaneous vertebroplasty may be performed for pain relief and reinforcement of the vertebral body, as in other lesions for which percutaneous vertebroplasty is used. In addition, percutaneous vertebroplasty may be used to devascularize the hemangioma to diminish operative blood loss.

8. How effective is percutaneous vertebroplasty in managing vertebrogenic pain?
About 85–90% of patients with osteoporosis experience dramatic or complete relief of pain within 72 hours after percutaneous vertebroplasty. In addition, 60–85% of patients with neoplastic vertebrogenic pain experience dramatic or complete relief of pain within 72 hours after percutaneous vertebroplasty.

9. What is the complication rate of percutaneous vertebroplasty?
About 1–2% of patients experience transient exacerbation of pain, which is usually dermatomal in distribution.

Three percent experience **minor complications,** including minor hemorrhage, transient exacerbation of vertebrogenic pain, minor cement symptoms, and asymptomatic cement pulmonary emboli.

Four percent experience **major complications,** including significant hemorrhage, infection or osteomyelitis, significant symptomatic pulmonary emboli, and irreversible nerve root or spinal cord injury

10. List the routes of cement extravasation related to percutaneous vertebroplasty. How common is cement extravasation?
- Epidural
- Paravertebral
- Foraminal (most symptomatic)

- Intradiscal (up to 5–10% of cases)
- Foraminal vein extravasation

The incidence of extravasation is reported to be 1–2% in patients with osteoporosis and 5–10% in patients with neoplastic processes.

11. How does percutaneous vertebroplasty alleviate pain?

The exact mechanism for pain relief is unknown. However, there are two possibilities:
1. Nerve receptor neurotoxicity due to the chemical effect of the cement.
2. Internal immobilization of the fracture, which reduces bone fragment motion and its associated pain.

12. Does the vertebral height increase (become restored) after vertebroplasty?

Injection of cement during percutaneous vertebroplasty may result directly in height restoration at the particular level of the vertebroplasty. This effect can be improved by treating patients under active hyperextension. However, the greatest overall height restoration results from the improved, more erect posture of the patient secondary to back pain relief.

13. What preparation is injected in fluoroscopically guided vertebroplasties?

Polymethylmethacrylate (PMMA) cement, admixed with 25–30% (by weight) of a radiopaque substance such as barium sulfate, tantalum, tungsten, or zirconium dioxide.

14. Describe the needle approaches and their uses in percutaneous vertebroplasty.

Transpedicular route: most commonly used. The lateral position of the needle usually requires a bilateral approach.

Parapedicular route: used in patients with small pedicles or for the thoracic vertebrae. The needle is more medial in position, which may permit the vertebroplasty to be completed with a unilateral approach. This route is associated with an increased incidence of pneumothoraces and renal injury.

Posterolateral route: should be used with caution above the level of L2 to reduce pleural injury.

Lateral and anterolateral route: required for cervical vertebroplasty.

15. How much cement should be instilled for a successful vertebroplasty?

The cement should be confined to the anterior 67–75% of the vertebral body. Biomechanical strength and stiffness can be achieved with approximately 2 ml of PMMA in the thoracic vertebra, 4 ml in the thoracolumbar region, and 6 ml in the lower lumbar vertebra.

16. Describe kyphoplasty. How is it different from vertebroplasty?

Kyphoplasty is an imaging-guided spinal intervention involving an inflatable balloon in the vertebral body. These procedures are designed to elevate the vertebral body endplates. Immediately after the deflation of the balloons, cement is injected into the void created by the balloon. The primary objective of kyphoplasty is vertebral body height restoration in addition to the objectives of vertebroplasty (pain relief by internal immobilization of the vertebral body).

17. What are the advantages of correcting kyphosis?

Kyphosis has been associated with undesirable gastrointestinal sequelae as well as reduction in the lung vital capacity. Kyphoplasty aims to improve indirectly the pulmonary and gastrointestinal functions of such kyphotic patients.

18. Summarize the results of kyphoplasty.

- Height restoration is achieved in 70–71% of patients.
- Vertebrae improve height by 25% to 62%; the degree of improvement depends on the age and degree of the initial compression fracture.

- The average increase in height of the anterior-to-mid portion of the vertebral body is 3.7–4.7 mm
- Major complication rates range from 1.0% to 2.4%.
- Improvement in vertebrogenic pain is seen in 90% of patients.

19. What are the advantages and major disadvantage of percutaneous bone biopsy compared with open surgical bone biopsy?
Advantages
- Avoids general anesthesia
- Lower cost
- Can be performed on an outpatient basis
- Diminished morbidity

Major disadvantage
- Provides reduced size and quality of tissue samples. However, sufficient material is usually provided for a diagnosis

20. Briefly discuss the planning of a percutaneous bone biopsy.
All biopsies of potentially malignant lesions should be planned in conjunction with the orthopedic surgeon in terms of approach and route of the needle since needle tract excision should be performed by the surgeon for a curative tumor resection.

Most aspiration biopsies are initially obtained in conjunction with a cytopathologist. If a diagnostic aspirate cannot be obtained, a core biopsy is required.

21. What is a trephine needle? How is it used?
Trephine needles are typically 12–14 gauge and have a serrated or smooth cutting edge used to penetrate through cortical bone. After cortical penetration the trephine needle can be used to aspirate biopsy fragments. Coaxial aspiration needle or core biopsies can be obtained with other needles.

22. Give examples of lesions that are best not biopsied or should be biopsied with caution if they occur in the vertebral column.
Expansile lesions such as aneurysmal bone cysts (ABCs) or giant-cell tumors are poor candidates for vertebral bone biopsies. **Hemorrhagic lesions** such as renal cell carcinoma and thyroid metastases can bleed and potentially compress the spinal cord.

23. List the bony lesions that may include radiofrequency ablation (RFA) in their management.
1. Osteoid osteomas (Fig. 2)
2. Painful skeletal metastases
3. Chondroblastomas
4. Chordoma
5. Epithelioid hemangio-endotheliomas

The first two are the most common indications for bone RFA.

24. Can RFA of vertebral tumors be combined with vertebroplasty of the same vertebra?
Vertebroplasty following vertebral RFA of a neoplastic process has been described. However, the experience is limited. Some authors have performed the vertebroplasty 3–7 days after the RFA session, and others perform both procedures sequentially in the same setting.

25. What is the advantage of combining the two procedures?
The vertebroplasty adds structure and support to the vertebral body following RFA, thus reducing the incidence of post-RFA vertebral collapse. In addition, some authors believe that RFA allows better cement distribution during the following vertebroplasty.

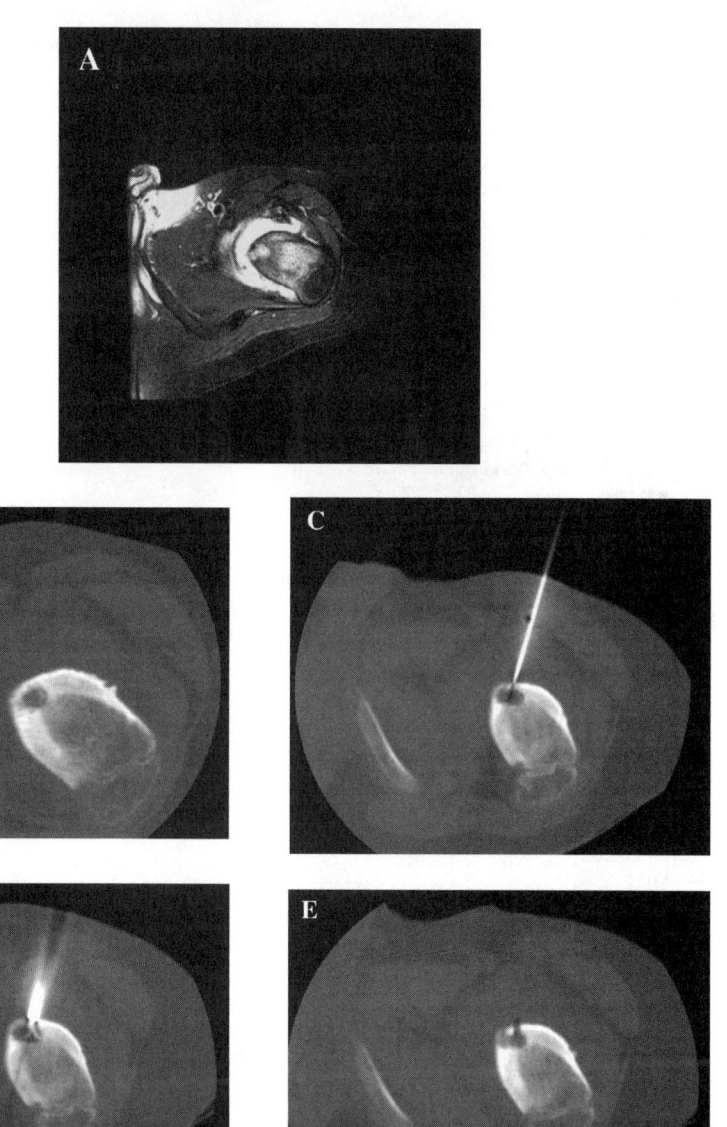

FIGURE 2. MRI (**A**) and CT (**B**) of left hip demonstrate a lesion characteristic of an osteoid osteoma. A drill was placed in the bone (**C**) over the lesion and an RFA probe (**D**) was placed. A biopsy of the nidus was obtained before ablation. Postablation scan (**E**) demonstrates a hole within the bone. The patient improved clinically.

26. List the inclusion and exclusion criteria for RFA with or without vertebroplasty.
Inclusion criteria
- Ineffective conventional treatment (radiation therapy)
- Pain refractory to analgesics
- High risk of neurologic deficit
- Increased risk of fractures

Exclusion criteria
- Osteoblastic neoplasms
- Paraplegia
- Coagulopathy

27. Summarize the results of RFA of vertebral metastases.
- Technical success rate: 100%
- Relative pain reduction rate: 74%
- Improved back pain-related disability: 27%
- Improved general health: 30%
- Stable general health: 60%
- Worse general health: 10%

28. Discuss the disadvantages of external beam radiation (conventional therapy) compared with RFA in treating painful skeletal metastases.

1. Higher levels of radiation required for local tumor control can expose the patient to an increased risk for pathologic radiation myelopathy (functional up to 3 months)

2. Radiation effects can take weeks to a month to provide adequate pain relief. RFA provides faster results.

3. Radiation therapy often has poor pain relief and frequent relapses compared with the initial data about RFA

29. Summarize the results of pain relief after RFA of skeletal metastases throughout the body (e.g., pelvis, ribs, sacrum).
Pain relief with adjunct pain management:
- Before RFA: 37% of patients
- 1week after RFA: 76% of patients
- 4weeks after RFA: 84% of patients
- 6months after RFA: 100% of patients who survived.

30. List the theories explaining the mechanism of pain relief of skeletal metastases after RFA.
- RFA (destruction) of local pain receptors
- Tumor debulking, which reduces tissue tension
- Tumor cell debulking, resulting in a reduction of pain mediators released by tumor cells
- Inhibition of osteoclast activity, which may cause pain

31. How are bone RFA sessions performed?
Bone RFA is usually performed under real-time CT guidance, although ultrasound guidance (particularly in the appendicular skeleton) has been described. If thick cortex needs to be traversed, a 14-gauge trephine needle is placed through the dense bone, followed by insertion of the RFA probe. If there is no thick cortical bone, the RFA probe is placed directly into the lesion.

32. What minimal distance between the RFA probe and the thecal sac is required to reduce the risk of spinal cord harm during vertebral RFA?
Harmful temperatures in the spinal cord have been documented at a distance of less than or equal to 5 mm between the probe and the thecal sac.

33. How can the risk of pathologic fractures following RFA of the appendicular skeleton be reduced?

Bones are at risk of pathologic fractures if the neoplastic process (benign or malignant) involves more than 50% of the cortex, particularly in weight-bearing bones. Percutaneous cementoplasty after treatment with RFA may reduce this risk and provide the added benefit of postprocedural safe ambulation as well as pain relief.

34. What factors may cause technical failures in RFA of osteoid osteomas?
- Inability to identify the lesion clearly under imaging during the procedure and/or poor positioning of the RFA probe
- Inability of the RFA probe to produce or reach ablative temperatures

35. List the indications for image-guided RFA of osteoid osteomas.
- Lesion visualized by fluoroscopy or CT
- Failed medical therapy
- Patient under consideraion for surgical treatment
- Failed previous surgery

36. Summarize the results of RFA of osteoid osteomas.
- Technical success: 89–100% (mean: 99%)
- Clinical success: 89–95% (mean: 90%)
- Recurrence rate: 0–50% (mean: 8%)

The recurrence rate (when mentioned) is 6–8% in large case series but has been reported in up to 50% of patients in a small case series of 9 patients.

37. What is the clinical success rate of RFA of osteoid osteomas that are recurrent after RFA and/or surgical excision?

The clinical success rate is 60% in this population compared with 90% in lesions treated with RFA de novo.

38. Define recurrence of osteoid osteomas and describe the features of lesions that are more likely to recur.

Recurrence is relapse of typical pain at the same site after a period of no pain. The vast majority of recurrences after RFA occur within a year after RFA. The standard accepted in the orthopedic literature is a minimum of two years to establish cure.

Large lesions are more likely to recur than smaller lesions.

39. What sites of osteoid osteomas are most amenable for RFA?

Weight-bearing bones, pelvis, upper arm, and forearm. RFA of the spine and hands has a higher rate of nerve injury. Furthermore, convalescence after hand surgery is shorter than after surgery of the lower extremity.

40. List the other percutaneous methods for treating osteoid osteomas.
- Percutaneous hollow needle excision
- Percutaneous nidus drilling and fragmentation, followed by ethanol injection
- Percutaneous interstitial laser photocoagulation

41. How many of the percutaneous bone biopsies of lesions suspected to be osteoid osteomas return positive?

From 36% to 73% of biopsies return positive. However, the clinical picture of pain that increases at night and is relieved with ibuprofen, coupled with radiographic findings, is almost always diagnostic. Many authors treat such lesions as osteoid osteomas without pathologic confirmation.

BIBLIOGRAPHY

1. Belkoff SM, Mathis JM, Jasper LE, et al: The biomechanics of vertebroplasty. The effect of cement volume on mechanical behavior. Spine 26:1537–1541, 2001.
2. Callstrom MR, Charboneau JM, Goetz MP, et al: Painful metastases involving bone: feasibility of percutaneous CT- and US-guided radiofrequency ablation. Radiology 224:87–97, 2002.
3. Clark W, El-Khoury GY: Percutaneous bone biopsies. In Thoracic and Visceral Non-vascular Interventions, Genitourinary Interventions. SCVIR Syllabus, 1997.
4. Cotton A, Deramond H, Cortet B, et al: Preoperative percutaneous injection of methyl methacrylate and N-butyl cyanoacrylate in vertebral hemangiomas. Am J Neuroradiol 17:137–142, 1996.
5. Do HM: Magnetic resonance imaging in the evaluation of patients for percutaneous vertebroplasty. Top Magn Reson Imag 11:235–244, 2000.
6. Dupuy D, Hong R, Oliver B, et al: Radiofrequency ablation of spinal tumors: temperature distribution in spinal canal. Am J Roentgenol 175:1263–1266, 2000.
7. Garfin SR, Yuan HA, Reiley MA: Kyphoplasty and vertebroplasty for the treatment of painful osteoporotic compression fractures. Spine 26:1511–1515, 2001.
8. Groenemeyer DH, Schirp S, Gevargez A: Image-guided radiofrequency ablation of spinal tumors: Preliminary experience with an expandable array electrode. Cancer J 8:33–39, 2002.
9. Jensen ME, Evans AJ, Mathis JM, et al: Percutaneous polymethylmethacrylate vertebroplasty in the treatment of osteoporotic vertebral body compression fractures: Technical aspects. Am J Neuroradiol 18:1897–1904, 1997.
10. Neeman Z, Wood BJ: Radiofrequency ablation beyond the liver. Tech Vasc Intervent Radiol 5:156–163, 2002.
11. Ortiz AO, Zoarski GH, Beckerman M: Kyphoplasty. Tech Vasc Intervent Radiol 5:239–249, 2002.
12. Ratliff J, Nguyen T, Heiss J: Root and spinal cord compression from methylmethacrylate vertebroplasty. Spine 26:E300–302, 2001.
13. Rosenthal DI, Hornicek FJ, Torriani M, et al: Osteoid osteoma: Percutaneous treatment with radiofrequency energy. Radiology 229:171–175, 2003.
14. Schaefer O, Lohrmann C, Herling M, et al: Combined radiofrequency thermal ablation and percutaneous cementoplasty treatment of a pathologic fracture. J Vasc Intervent Radiol 13:1047–1050, 2002.
15. Schaefer O, Lohrmann C, Markmiller M, et al: Technical innovation: Combined treatment of a spinal metastasis with radiofrequency heat ablation and vertebroplasty. Am J Roentgenol 180:1075–1077, 2003.
16. Silverman SL: The clinical consequences of vertebral compression fracture. Bone 13:S27-S31, 1992.
17. Venbrux AC, Montague BJ, Murphy KPJ, et al: Image-guided percutaneous radiofrequency ablation for osteoid osteomas. J Vasc Intervent Radiol 14:375–380, 2003.
18. Zoarski GH, Snow P, Olan WJ, et al: Percutaneous vertebroplasty or osteoporotic compression fractures: quantitative prospective evaluation of long-term outcomes. J Vasc Intervent Radiol 13:139–148, 2002.
19. Zoarski GH, Stallmeyer MJB, Obuchowski A: Percutaneous vertebroplasty: A to Z. Tech Vasc Intervent Radiol 5:223–238, 2002.

38. IMAGE-GUIDED BIOPSY
Wael E. A. Saad, MBBCh

1. How is the gauge (size number) of the biopsy needle determined?
The number of needles that can be stacked across one inch is the gauge of the needle; i.e., if you can put 18 needles of the same size adjacent to one another in a space spanning 1 inch, the gauge of those needles is 18. Therefore, the larger the gauge, the thinner the needle.

2. List the types of percutaneous needle biopsies.
- Aspiration technique
- Menghini-type cutting needle technique
- Tru-Cut technique

3. Describe the aspiration technique.
The needle (which is usually 20 gauge or thinner) is adjacent to the target. Suction is then applied, and the needle is inserted into the lesion as numerous, repetitive, short, rapid passing movements are made through the lesion. The sample/aspirate is collected in the attached syringe.

4. Describe the capillary method of aspiration needle biopsy.
This method is similar to the aspiration technique, but no suction is applied by a syringe to the skinny needle being used. This method is preferred by some physicians when the sample/aspirate is bloody (e.g., cases of thyroid disease).

5. Describe the Menghini -type cutting needle technique.
This method involves making one pass under aspiration using a core biopsy needle. The needle is hollow, and its bevel is sharpened.

6. Describe the Tru-Cut method.
The needle is coaxial with an inner tissue stylet and an outer cutting cannula. The needle tip is first placed immediately proximal to the target lesion. The stylet is advanced into the lesion, and the cutting cannula is moved over the stylet, thus shaving the tissue sample.

7. How many needle passes by an 18-guage and a 20-gauge needle are required to obtain the same sample size obtained by one pass using a 14-gauge needle?
- 3 passes for the 18-gauge needle
- 6 passes for the 20-gauge needle

8. When is it advantageous to use aspiration needles (20-gauge and thinner) instead of core biopsy needles (18-gauge and thicker)?
When only a confirmatory diagnosis of malignancy is required and a high level of safety is desired.

9. Does core biopsy needle size in liver biopsies affect bleeding rates?
Yes: 14- and 16-gauge needles have a higher bleeding rate than 18- and 20-gauge needles.

10. What can be done to reduce the bleeding risks after core needle biopsies?
Prebiopsy correction of coagulopathies and discontinuing antiplatelet medications (such as aspirin) 7 days before the biopsy. In addition, embolization of the biopsy track with gelfoam can be considered.

11. If a mass is suspected to be a lymphoma by imaging criteria, what kind of samples should be obtained in addition to core samples?
Aspiration samples should be obtained for flow-cytometry evaluation.

12. What is the major predisposing factor for developing a pneumothorax after a lung biopsy?
Emphysema.

13. Describe the methods used to reduce the risk of pneumothorax development after lung biopsies.
- Minimize the size of the needle. Aspiration needle biopsy is usually satisfactory for sampling routine primary lung masses (Fig. 1).
- Minimizing the pathway through the aerated lung parenchyma by planning the trajectory of the needle and preferring to traverse consolidations and fibrous attachments.
- Avoiding obvious blebs.
- Minimize the number of needle passes through the pleura.

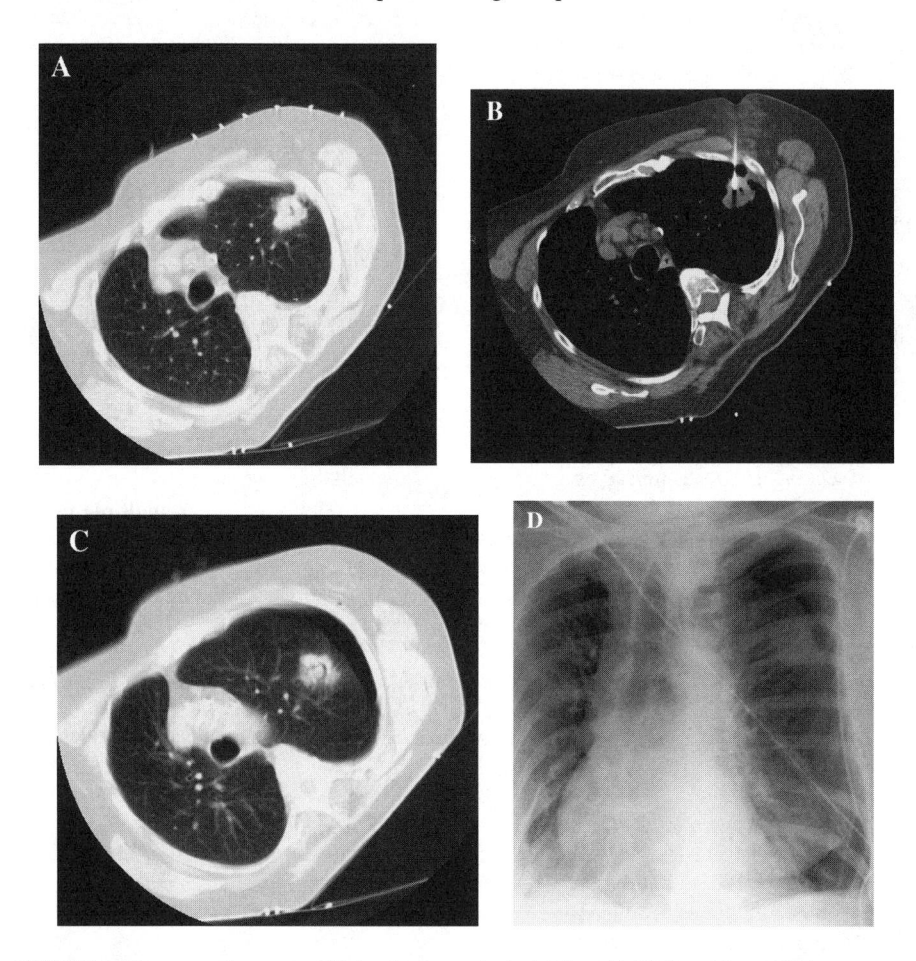

FIGURE 1. Biopsy was done under CT for a lung mass in the left lung (**A, B**). Post-biopsy CT demonstrates a pneumothorax (**C**). The patient was clinically stable. One hour after biopsy a film showed an increasing pneumothorax (**D**). The patient became increasingly short of breath. A chest tube was placed (**E**) with near immediate resolution (**F**). The chest tube was pulled in 48 hours with no residual pneumothorax (**G**).

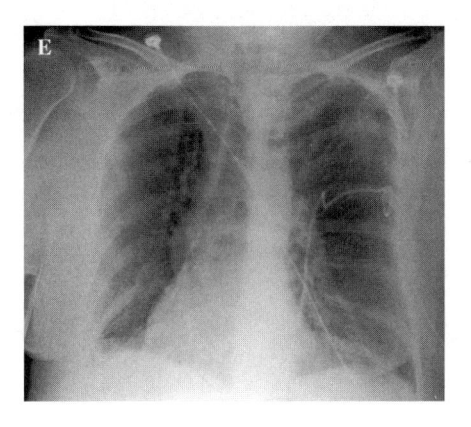

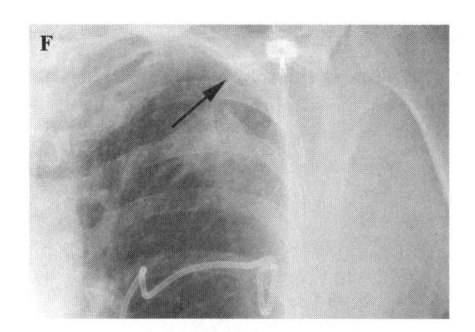

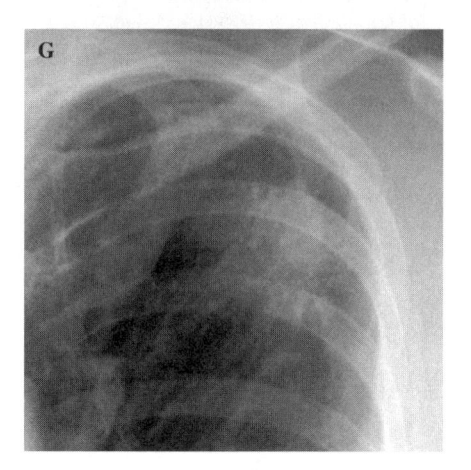

FIGURE 1. (continued)

14. **How can you minimize the needle passes through the pleura when multiple needle passes are required to obtain an adequate sample from the target mass?**
    A coaxial system can be used by placing one larger needle through the pleura and making multiple needle passes through that needle with a thinner needle, thus creating one needle pass through the pleura and multiple passes through the target lesion.

15. **List the contraindications for transthoracic needle biopsy.**
    Absolute: totally uncooperative patient.
    Relative: severe bullous emphysema, pulmonary hypertension, uncorrectable coagulopathy.

16. **How can the visceral pleural be avoided during biopsy of a postmediastinal mass via a paravertebral approach?**
    Injecting saline and/or lidocaine solution into the paraspinal soft tissues elevates the pleura off the spine and provides a route through which a posterior mediastinal mass can be biopsied.

17. **List the complications encountered after lung biopsies.**
    - Pneumothorax (10–60%)
    - Pneumothorax requiring a chest tube (8%)
    - Hemoptysis (5%)
    - Infection (rare)

- Neoplastic seeding of needle tract (rare)
- Air embolism (rare)
- Mortality (0.01–0.05%)

18. Describe the preferred target area in the kidney for a "random" renal parenchymal biopsy.

The ideal site is an area that will yield an adequate cortical sample with minimal risk of bleeding (Fig. 2). The target area should be superficial and avoid the medullary region where larger vessels reside. The best area fulfilling the above description is the lateral cortex of the lower pole of the kidney.

19. How can renal masses be biopsied to evaluate for primary malignancy?

Renal masses should not be biopsied for fear of seeding and thus advancing the staging of the neoplasm. Multimodality imaging with or without imaging follow-up is accurate enough to determine suspicious lesions that should be resected (partial or total nephrectomy) without biopsy.

20. With all other factors equal, which is more likely to bleed—a renal biopsy or a liver biopsy?

Despite the best techniques, bleeding is more common with renal parenchymal biopsies and is frequently visualized around the organ by ultrasound or CT.

21. List the advantages and disadvantages of the use of ultrasound in percutaneous biopsies.
Advantages
- Realtime
- Multiplanar
- Portable
- Readily available

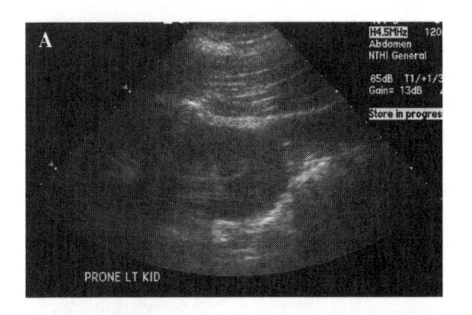

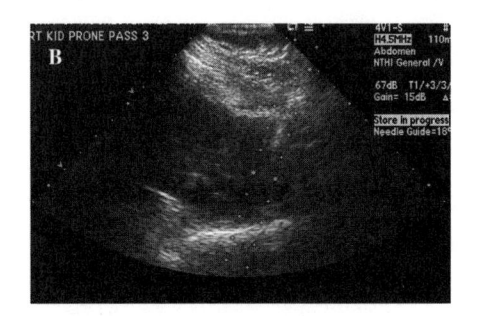

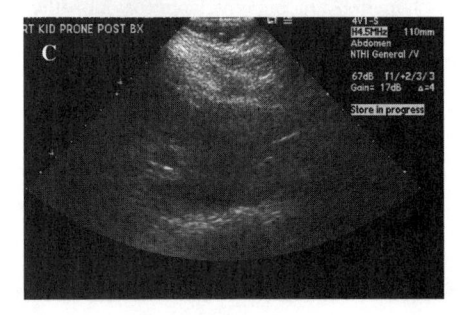

FIGURE 2. Ultrasound image of a native right kidney before biopsy (**A**). The needle is placed through the guide just through the capsule (**B**). It is important to aim the guide so that the needle will travel through the renal cortex. After the biopsy gun is fired, the kidney must be re-imaged to exclude bleeding complications (**C**).

- Safer/lack of radiation
- Time-saving

Disadvantages
- Operator-dependent
- Limited by overlying bone, gas, and lung

22. Discuss the advantages and disadvantages of freehand and needle-guide techniques during ultrasound-guided percutaneous biopsies.

Freehand technique is technically demanding and requires experience. However, it provides flexibility, allowing the operator to select the appropriate needle entry site to reduce the length of the needle path, avoid overlying structures, and optimize needle visibility. In addition, freehand technique allows real-time probe adjustments to compensate for needle deviation and/or patient movement.

23. List the indications for percutaneous liver biopsy.

Diffuse disease
- Chronic hepatitis
- Cirrhosis
- Metabolic liver disease
- Hepatic transplant rejection

Focal disease
- Liver mass in patients with or without known malignancym (Fig. 3)
- Liver mass in cirrhotic patients

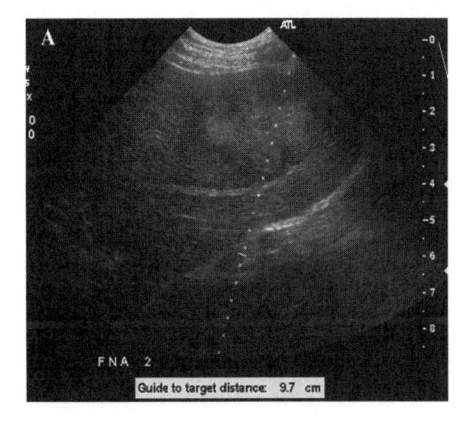

FIGURE 3. A mass is seen on ultrasound (**A**). The biopsy guide is turned on (**B**), and the needle is advanced under real time. The needle is seen at the edge of the mass *(arrow)*. After the core biopsy is obtained, it is important to re-image the liver to exclude any immediate complications (**C**). Bleeding is the most frequent complication. Pain at the skin site is normal; however, if the patient complains of internal abdominal pain after a biopsy, an immediate CT scan should be obtained to exclude bleeding or a biliary leak.

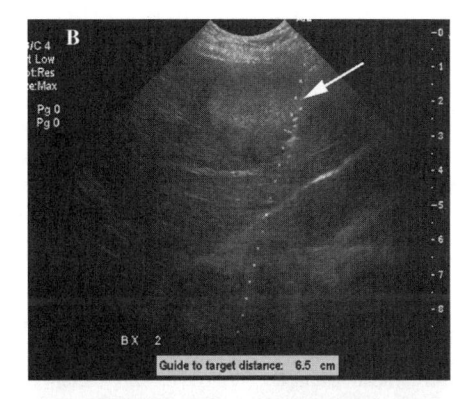

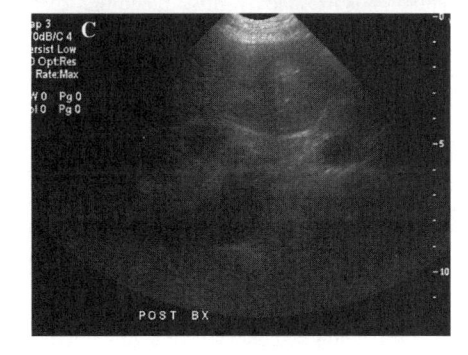

24. What lesions can be unsafe (relative contraindications) for percutaneous liver biopsies?
- **Hemangiomas** are vascular and can bleed if biopsied. In addition, they are difficult to diagnose pathologically from aspiration samples. Tagged red blood cell scans and MR are specific for this diagnosis, especially if the lesion does not exhibit rapid growth and/or malignant features on imaging follow-up.
- **Vascular tumors** (e.g., carcinoids) in a subcapsular location.

25. List the advantages and major disadvantage of a subcostal approach to liver biopsies compared with an intercostal approach.
Advantages
- A subcostal approach avoids the pleural surface and thus reduces related pleural complications.
- A subcostal approach avoids the intercostal neurovascular bundle and thus reduces puncture site hematomas. Furthermore, the subcostal approach is generally felt to be less painful.

Major disadvantage
- A subcostal approach may have a longer needle path to the target lesion compared with an intercostals approach, and some lesions may not be optimally visualized.

26. Describe the preferred route for biopsy of a hepatic subcapsular mass.
Adirect orthogonal needle biopsy is usually not advised because of the increased risk of bleeding (especially vascular lesions) and the potential for capsular/peritoneal tumor seeding. An effort should be made to select a path that interposes at least 2–3 cm of liver parenchyma between the puncture site on the liver surface and the lesion. This can be achieved by modifying the direction of the ultrasound beam.

27. Summarize patient management after liver biopsy.
A gray-scale and Doppler ultrasound evaluation is performed to rule out frank hemorrhage or a growing subcapsular hematoma. The patient is monitored for 4 hours, preferably lying on his or her right side,especially if an intercostal approach was taken. This position helps tamponade any postprocedural hemorrhage.

28. What is the complication rate after liver biopsies? What conditions predispose patients to a higher complication rate?
The complication rate is 0.1–1.0%. Complications are relatively more common in patients with severe disease, coagulopathy, ascites, and biopsy of hypervascular lesions.

29. What is the most common complication after percutaneous liver biopsy? When should the interventionalist be concerned?
Pain is the most common complication and is experienced when the biopsy needle traverses the liver capsule and/or injures the subcostal nerve plexus. Pain is usually experienced at the puncture site but can be referred to the left shoulder if the needle passes the diaphragm or the diaphragm is irritated by minor bleeding.

The interventionalist should become concerned if pain persists, especially if peritoneal signs are found. Obviously, signs of hypovolemia should prompt fluid resuscitation and investigative imaging.

30. List the indications for percutaneous pancreatic biopsies.
- Confirm diagnosis of pancreatic adenocarcinoma (accuracy of 80–95%).
- Characterize other pancreatic lesions such as pseudocysts and abscesses.
- Differentiate chronic pancreatitis from neoplasm (Fig. 4).
- Evaluate for rejection in pancreatic transplants.

31. What is the preferred imaging modality for guiding pancreatic biopsies?
As in any percutaneous image-guided biopsy, the imaging modality that best demonstrates the lesion is preferred. CT localization may be preferred in cases of pancreatic biopsy because it

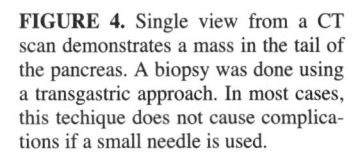

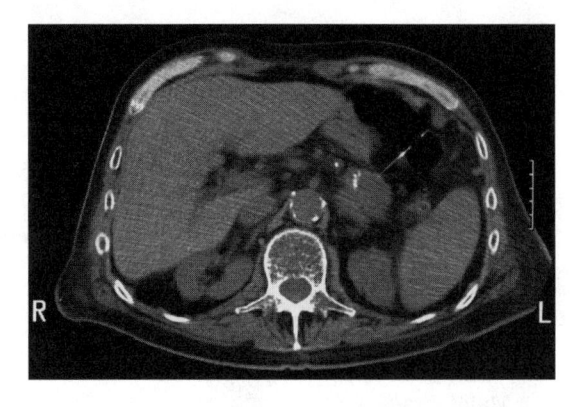

FIGURE 4. Single view from a CT scan demonstrates a mass in the tail of the pancreas. A biopsy was done using a transgastric approach. In most cases, this techique does not cause complications if a small needle is used.

offers the option of anterior or posterior approach, and CT often demonstrates pancreatic lesions that are not clearly defined by ultrasound. Ultrasound is particularly handicapped in lesions that are close to bowel (due to overlying bowel gas). If the lesion is visualized by ultrasound, ultrasound is preferred due to its versatility.

32. What trajectories are used for percutaneous biopsy of the the pancreas?
Numerous trajectories have been described, including transperitoneal and retroperitoneal trajectories. The pancreas is a deep-seated organ that is difficult to biopsy without traversing other viscera. Transhepatic, transgastric, and transduodenal biopsies have been described without consequences. In fact, the former two routes are preferred by many interventionalists.

33. List the complications that can occur after percutaneous pancreatic biopsies.
The complication rate is approximately 1%. Complications may include mesenteric hematomas, pancreatic duct injury, and injury to surrounding organs. The most common causes of mortality are pancreatitis and sepsis.

34. What is the preferred image guidance modality for adrenal biopsies?
CT is preferred for small adrenal lesions, and ultrasound is preferred for larger lesions.

35. List the complications arising from percutaneous adrenal biopsies.
The complication rate is 5.3–8.4%, and 40–45% of these complications are considered major. The following is a list of the more common complications:
- Adrenal hemorrhage
- Pneumothorax
- Hepatic or renal hemorrhage
- Pancreatitis
- Track seeding
- Adrenal abscesses

36. What size of percutaneous transhepatic biliary tract is required for a transhepatic biliary biopsy?
A9-French tract is enough for a fluoro-guided transhepatic biopsy. However, a 16-French tract is required for a choledochofibroscope-guided biopsy.

37. List the techniques used to perform transhepatic biliary biopsies.
Fluoroscopically
- Aspiration cytology
- Brush/scrape biopsy
- Needle biopsy
- Atherectomy biopsy technique

Endoscopically
- Brush/scrape biopsy
- Biopsy forceps (bioptome)

38. Which two techniques are least traumatic in detecting malignancy? What are their sensitivities?

The least traumatic techniques are usually the least sensitive. Obviously, aspiration is the least traumatic method, and its sensitivity is approximately 34%. Next is the brush/scrape biopsy technique, which has a sensitivity of 60–68%.

39. What other visceral structure can be biopsied using the brush technique?

The ureters and urethra.

40. Describe the brush biopsy technique.

The brush is not advanced bare. A vascular sheath is advanced over a wire, and the brush is advanced through the sheath to the level of the target lesion. The brush is then unsheathed by pulling back the sheath and exposing the brush. The brush is passed to and fro reciprocally and then re-sheathed. The brush is then removed, the brush wire is cut, and the brush is sent to the pathology lab in total.

41. Which organs can be biopsied from a transvenous approach?
- Liver (Fig. 5)
- Sometimes kidney
- Transvenous adrenal or parathyroid vein sampling is not tissue sampling; hence, it is not a biopsy. It is instead a method of venous blood sampling to evaluate for functional tumors

42. When are transjugular hepatic or renal biopsies needed?

These techniques are for diffuse disease involving these organs; they are not for focal lesions. The transjugular route is used in patients with coagulopathy and an increased risk for bleeding.

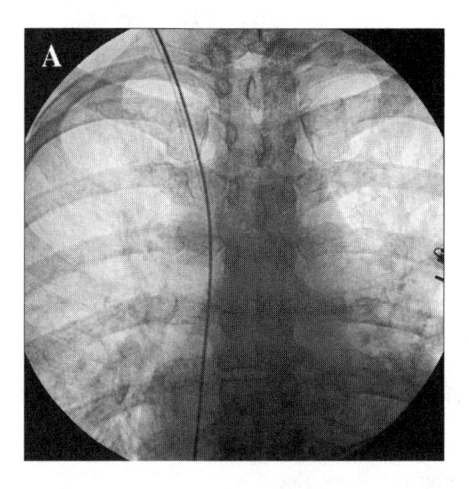

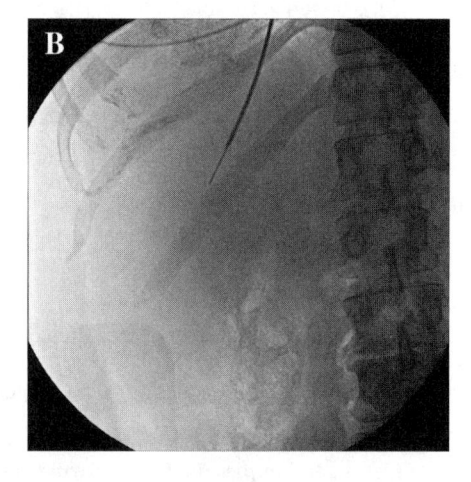

FIGURE 5. A transjugular liver biopsy was requested to reduce the risk of bleeding in a patient with a high international normalized ratio (INR). Initial access is gained from the jugular vein (**A**). A guiding sheath and needle are guided into the right or middle hepatic vein. The guide is turned anterior and medial to a TIPS procedure. The needle is placed in the proximal vein to avoid liver capsule puncture. The spring-loaded needle (18-gauge) is then fired (**B**). Usually two to three passes are required for adequate tissue.

43. List the advantages and disadvantages of transjugular liver biopsies.

Advantages
- Reduced risk of bleeding complications
- Opportunity to measure hepatic pressures, which assess for portal hypertension
- Opportunity to perform hepatic venography, which can give some idea about the degree of cirrhosis, if any

Disadvantage
- Reduced needle gauge (20–21 gauge) requiring multiple needle passes to obtain an adequate tissue sample comparable to that obtained by a percutaneous core biopsy

BIBLIOGRAPHY

1. Brandt KR, Charboneau JW, Stephens DH, et al: CT- and US-guided biopsy of the pancreas. Radiology 187:99–104, 1993.
2. Burbank F, Kayek K, Belville J, et al: Image-guided automated core biopsies of the breast, chest, abdomen and pelvis. Radiology 191:165–171, 1994.
3. Carrasco CH, Richili WR, Lawrence DD, Waugh KA: Adrenal biopsy. In Thoracic and Visceral Nonvascular Interventions, Genitourinary Interventions. SCVIR Syllabus, 1997.
4. Chopra S, Esola CC, Dodd GD III: Percutaneous liver biopsy. In Thoracic and Visceral Nonvascular Interventions, Genitourinary Interventions. SCVIR Syllabus, 1997.
5. Cope C, Marinelli DL, Weinstein JK: Transcatheter biopsy of lesions obstructing the bile ducts. Radiology 169:555–556, 1988.
6. Dodd GD III, Esola CC, Memel DS, et al: Sonography: The undiscovered jewel of interventional radiology. Radiographics 16:1271–1288, 1996.
7. Gazelle GS, Haaga JR, Rowland DY: Effect of needle gauge, level of anticoagulation, and target organ on bleeding associated with aspiration biopsy. Work in progress. Radiology 183:509–513, 1992.
8. Haaga JR: Interventional CT-guided procedures. In Haaga JR, Lanzieri CF, Sartoris DJ, Zerhouni EA (eds): Computed Tomography and Magnetic Resonance Imaging of the Whole Body, 3rd ed. St. Louis, Mosby, 1994.
9. Haaga JR: Overview of biopsy technique and biopsy needles. In Thoracic and Visceral Nonvascular Interventions, Genitourinary Interventions. SCVIR Syllabus, 1997.
10. Hall-Craggs MA, Lees WR: Fine-needle aspiration biopsy: pancreatic and biliary tumors. Am J Roentgenol 147:399–403, 1986.
11. Jackson JE, Adam A, Allison DJ: Transjugular and plugged liver biopsies. Baillieres Clin Gastroenterol 6:245–258, 1992.
12. Mody MK, Kazerooni EA, Korobkin M: Percutaneous C7-guided biopsy of adrenal masses: Immediate and delayed complications. J Comput Assist Tomogr 19:434–439, 1995.
13. Reading CC, Charboneau JW, James EM, Hurt MR: Sonographically guided percutaneous biopsy of small (3cm or less) masses. Am J Roentgenol 151:189–192, 1988.
14. Smith TP, McDermott VG, Ayoub DM, et al: Percutaneous transhepatic liver biopsy with tract embolization. Radiology 198:769–774, 1996.
15. Teplick SK, Haskin PH, Kline TS, et al: Percutaneous pancreaticobiliary biopsies in 173 patients using primarily ultrasound fluoroscopic guidance. Cardiovasc Intervent Radiol 11:26–28, 1998.
16. Welch TJ, Sheedy PF, Johnson CD, et al: C7-guided biopsy: Prospective analysis of 1000 procedures. Radiology 171:493–496, 1989.

INDEX

Boldface type indicates entire chapter.

Abdomen
  abscess drainage within, 293–294, 295
  traumatic injury to
    percutaneous interventions for, 142
    splenic, 143
Abele, John, 1, 3
ABI. *See* Ankle-brachial index
Ablation therapy, percutaneous
  for bony lesions, 314–317
  for hepatic tumors, 149–150, 150, 152
  laser, for varicose veins, 218–219
  radiofrequency techniques in, 149, 150, 152, 314–317
  thermal techniques in, 149–151
Ablative margins, 150
Abortion, spontaneous, uterine fibroids-related, 129
Abscesses
  cerebral, pulmonary arteriovenous malformation-related, 202–203
  drain and catheter management in, 304–305
  hepatic
    aspiration of, 295–296
    drainage of, 295, 296
    pyogenic, 295–296
  intraabdominal, drainage of, 293–294, 295
  pancreatic, drainage of, 299–301, 305
  pelvic
    drainage of, 297–299, 305
    endocautery of, 299
    prevalence and causes of, 297
  pulmonary, 302
Accunet, 90
Achalasia, treatment of, 261
Acquired immunodeficiency syndrome (AIDS). *See also* Human immunodeficiency virus (HIV) infection
  sclerosing cholangitis associated with, 270
Adductor hiatus, 32
Adenoma, hepatic, 113
Adenomyosis, 138
Adenoviruses, as viral vectors, 22
Air embolism
  lung biopsy-related, 322
  venous access-related, 160
Airway management, in contrast reactions, 7
Albuterol inhalers, as contrast reaction treatment, 9
Alcohol, as sclerosing agent, 19
Alcohol abuse, as stroke risk factor, 84
Allen test, 32
Allergic reactions
  to contrast agents, 5, 7
  to sclerosants, 217
Alpha agonists, as contrast reaction treatment, 9
Amenorrhea, uterine fibroid embolization-related, 136
Aminophylline, as contrast agent-related bronchospasm treatment, 9
Amplatz, Kurt, 2
Ampullary cancer, percutaneous transhepatic cholangiographic imaging in, 268

Amputations, lower-extremity, arteriovenous malformation-related, 41
Anaphylactoid reactions, to contrast agents, 7
Ancure endoluminal grafts, 48
AneuRx endoluminal grafts, 48
Aneurysms. *See also* Pseudoaneurysms
  aortic, 47–53
    abdominal, stent graft placement in, 16
    endoluminal graft repair of, 47–50
    endovascular leaks in, 49–52
    gender differences in, 47
    located below the renal arteries, 47
    rupture risk in, 47
    thoracic, 65
  evaluation of parent artery in, 115
  polyarteritis nodosa-related, 56, 109
  of popliteal artery, 32
  Rasmussen, as bronchial system hemorrhage cause, 96
  splenic, 143
  of "true" carotid artery, 91
  of ulnar artery, 32
  visceral, 114–115
    saccular, 115–116
Angiogenesis, 21
Angiography
  aortic, normal findings in, 29
  of arterial injuries, 140, 141
  of arteriovenous malformations, 42, 43
  balloon, "waist" in, 19
  blood pressure control during, 5
  of bronchial arteries, **92–98**
  with carbon dioxide, 3
  of carotid artery, as high-risk procedure, 82
  coding in, 24–25
  contrast agent administration in, 71
  first clinical use of, 1
  hand-injection digital subtraction, 19
  of hemangiomas, 36
  of hepatic artery, 112
  of lower extremities, 69, 70–71
  mesenteric, **113–123**
  patient positioning during, 6
  for peripheral vascular disease diagnosis, 69, 70–71
  of polyarteritis nodosa, 109
  prior to visceral aneurysm treatment, 115
  problems encountered during, 71
  pulmonary
    indications for, 197
    of pulmonary embolism, 197–198, 199–200
  renal, 103–104
    catheters for, 104
    diagnostic and therapeutic indications for, 100
  of renal artery stenosis, 101
  of transplant renal artery stenosis, 242
  of vascular malformations, 36
Angioguard filter, 90
Angioplasty
  as acute renal artery occlusion cause, 110

329

Angioplasty (*cont.*)
  aortic intrarenal, as peripheral vascular disease treatment, 73–74
  carotid, periprocedural complication rate in, 85
  complications of, 85, 104
  femoropopliteal, 76
  as hepatic artery stenosis treatment, 247, 248
  iliac, 53, 75–76
  as inferior vena cava syndrome treatment, 193
  infrapopliteal, 76, 77
  percutaneous transluminal balloon
    as chronic mesenteric ischemia treatment, 122
    as fibromuscular dysplasia treatment, 106, 108
    as hemodialysis fistula treatment, 175, 176
    history of, 1
    as iliac artery lesion treatment, 53
    as peripheral vascular disease treatment, 72–73
    prior to carotid artery stenting, 86, 87
    as renal artery stenosis treatment, 101, 103, 104, 243–244
    as superior vena cava syndrome treatment, 188
    as transplant renal artery stenosis treatment, 243–244
  of portal vein, in liver transplant recipients, 249
  renal, contraindications to, 103
Angioseal, 154, 155
Ankle-brachial index (ABI), 70
  in claudication, 46
  definition of, 44, 53
Anomalous pulmonary venous return
  partial (PAPVR), 34
  total (TAPVR), 33
Anorectal varices, 230
Anterior tibial vein, 34
Anticoagulation therapy
  contraindications to, 184–185
  for deep venous thrombosis, 184–185, 200, 205
  for inferior vena cava syndrome, 191
  for pulmonary embolism, 200, 205
  for superior vena cava syndrome, 186
Antiemetics, 135
Antiplatelet medications, as stroke treatment, 84
Antithrombin III deficiency, as deep venous thrombosis risk factor, 182
Anxiety, contrast agents-related, 8
Aorta
  angiographic evaluation of, bony landmarks in, 31–32
  thoracic, normal size of, 65
  traumatic rupture of, 65
    endograft repair of, 65, 67
Aortic arch
  atheromata of, as stroke risk factor, 83
  clinically important variants in, 28
Aortic coarctation
  collateral pathways in, 28
  development of, 27–28
Aortic dissection, 62–65
  classification of, 62, 63, 64
  as mesenteric ischemia cause, 120
Aortic fenestration, 63

Aortic occlusion
  collateral pathways in, 29
  infrarenal, 30
Aortic stenosis
  infrarenal aortic angioplasty treatment of, 74
  infrarenal aortic stenting treatment of, 74–75
Aortic transection, ductus diverticulum misdiagnosed as, 27
Aortography
  abdominal
    of fibromuscular dysplasia, 102
    prior to renal artery embolization, 112
    prior to visceral aneurysm treatment, 114
    of renal artery stenosis, 101, 102
    "string of beads" sign on, 107
  regional, prior to visceral aneurysm treatment, 114
Aortoiliac disease. *See also* Iliac arteries
  significant, 53
  stent treatment of, 53–55
    postoperative follow-up in, 54–55
Appendix perforation, as pelvic abscess cause, 297
Arc of Barkow, 30, 31
Arc of Buhler, 30, 31
Arc of Riolan, 30, 31
Arrhythmias
  contrast agents-related, 7, 8
  during venous access, 160
Arteri Bate floating catheter, 91
Arteries. *See also* specific arteries
  "evaluating the importance and vitality" of, 115
  occlusion of, 78–81
    "five Ps" of, 79
  lower-extremity, 78–81
  as mesenteric ischemia cause, 120
  with significant collateralization, 115
  traumatic injuries to, 139–142
    of the extremities, 144–145
    of the head and neck, 145
    hepatic, 143
    pelvic, 139–140
    renal, 144
Arteriography
  of bronchial artery, 96
  for massive hemoptysis evaluation, 92, 94, 96
  of celiac artery, in chemoembolization, 148
  of pelvic arterial injuries, 139, 140, 142
  of superior mesenteric artery, in chemoembolization, 148
  of upper gastrointestinal hemorrhage, 119
Arteriotomy, groin puncture site care in, 153
Arteriovenous access. *See also* Venous access
  in hemodialysis, **171–180**
  catheter use in, 165–167, 168, 170, 171, 180
  fistula use in, 167, 171–179
  steal phenomenon in, 172–174
Arteriovenous bridge grafts, for hemodialysis access, 171
Arteriovenous malformations, 35–36, 40–43
  ethanol-induced thrombosis of, 39
  high-flow, 40
  prognosis in, 41

Arteriovenous malformations *(cont.)*
  treatment of, 41, 42
  intrahepatic, endoluminal embolization of, 117
  pelvic, 40–41
  pulmonary, 200–203
    as bronchial system hemorrhage cause, 96, 97
  renal, 110, 111
    treatment of, 41, 42–43
  uterine, 42
Arteritis
  giant-cell, 56, 58
  Takayasu, 56, 57
Ascites, 233
  refractory, 236
Aspergilloma, as massive hemoptysis cause, 92, 93
  bronchial artery embolization treatment of, 96
  rebleeding from, 96
Asphyxiation, massive hemoptysis-related, 92, 96
Aspiration. *See also* Biopsy, aspiration needle; Drainage
  of pyogenic hepatic abscesses, 295–296
  technique of, 319
Aspirin, as stroke treatment, 84
Asymptomatic Carotid Atherosclerosis Study, 83
Atherosclerosis
  aortic, 73, 74, 75
  brachiocephalic, as stroke cause, 83
  as carotid artery stenosis cause
    calcified plaques-related, 84
    treatment of, 85–91
    ulcerated plaques-related, 83–84
  as mesenteric ischemia cause, 120
  as peripheral vascular disease cause, 71–78
  as renovascular disease cause, 99–100
  vascular gene therapy for, 21
  visceral aneurysm-associated, 114
Atherosclerotic plaques
  calcified, 84
  pathologic features of, 83
  ulcerated, 83–84
Atropine, as contrast reaction treatment, 9
Axillary artery
  in giant-cell arteritis, 58
  in massive hemoptysis, 92

Back pain, vertebroplasty treatment of, 311–313
Bacteremia, percutaneous transhepatic cholangiography-related, 269
Balkan sheaths, 14
Balloon dilation. *See also* Angioplasty, percutaneous transluminal balloon
  biliary
    biliary drain removal after, 309
    of biliary strictures, 271–272, 273
  esophageal, 2582–59
    as achalasia treatment, 261
    as benign esophageal stricture treatment, 261
  transhepatic, in liver transplant recipients, 282
Balloon inflation, pain associated with, 4
Baum, Stanley, 3
Beta-agonist inhalers, as contrast reaction treatment, 8, 9

Bile, infected, in biliary obstruction, 269
Bile ducts
  common
    bile leak at, 268
    pancreatic cancer-related obstruction of, 275
  left, obstruction of, 269
Bile duct stones, 271, 272
  coexistent with biliary strictures, 272
Biliary cast syndrome, 280, 281
Biliary drainage. *See* Drainage, biliary
Biliary drains. *See* Drains, biliary
Biliary leaks
  at common bile duct, 268
  liver biopsy-related, 323
  liver transplantation-related, 280
Biliary stents, 275, 279
Biliary strictures, 271
  balloon dilation of, 271–272, 273
  coexistent with bile stones, 272
  liver transplantation-related, 280, 281–282
  malignant, 275
  postlaparoscopic cholecystectomy, 272
  stent placement in, 275
Biliary tract
  stent placement in, 275
  upsizing of, 278
Biliary tree, decompression of, as hilar disease treatment, 275–276
Biopsy
  adrenal, 325
  aspiration needle, 319–327
    capillary method, 319
    for detection of malignancy, 326
    Menghini-type cutting needle method, 319
    Tru-Cut method, 319
  biliary
    endobiliary, 275
    transhepatic, 325–326
  of bone, 314
    in osteoid osteoma, 317
    pain associated with, 4
  brush/scrape method, 326
  core needle, as hemorrhage cause, 319
  endometrial, 127
  image-guided, **319–327**
  of liver, 323–324
    needle size in, 319
    transjugular, 2, 326, 327
  of lung, complications of, 320–322
  of lymphoma, 320
  of pancreas, 324–325
  renal, 322
    as arteriovenous fistula cause, 112
    transjugular, 326
  of renal transplants, vascular complications of, 280
  transthoracic, 320–322
    contraindications to, 321
    ultrasound use in, 322–323
Biospheres, use in chemoembolization, 148
Bladder cancer, percutaneous nephrostomy in, 287, 288

332 INDEX

Bleomycin, as malignant pleural effusion treatment, 301
Blood pressure. *See also* Hypertension; Hypotension
  portal, 225
  segmental, 44
Blood pressure control, during angiographic procedures, 5
Blood pressure measurement, history of, 44
Blood urea nitrogen (BUN), 5
  implication for contrast agent administration, 72
Blue toe syndrome, 74–75
Bony lesions, radiofrequency ablation therapy of, 314–317
Boston Scientific, 3
Bovine arch, 82
Bowel obstruction, distal, effect on enterocutaneous fistula healing, 294
Boyd's perforator veins, 34
Brachiocephalic artery occlusion, as subclavian steal syndrome cause, 61
Brachiocephalic vein
  ipsilateral, occlusion or stenosis of, 188
  occlusion of, 179
  right, thrombosis of, 187
  in superior vena cava syndrome, 188–189
Bradycardia
  carotid artery stenting-related, 87
  contrast agents-related, 8
  with bronchospasm, 10
Brain abscess, pulmonary arteriovenous malformation-related, 202–203
Brain infarction, pulmonary arteriovenous malformation-related, 202
Brain injury, as indication for inferior vena cava filter placement, 209, 210
Bronchial arteries
  anatomy and function of, 92
  angiography of, **92–98**
  in chronic pulmonary disease, 96
  embolization of, 92–98
  normal diameter of, 96
  occlusion of, 96
  usual branching pattern of, 29
Bronchiectasis, as massive hemoptysis cause, 92
Bronchospasm, contrast agents-related, 8, 9
  with bradycardia, 10
  with tachycardia, 9
Budd-Chiari syndrome, 227–228
  definition of, 227
  as portal hypertension cause, 226
  transjugular intrahepatic portosystemic shunt treatment of, 236, 238–239
Buerger's disease, 56, 59–60
Burns, as deep venous thrombosis risk factor, 182
(N)-Butyl cyanocrylate, as embolization agent, 139

Calf muscle pump, 215
Cancer. *See also* specific types of cancer
  as deep venous thrombosis cause, 182
  as superior vena cava syndrome cause, 186–188
Caput medusae, 230

Carbon dioxide, as angiographic contrast agent, 3
Carcinoid tumors, liver metastases from, 149
Cardiac arrest, venous access-related, 160
Cardiovascular disease
  gene therapy for, 21
  as stroke risk factor, 84
Caroli disease, as cholangiocarcinoma risk factor, 270
Carotid arteries. *See also* Common carotid artery; External carotid artery; Internal carotid artery
  aneurysms of, 91
  carotid endarterectomy dissection of, 87
  internal jugular venous access-related, 161
  stenosis of
    asymptomatic, stroke rate in, 83
    calcified atherosclerotic plaques-related, 84
    treatment of, 85–91
    ulcerated atherosclerotic plaques-related, 84
  stenting of, 86, 87, 88–89
    balloon angioplasty predilation prior to, 86, 87
  width of, 84
Carotid artery disease, as atherosclerotic renal artery disease cause, 99
Carotid dissection, carotid endarterectomy-related, 87
Carotid endarterectomy (CEA), 82
  as carotid artery atherosclerotic stenosis treatment, 85–91
  carotid guiding sheath placement in, 85–86
  complications of, 87
  indications for, 85, 89
  neuroembolic protection device use in, 89, 90–91
Carotid Revascularization Endarterectomy *versus* Stenting Trial (CREST), 90
Carotid stents, 87, 88–89
  balloon angioplasty predilation prior to placement of, 86, 87
  complications of, 88, 89, 90
  as high-risk procedure, 82
  periprocedural complication rate for, 85
  thrombosis of, 89
Catheterization, nonselective arterial, 24
Catheters
  angiographic
    "forming" of, 19
    primary and secondary curves of, 13
    typical size of, 12
  Arteri Bate floating, 91
  balloon dilation, development of, 1
  central venous
    cuffed, for hemodialysis access, 171, 180
    peripherally inserted central (PICC), 33, 163
    thrombosis of, 164
  choice of, 13
  for drainage
    biliary, 308
    in fistulous tracts, 305
    flushing of, 304
    output blockage in, 304
  Foley, in uterine fibroid embolization, 134
  general care and positioning of, 309–310

Catheters *(cont.)*
  guiding, 14
  for hemodialysis access, 165–167
    cuffed central venous, 171, 180
    malfunction of, 168, 170
    indwelling, in superior vena cava syndrome, 189, 190–191
    insertion of, pain associated with, 4
    management of, **304–310**
    in pelvic lymphocele management, 306–307
    re-establishment of percutaneous tract for, 307
    side-hole, differentiated from end-hole catheters, 12, 13
    transgluteal, in pelvic abscess drainage, 297, 298
  in venous access
    malfunction of, 168–170
    thrombosis of, 168
Cavagraphy, inferior vena cava, 205
Caval interruption. *See also* Inferior vena cava interruption
  as deep venous thrombosis treatment, 185
Cecostomy, percutaneous, 265
Cefazolin, 148
Cefazoline, 135
Celiac artery
  arteriography of, in chemoembolization, 148
  occlusion of, 57
  traumatic injury to, 140
Celiac axis
  anatomic variants of, 28–29
  aneurysm of, 114
  in contrast extravasation, 118
  in mesenteric ischemia, 121
Cement extravasation, in percutaneous vertebroplasty, 312–313
Central lines
  cuffed, for hemodialysis access, 171, 180
  peripherally inserted central catheters (PICC), 33, 163
  thrombosis of, 164
Central nervous system injury, as deep venous thrombosis risk factor, 182
Cerebral protection devices, 89, 90–91
Cervical cancer
  screening for, 136–137
  as ureteral obstruction cause, 289
Chemoembolization, transcatheter arterial
  as hepatocellular carcinoma treatment, 146–149
  as liver metastases treatment, 149
Chemotherapy, for superior vena cava syndrome, 186
Chemotoxic reactions, to contrast agents, 7
Chest pain, bronchial artery embolization-related, 97
Chest tubes, for pneumothorax management, 301, 305
Chest x-rays, for pulmonary embolism evaluation, 198
Chiba needles, 271, 273, 286
Children
  carotid artery width in, 84
  contrast reactions in, 8–9

Children *(cont.)*
  liver transplantation in, 233
    hepatic artery thrombosis associated with, 245
  renovascular hypertension in, 106
Childs-Pugh Classification, of liver disease prognosis, 228–229, 235
Cholangiocarcinomas
  classes of, 270
  as hepatic segmental atrophy cause, 270
  Klatskin tumors as, 269, 270, 275
  risk factors for, 270
  sclerosing cholangitis associated with, 270
Cholangiography, percutaneous transhepatic, 268–272
  antibiotic prophylaxis with, 271
  as hemorrhage cause, 276
  left-lobe subxiphoid approach in, 270, 271, 274–275, 276–277
  needle insertion technique in, 271, 273–274
  right intercostal approach in, 268
  right-lobe midaxillary approach in, 270
  with transhepatic endoscopy, 273–274
Cholangitis
  ascending pyogenic, 295
  sclerosing, 270
    as cholangiocarcinoma risk factor, 270
    liver transplantation-related, 280, 281
    primary, 270, 271, 273, 280, 281
    secondary, 270
Cholecystitis, nontarget embolization-related, 18
Choledochojejunostomy, posttransplant biliary strictures-related, 280
Choledoscopes, biliary tract accommodation of, 278
Choledoscopy, 278
Chondroblastomas, 314
Chordomas, 314
Cirrhosis
  definition of, 227
  liver transplantation treatment of, 233
  pathologic classification of, 227
  as portal hypertension cause, 226
  upper gastrointestinal varices associated with, 231
Cisplatin, 146
Claudication
  ankle-brachial index in, 46
  buttock
    Leriche syndrome-related, 75
    right common iliac artery occlusion-related, 73
  definition of, 70
  exercise testing in, 46
  intermittent, 50
Clonorchis sinensis infections, as cholangiocarcinoma risk factor, 270
Clopidigrel, as stroke treatment, 84
Coagulation, radiofrequency electrode-induced, 150
Coagulation disorders, as deep venous thrombosis risk factor, 182
Cockett's perforator veins, 34
Coding, in interventional radiology, **24–26**
Coils, as embolization agents
  Gugliemo detachable, 139

Coils, as embolization agents *(cont.)*
  renal microcoils, 144
  thrombogenicity of, 17
  Tornado, 18
  in traumatic injuries, 139
Colitis, ulcerative, sclerosing cholangitis associated with, 270
Colon
  perforation of
    during colonic stenting, 265
    as colonic stenting contraindication, 264
  pseudo-obstruction of, 265
Colon cancer
  liver metastases from, 149
  stent treatment of, 263–264
Colonic stents, 263–265
Colonic strictures, 263
Common carotid artery
  anatomic relationship to internal jugular vein, 160
  aneurysms of, 91
  origin of, 82
Common femoral vein, 34
Computed tomography
  of abdominal trauma, 142
  discovery of, 2
  for lung biopsy guidance, 320
  for pancreatic biopsy guidance, 324–325
  for percutaneous drainage guidance
    of hepatic abscesses, 296
    of intraabdominal abscesses, 293, 294
    of pancreatic fluid, 299
    of pleural fluid, 301
  prior to vertebroplasty, 312
  of pulmonary embolism, 199
Computed tomography angiography
  of peripheral vascular disease, 70
  of renal artery stenosis, 100
Congestive heart failure, as deep venous thrombosis risk factor, 182
Connective tissue disease, vasculitis associated with, 56
Constipation, uterine fibroids-related, 129
Consultation services, inpatient, codes for, 26
Contrast agents
  administration of, 71
  extravasation of, 10, 118
  in hand-injection digital subtraction angiography, 19
  in inferior vena cava filter placement, 212, 214
  in lower-extremity angiography, 70, 71
  low-osmolarity, nonionic, 198
  for patients with poor renal function, 5
Contrast reactions, **7–10**
  allergic reactions, 5, 7
  bronchospasm, 8, 9
    with bradycardia, 9
    with tachycardia, 10
  definition of, 7
  in pediatric patients, 8–9
  prevention of, 7
  severity of, 8
  treatment of, 7, 8–10

Cook, Inc., 2
Cook, William, 1, 2
Cope loops, 304
"Corkscrew collaterals," 59
Coronary artery disease
  as atherosclerotic renal artery disease cause, 99
  as thoracic aneurysm cause, 65
Coronary vein, in transjugular intrahepatic portosystemic shunt procedure, 234
Corticosteroids, as contrast reaction treatment, 8
Cough
  contrast agents-related, 8
  superior vena cava syndrome-related, 186
CPT (current procedural terminology coding method), 24
  modifiers in, 25
Creatinine
  implication for contrast agent administration, 71, 72
  as liver disease prognostic indicator, 229
Crohn's disease, colonic stenting in, 263
Cruveilheir-von Baumgarten syndrome, 230
Cryoplasty, as peripheral vascular disease treatment, 73, 77
Cryptosporidium infection, as AIDS-related sclerosing cholangitis cause, 270
Current procedural terminology (CPT) coding method, 24
  modifiers in, 25
(N-butyl)-Cyanocrylate, as embolization agent, 139
Cystic fibrosis
  bronchial artery embolization in, 96
  as massive hemoptysis cause, 92
Cysts
  aneurysmal bone, 314
  echinococcal hepatic, 295, 297
Cytomegalovirus infection
  as AIDS-related sclerosing cholangitis cause, 270
  as transplant renal artery stenosis cause, 241, 242
Cytosine deaminase, 21

Dandy, Walter, 1
DeBakey classification system, for aortic dissection, 62, 64
De Cavalho, Lopo, 1
Deceleration injuries, as aortic rupture cause, 65
Diabetes mellitus
  as atherosclerotic renal artery disease cause, 99
  as peripheral vascular disease cause, 53, 69, 70, 71
  as stroke risk factor, 84
Diarrhea, "dumping syndrome"-related, 256, 306
Dieulafoy lesions/erosions, 119
Diphenhydramine, as contrast reaction treatment, 8
DIPS (direct intrahepatic portosystemic shunts), 239–240
Disc disease, implication for vertebroplasty performance, 312
Distal occlusion devices, 90
Diuretics
  as contrast reaction treatment, 8
  potassium-sparing, as ascites treatment, 236

Diverticulitis, colonic stenting in, 263
Diverticulum of Kommerell, 27
Dodd's perforator veins, 34
Doppler frequency shift (F_d), calculation of, 46
Doppler ultrasound
　of deep venous thrombosis, 200
　in noninvasive vascular testing, 44
　prior to arteriovenous hemodialysis access, 171
　of testicular varicoceles, 223
　in transjugular intrahepatic portosystemic shunt patients, 239
　of transplant renal artery stenosis, 242
　of varicose veins, 216
　of vascular malformations, 37–38
　waveforms in, 45
Doppman, John, 2
Dotter, Charles, 1, 2
Double-flushing, 12
Down's syndrome, 37
Doxorubicin, 146
Doxycycline, as malignant pleural effusion treatment, 301
Drainage
　biliary
　　in children, 282
　　in liver transplant recipients, 282
　of enterocutaneous fistulas, 294
　of hepatic abscesses, 295, 296
　of hepatic echinococcal cysts, 197
　of intraabdominal abscesses, 293–294, 295
　of pancreatic fluid, 299–301, 305
　of pelvic abscesses, 297–299
　　pain associated with, 305
　of pelvic lymphoceles, 302–303, 306–307
　of pleural fluid, 301–302
　of pulmonary abscesses, 302
　trocar technique for, 18, 293
Drains
　biliary, 271, 272
　　changing of, 307
　　external, 307
　　functional types of, 278–279
　　as hemobilia cause, 309
　　indwelling, removal of, 272–273
　　internal-external, 307, 309
　　leakage from, 309
　　placement of, 274
　　removal of, 272–273, 309
　　U-shaped, 309
　general care and positioning of, 309–310
　percutaneous abscess
　　flushing of, 304
　　management of, 304–305
　　removal of, 305
　　sinogram evaluation of, 304
　　re-establishment of percutaneous tract for, 307
Drug delivery devices, for endovascular use, 22
Ductopenia, liver transplantation-related, 280, 282–283
Ductus diverticulum, 27
Duett vascular closure device, 156–157
"Dumping syndrome," 256, 306

Duplex ultrasound
　of deep venous thrombosis, 183
　of peripheral vascular disease, 70
　of renal artery stenosis, 100
　of varicose veins, 216
Dysphagia
　benign postoperative, 259, 260
　malignant, 258–259
　superior vena cava syndrome-related, 186
Dysplasia, fibromuscular
　abdominal aortography of, 107
　definition of, 56
　as pediatric renovascular hypertension cause, 106
　as renal artery stenosis cause, 99, 100, 102, 104
　"string of beads" angiographic appearance of, 56, 60, 106, 107
　treatment of, 106, 108
　types of, 56, 60
　visceral aneurysm-associated, 114
Dysrhythmias. *See* Arrhythmias

Edema
　facial, contrast agents-related, 8, 9
　laryngeal
　　contrast agents-related, 8, 9
　　superior vena cava syndrome-related, 186
　lower-extremity, inferior vena cava syndrome-related, 191
　pulmonary
　　contrast agents-related, 10
　　renovascular disease-related, 99
Edmonton suspension, 251
Elderly persons, peripheral vascular disease in, 69
Embolectomy
　as meniscal embolism treatment, 80
　as pulmonary embolism treatment, 200
Embolism. *See also* Thromboembolism
　as acute mesenteric ischemia cause, 121
　as acute renal artery occlusion cause, 110
　of lower-extremity arteries, 78, 79, 80
　as mesenteric ischemia cause, 120
　pulmonary
　　angiographic findings in, 197–198, 199–200
　　causes of, 197
　　chest x-ray findings in, 198
　　clinical symptoms of, 197
　　computed tomographic findings in, 199
　　deep venous thrombosis-related, 181, 182
　　early diagnosis of, 197
　　evaluation of, 197
　　Greenfield filter-related recurrence of, 209
　　incidence of, 205
　　as infarction cause, 198
　　inferior vena cava interruption treatment of, **206–215**
　　life-threatening massive, 200
　　nonfatal incidence of, 205
　　polytetrafluoroethylene graft-related clots as cause of, 16
　　treatment of, 200, **206–215**
　of superior mesenteric artery, 121–122

Embolization
  as aneurysm treatment
    parent artery evaluation in, 115
    for saccular visceral aneurysms, 116
  as arterial injury treatment, 139, 140, 141, 142
    in hepatic injuries, 143
  of biopsy tracts, 319
  of bronchial arteries, 92–98
  cerebral, as carotid stenting complication, 88, 89, 90
  direct percutaneous, 116
  as extremity injury treatment, 144–145
  of gastroduodenal artery, 119
  as head and neck injury treatment, 145
  hepatic
    as bleeding varices treatment, 2
    of hepatic arterial injuries, 143
    as hepatic arteriovenous malformation treatment, 117
    in hepatic injuries, 143
  nontarget, 17–18
  pelvic, as arterial injury treatment, 140, 141, 142
  as pseudoaneurysm treatment, 115
  as pulmonary arteriovenous malformation treatment, 200–202
  renal, 144
    of arteriovenous fistulas, in renal transplants, 280
    of renal artery, 110–111
      abdominal aortogram prior to, 112
      agents for, 111
      transcatheter, 111
  of splenic artery, 143–144
    as liver transplant ischemia treatment, 248
  of testicular vein, **220–224**
  transcatheter, as liver injury treatment, 142–143
  as upper gastrointestinal hemorrhage treatment, 117–119
  of uterine artery, **124–138**
    arterial anatomic variants in, 31
    bilateral, 129, 130
    embolic agents for, 133, 134
    inadvertent leiomyosarcoma embolization during, 137
    medications used in, 134–135
    of pedunculated fibroids, 138
    uterine fibroid, 124
Embolization agents. See also Coils; Gelfoam; Polyvinyl alcohol
  distal differentiated from proximal, 17
  as nontarget embolization cause, 17–18
  temporary differentiated from permanent, 17
Embospheres, 133, 134
E&M (evaluation and management) codes, 24, 25–26
EMLA cream, 135
Emphysema, as lung biopsy-related pneumothorax risk factor, 320
Empyema, fibrinopurulent, 305
Encephalopathy
  contrast, carotid artery stent-related, 87
  transjugular intrahepatic portosystemic shunt-related, 235, 237

Endocautery, of pelvic abscesses, 299
Endoluminal therapy, for arteriovenous malformations, 41, 42, 43
Endometrial cancer, 136–137
Endoprostheses, as biliary stricture treatment, 275
Endoscopy
  percutaneous transhepatic biliary, 278
  transhepatic, as adjunct to biliary interventions, 273–274
Endothelium, vascular, use in gene therapy, 21
Endotracheal stents, 257
Endovascular therapy
  for inferior vena cava syndrome, 191–193
  for superior vena cava syndrome, 188–189
  for thoracic aneurysms, 65, 66
  for upper gastrointestinal hemorrhage, 117
Epidermoid cancer, as superior vena cava syndrome cause, 186
EPI filter wire, 89, 90
Epinephrine, as contrast reaction treatment, 8, 9
Erectile dysfunction, aortic stenosis-related, 74, 75
Esophageal balloon tamponading, 232
Esophageal cancer
  as contraindication to esophageal stents, 261
  esophagorespiratory fistulas associated with, 259–260
  stent treatment of
    delayed complications of, 261–262
    "funnel phenomenon" of, 262
Esophageal stents, 259–262
Esophageal strictures, 261
Esophagogastroduodenoscopy, 117
  flexible, 231
Esophagus
  benign strictures of, 261
  malignant narrowing of, 261
  stenting/laser therapy-related perforation of, 261
Ethanol
  as liver tumor treatment, 152
  as vascular malformation treatment, 39–40
Ethiodol, use in chemoembolization, 148
E-Trgs Filter, 91
Evaluation and management (E&M) codes, 24, 25–26
Excluder endoluminal graft, 48
External carotid artery
  branches of, 82
  embolization of, 145
  in stroke, 82
  width of, 84
External spermatic vein, 220
Extravasation
  of cement, in percutaneous vertebroplasty, 312–313
  of contrast agents, 10, 118
  hepatic, embolization of, 142
  pelvic, 141
  from popliteal artery, 144
  renal, 144
  renal transplant biopsy-related, 280
Extremity pressure measurements, 44
Eye injury, as indication for vena cava filter placement, 209

INDEX

Factor V Leiden, as deep venous thrombosis risk factor, 182
Fallopian tubes
  blockage of, as infertility cause, 290, 292
  recanalization of, 290, 292
Fat, epiploic, as pancreatic islet cell deposition site, 250
Femoral access, for renal angiography, 104
Femoral artery
  common, embolus to, 78
  femoral venous access-related puncture of, 163
  occlusion of, femoropopliteal angioplasty treatment of, 76
  right, endoluminal treatment of, 217–218
  superior, cryoplasty of, 77
Femoral bypass grafts, occluded axillary vessels in, 79
Femoral vein access, 163
Femoropopliteal interventions, indications for, 76
Fentanyl, 4
Fever, uterine fibroid embolization-related, 135–136
Fibrin glue, as fistulous tract treatment, 294
Fibrin sheaths, as venous catheter thrombosis cause, 168
Fibrin sheath stripping, of malfunctioning catheters, 169–170
Fibroids, uterine. *See* Leiomyomas
Fibrosis, retroperitoneal, 270
Fistulas
  arteriobiliary, embolization of, 142
  arteriocalyceal, renal transplant biopsy-related, 280
  arteriovenous, 110, 111, 112
    embolization of, 142, 144
    renal transplant biopsy-related, 280
    splenic, as portal hypertension cause, 226
  enterocutaneous, drainage of, 294, 295
  esophagorespiratory, 259–260
  for hemodialysis access, 167, 171–179
    aradial-cephalic wrist (Brescia-Cimino), 171
    arteriovenous polytetrafluoroethylene, 171, 174, 175
    brachiocephalic elbow, 171
    graft, 171, 172, 174–175, 176
    native, 171–172, 175, 176
    stenosis/thrombosis of, 172, 173, 174, 175, 176–179
    transposed brachial-basilic native, 171
  hepatoportal, 226
  of pancreatic duct, 301
Fluid collections, percutaneous management of, **293–303**
  hepatic abscesses, 295–296
  pancreatic abscesses/fistulas, 299–301, 305
  pelvic abscesses, 297–299
  pleural effusions, 301–302
Flumazepil, 4
Fluoroscopy, contraindication in testicular vein embolization, 221
Focal nodular hyperplasia (FNH), 114
Foreign bodies, in the pulmonary arteries, 202
  removal of, 204

Fractures
  as deep venous thrombosis risk factor, 182
  as indication for vena cava filter placement, 209
  pathologic, radiofrequency ablation therapy-related, 317
  of ribs, 143
  vertebral compression, 311
French (F), to one millimeter, 11
Frontal lobotomy, 1
"Funnel phenomenon," 262
Furosemide, 236
  as contrast reaction treatment, 8

Gastric artery, aneurysm of, 114
Gastritis, erosive, 231
Gastroduodenal artery
  aneurysm of, 114
  in chemoembolization, 148
  collateralization of, 115
  embolization of, 119
  as gastrointestinal hemorrhage cause, 117, 119
  normal, 29
Gastroduodenal lesions, stent treatment of, 262–265
Gastroduodenal obstruction, malignant, stent treatment of, 262
Gastroduodenal stents, 262–265
Gastroepiploic artery
  aneurysm of, 114
  normal, 29
Gastroesophageal lesions, stent treatment of, 260
Gastrointestinal interventions, **253–267**
Gastrointestinal tract, anatomic connection to liver, 225
Gastropexy, sutures used in, 253, 254
Gastrostomy tube feeding, differentiated from jejunal tube feeding, 306
Gastrostomy tubes, 253–257
  blockage of, 306
  comparison with nasogastric tubes, 255
  complications of, 255–256
  contraindications to, 253–254
  as esophageal stricture treatment, 261
  fallen, 307
  jejunal extensions to, 254, 255
  leakage from, 306
  malpositioned in the duodenum, 306
  mushroom retention devices in, 256
  placement of, 254
  radiologically-placed, 255–256
Gelfoam
  as arteriovenous malformation treatment, 32
  as embolization agent, 146, 148
    advantages of, 17
    in biopsy tracts, 319
    in renal embolization, 144
    in traumatic injuries, 139, 142
    in uterine artery embolization, 133, 134
Gene expression, 22
Genes, reporter, 22
Gene therapy, **21–23**
Genitourinary interventions, **285–292**

INDEX

Giant-cell tumors
  percutaneous vertebroplasty of, 312
  vertebral bone biopsy contraindication in, 314
Gianturco, Cesare, 2
Glue, fibrin, as fistulous tract treatment, 294
"Glue," 139
Gonadal arteries, as renal artery variants, 99
Gonadal veins
  as endoluminal therapy administration site, 224
  left, insertion into circumaortic renal vein, 223
  in testicular vein embolization, 223, 224
  venous collaterals of, 223
Gonadotropin-releasing hormone agonists, as uterine fibroids treatment, 125, 132
Graft bypass surgery, as peripheral arterial occlusive disease treatment, 78
Grafts
  endoluminal, 48
    for aortic aneurysm repair, 47–50
    for aortic rupture repair, 65, 67
    for hemodialysis arteriovenous access, 171, 172, 174–175, 176
  polytetrafluoroethylene
    for hemodialysis arteriovenous access, 171, 174, 175
    as pulmonary embolism cause, 16
    Trerotolo device placement in, 16
Greater saphenous vein
  endovenous laser therapy of, 218
  sonographic features of, 34
  varicose veins-related obliteration of, 217
Greater saphenous venous system, 34
Great vessel injury, diverticulum of Kommerell misdiagnosed as, 27
Greenfield embolectomy device, 200
Greenfield filters, 16, 209
Groin puncture site
  in arteriotomy, 153
  clot formation at, 6
Gruentzig, Andreas, 1, 3
Guidewires
  Amplatz, 11
  Bentson, 11
  characteristics of, 19
  glide/Terumo, 11, 12
  mandril of, 11
  Rosen, 11
Gun shot wound, to the popliteal artery, 144

Hales, Steven, 44
Hampton's hump, 198
Hawkins, Irvin F., 3
HCFA (Health Care Financing Administration), 24
Headaches
  contrast agents-related, 8
  superior vena cava syndrome-related, 186
Head and neck cancer, metastatic to gastrostomy tube exit site, 256
Head injury, embolization treatment of, 145
Health Care Financing Administration (HCFA), 24
Health Insurance Portability and Accountability Act (HIPPA), 26

Hemangio-endotheliomas, epitheloid, 314
Hemangiomas
  cavernous, 113
  classification of, 35
  differentiated from vascular malformations, 36
  growth of, 35
  as liver biopsy contraindication, 324
  natural history of, 35
  vertebral, percutaneous vertebroplasty treatment of, 312
Hematomas
  at arteriotomy groin puncture site, 153
  femoral artery puncture-related, 163
  perinephric, renal transplant biopsy-related, 280
Hemicolon cancer, colonic stenting in, 263
Hemobilia
  percutaneous biliary drain-related, 309
  percutaneous transhepatic cholangiography-related, 276
Hemodialysis, arteriovenous access in, 167, 171–179, **171–180**
  catheters for, 165–167
    cuffed central venous, 171, 180
    malfunction of, 168, 170
  fistulas for, 167, 171–179
    aradial-cephalic wrist (Brescia-Cimino), 171
    arteriovenous polytetrafluoroethylene, 171, 174, 175
    brachiocephalic elbow, 171
    graft, 171, 172, 174–175, 176
    native, 171–172, 175, 176
    stenosis/thrombosis of, 172, 173, 174, 175, 176–179
    transposed brachial-basilic native, 171
  steal phenomenon in, 172–174
Hemoperitoneum, 143
Hemoptysis, massive, 92–98
Hemorrhage
  arteriovenous malformation-related, 40
  core needle biopsy-related, 319
  during drainage catheter exchange, 305
  gastroesophageal, 231, 232
  gastrointestinal, 232
  liver biopsy-related, 322, 323
  percutaneous transhepatic cholangiography-related, 276
  renal biopsy-related, 322
  upper gastrointestinal, 117–119
    in portal hypertension, 117, 231
  variceal, 236, 237–238
Heparin
  action mechanism of, 184
  as deep venous thrombosis prophylaxis and treatment, 184
  low-molecular-weight, 184
Hepatic artery
  aneurysm of, 114
  chemoembolization of, 146
  embolization of, 117
  intrahepatic collateralization of, 115
  normal, 29

Hepatic artery *(cont.)*
  pseudoaneurysm of, cholangiography-related, 276, 277
  stenosis of
    in liver transplants, 247–248
    posttransplant biliary stricture-related, 280
  thrombosis of
    in liver transplants, 245–247
    posttransplant biliary cast syndrome-related, 280
    posttransplant biliary stricture-related, 280
Hepatic artery stents, 244
Hepatic mass, benign, arteriographic characteristics of, 113
Hepatic portal circulation, 225
Hepatic tumors
  hypervascular, as transjugular intrahepatic portosystemic shunt contraindication, 239
  interventional radiology-based treatment of, **146–152**
Hepatic vein, stenosis of, in liver transplants, 249
Hepatitis, as portal hypertension cause, 226
Hepatitis B, polyarteritis nodosa associated with, 56, 120
Hepatobiliary interventions, **268–279**
Hepatocellular carcinoma, 146, 228
  arteriographic characteristics of, 113
  chemoembolization treatment of, 146–149
  as persistent ascites cause, 236
Hepatocyte growth factor, 21
Hepatocytes, 225
Hepatorenal syndrome, 236–237
Hess, Walter Rudolf, 1
Hilar disease, intrahepatic biliary tree decompression in, 275–276
HIPPA (Health Insurance Portability and Accountability Act), 26
Homan's sign, 181–182
Homocysteine, as peripheral vascular disease cause, 69
Hormonal therapy, for uterine fibroids, 125, 126
Horner's syndrome, 163
Hospital care, codes for, 26
Hounsfield, Godfrey Newbold, 2
Human immunodeficiency virus (HIV) infection, bronchial artery embolization in, 97
Hunt, Ramsay, 82
Hunterian perforator veins, 34
Hydronephrosis, uterine fibroids-related, 128
Hydrothorax
  hepatic, 302
  as transjugular intrahepatic portosystemic shunt indication, 236
Hypercholesterolemia
  as peripheral vascular disease risk factor, 50, 69, 70, 71
  as stroke risk factor, 84
  vascular gene therapy for, 21
Hyperplasia
  focal nodular (FNH), 114
  intimal, 16
Hypertension
  as aortic dissection risk factor, 62

Hypertension *(cont.)*
  as atherosclerotic renal artery disease cause, 99
  contrast agents-related, 8, 10
  as peripheral vascular disease cause, 50, 69, 71
  portal, **225–240**
    in children, 226
    clinical findings in, 228
    liver transplantation treatment for, 233
    mortality causes in, 228
    pathogenesis of, 225–226
    portosystemic anastomoses development in, 229–231
    sinusoidal classification of, 227
  pulmonary, angiographic findings in, 198
  renal embolization-related, 144
  renovascular, 99, 101
    in children and young adults, 106
  as stroke risk factor, 84
  superior vena cava syndrome-related, 186
  as thoracic aneurysm risk factor, 65
  vascular gene therapy for, 21
Hypophyseal portal circulation, 225
Hypotension, contrast agents-related, 8, 9, 10
Hypothenar hammer syndrome, 32
Hysterectomy, as uterine fibroids treatment, 124, 125, 126–128
Hysterosalpingography, 289, 290

ICD9 (International Classification of Disease, Ninth Edition), 24
Iliac arteries
  occlusion of
    collateral pathways in, 29
    oral contraceptives-related, 192
    stent treatment of, 53
  stenosis of, iliac angioplasty treatment of, 75–76, 78
Iliac stents, 53, 54, 55, 192
  patency rate for, 53
Iliac veins, external, 34
Implantable ports, 164–165
  malpositioning of, 169
Infarction, cerebral, pulmonary arteriovenous malformation-related, 202
Infection, as visceral aneurysm and pseudoaneurysm cause, 114
Inferior adrenal arteries, as renal artery variant, 99
Inferior mesenteric artery
  endoleak at, 51
  normal branching pattern of, 31
Inferior mesenteric vein, in hepatic portal circulation system, 225
Inferior phrenic artery
  in massive hemoptysis, 92
  as renal artery variant, 99
Inferior vena cava
  duplication of, 33
  Greenfield filter placement in, 16
  hemodialysis catheter-related thrombosis of, 166–167
  as megacava, 210
  stenosis of, in liver transplants, 249, 250
Inferior vena cava filters, 33, 160

Inferior vena cava interruption, **206–215**
  filter migration in, 206
  filter penetration in, 207
  filter placement in, 205–206, 207–208
    complications of, 209
    contraindications to, 208
    contrast agents for, 212, 214
    infrarenal, 206, 207–208
    modalities for, 212
    prophylactic, 209, 210
    suprarenal, 206, 208
  filter types used in
    bird's nest, 2, 210
    optional retrievable, 211, 212, 213
    permanent, 212, 213
    temporary, 211
  inferior vena cava cavagram prior to, 205
Inferior vena cava syndrome, 189, 191–193
Infertility
  female, 290
    fallopian tubal occlusion-related, 290, 292
    uterine fibroids-related, 129
  male, varicocele-related, 220, 223
Inflammation, as visceral aneurysm and pseudoaneurysm cause, 114
Inflammatory bowel disease, as cholangiocarcinoma risk factor, 270
Inpatient consultation services, codes for, 26
Inpatients, post-procedural care for, 6
Instruments and equipment, in interventional radiology, **11–20**
Insulin independence, following pancreatic islet cell transplantation, 250, 251
Intercostal artery, in massive hemoptysis, 92
Internal carotid artery
  anatomic portions of, 82
  distal, stent-related kinking and spasms in, 87
  endoluminal interventions in, 84
  width of, 84
Internal jugular vein, anatomic relationship to common carotid artery, 160
Internal jugular vein access, 160–163, 165
  catheter occlusion in, 168
  central approach technique in, 161
  contraindications to, 161, 162
  for hemodialysis catheters, 165
  for implantable ports, 164
  inferior vena cava filters in, 160
  micropuncture technique in, 161, 163
Internal mammary artery
  in massive hemoptysis, 92
  thyroidea, 28
Internal pudendal artery, in pelvic trauma, 140
Internal spermatic vein, 220
International Classification of Disease, ninth edition (ICD9), 24
International normalized ratio (INR), 5
  assessment prior to arterial access, 71
Intersocietal Commission for the Accreditation of Vascular Laboratories (ICAVL), 45
Interventional radiology
  "father" of, 1

Interventional radiology *(cont.)*
  history and famous people of, **1–3**
  instruments and equipment in, **11–20**
Ischemia
  categorization of, 79
  cerebral, carotid artery stenting-related, 87
  in liver transplants, 248
  lower-extremity, 79
  mesenteric, 120–121, 122
  vascular gene therapy for, 21

Jejunal tube feeding, differentiated from gastrostomy tube feeding, 306
Jejunostomy tubes, 257

Kasabach-Merritt syndrome, 37, 113
Kidney. *See also* Renal entries
  arteriovenous malformations in, 110, 111
  in polyarteritis nodosa, 109
  "protected" differentiated from "unprotected," 110
  vascular anatomy of, 99
"Kissing" balloon technique, 78, 108, 109
Klatskin tumors, 269, 270, 275
Klippel-Trenaunay syndrome, 37
Kyphoplasty, 313–314
Kyphosis, kyphoplasty treatment of, 313–314

Laboratory tests, prior to interventional radiology procedures, 5
Laparotomy, emergency, 142
Larynx, edema of
  contrast agents-related, 8, 9
  superior vena cava syndrome-related, 186
Laser therapy
  comparison with esophageal stents, 260–261
  for varicose veins, 218–219
Lateral sacral vessels, in pelvic trauma, 140
Lateral venous system, 34
Left bronchial tree, 92
Left bundle-branch block, implication for pulmonary angiography, 197–198
Left gastric vein, in hepatic portal circulation system, 225
Left hypogastric artery, traumatic injury to, 141, 142
Left renal vein, retroaortic, 209
Leiomyomas
  arterial supply to, 31
  pedunculated, 138
  uterine artery embolization treatment of, **124–138**
    arterial anatomic variants in, 31
    bilateral, 129, 130
    embolic agents for, 133, 134
    inadvertent leiomyosarcoma embolization during, 137
    medications used in, 134–135
    of pedunculated fibroids, 138
    volume measurement of, 136
Leiomyosarcomas, 137
Leptin, 21

Leriche syndrome, 75
Lesser saphenous venous system, 34
Leucotomy, 1
Lidocaine anesthesia, tumescent/infiltrative, 218
Life expectancy, peripheral vascular disease-related decrease in, 69
Liposomes, 23
Lithotripsy, percutaneous intracorporeal electrohydraulic, 272
Liver
  abscesses of
    aspiration of, 295–296
    drainage of, 295, 296
    pyogenic, 295–295
  adenoma of, 113
  biopsy of, 323–324
    transjugular approach in, 326, 327
  connection to gastrointestinal tract, 225
  echinococcal cysts of, 295, 297
  hydrothorax of, 302
  portal circulation in, 225
  subcapsular mass in, biopsy of, 324
  traumatic injuries to, transcatheter embolization of, 142–143
Liver disease
  polycystic, as transjugular intrahepatic portosystemic shunt contraindication, 239
  prognostic classification of, 228–229
Liver failure
  after transjugular intrahepatic portosystemic shunt placement, 237
  transcatheter arterial catheterization-related, 147, 148
Liver metastases, transcatheter arterial embolization treatment of, 149
Liver transplantation
  arteriovenous malformation embolization-related, 117
  biliary complications of, 280–283
  as Budd-Chiari syndrome treatment, 238–239
  in children, 233
  as cirrhosis treatment, 233
  as hepatic hydrothorax treatment, 302
  as portal hypertension treatment, 233
  as primary sclerosing cholangitis treatment, 273
Liver transplant recipients
  hepatic pseudoaneurysms in, 116
  transjugular intrahepatic portosystemic shunts in, 240
Liver transplants
  hepatic vein stenosis in, 247, 249
  hepatic vein thrombosis in, 245–247
  inferior vena cava stenosis in, 249, 250
  portal vein stenosis in, 249
  portal vein thrombosis in, 248–249
  renal artery stenosis in, 242
Liver tumors. *See* Hepatic tumors
Lower extremity
  deep/draining venous system of, 34, 215
  peripheral arterial occlusive disease of, 78
  venous reflux patterns in, 216
Lunderquist, Anders, 2

Lung
  abscess of, 302
  arteriovenous malformations in, 200–203
  as bronchial system hemorrhage cause, 96, 97
  embolism of. *See* Embolism, pulmonary
Lung cancer, as superior vena cava syndrome cause, 186
Lung transplantation, as tracheobronchial stenosis cause, 258
Luxury perfusion, carotid artery stenting-related, 87
Lymphatic malformations, syndromes associated with, 37
Lymphoceles, pelvic
  catheter therapy/management of, 306–307
  drainage of, 302–303, 306–307
Lymphoma, biopsy of, 320

Maffucci syndrome, 37
Magnetic resonance imaging
  of deep venous thromboses, 183–184
  in gene therapy, 22
  of peripheral vascular disease, 70
  of renal artery stenosis, 100
  for uterine artery embolization evaluation, 128
  of vascular malformations, 37
  of vertebral compression, 311–312
Mallory-Weiss tears, 117
Marfan syndrome, as aortic dissection risk factor, 62
Marginal artery of Drummond, 30, 31
May-Thurner syndrome, 193–194
Medial degeneration, visceral aneurysm-related, 114
Median arcuate syndrome, 120–121, 122
Medi-Tech, 3
MedNova Neuroshield, 90
Megacava, 210
Meniscus, embolism of, 80
Menometrorrhagia, definition of, 128
Menopause, premature, 127
Menorrhagia
  causes of, 126
  definition of, 128
Meperidine, 4
Mesenteric angiography and intervention, **113–123**
Mesenteric dissection, as mesenteric ischemia cause, 120
Mesenteric ischemia, 120–121, 122
Metastases
  hepatic, transcatheter arterial embolization treatment of, 149
  inferior vena cava filter use in, 207
  as superior vena cava syndrome cause, 186
  vertebral, radiofrequency ablation treatment of, 316
Methylprednisolone, as contrast reaction treatment, 8
Metoclopramide, 135
Metronidazole, 148
Microaneurysms
  saccular, polyarteritis nodosa-related, 120
  in splanchnic vessels, 119

Microbubbles, 23
Microcatheters, 20
Microcoils, as renal embolization agents, 144
Midazolam, 4
Middle meningeal artery, origin of, 82
Middle spermatic vein, 220
Mitomycin C, 146
Mobin-Uddin filter, 205
Molecular imaging, 21
Moniz, Egas, 1
Motor vehicle accidents
 as abdominal trauma cause, 143
 as aortic rupture cause, 65, 67
 as arterial injury cause, 140, 141, 142
Mucomyst, 71
Musculoskeletal interventions, **311–318**
Myeloma, percutaneous vertebroplasty treatment of, 312
Myocardial infarction, as deep venous thrombosis risk factor, 182
Myomectomy, as uterine fibroid treatment, 125, 127

Naloxone, 4
Nasogastric tubes, comparison with gastrostomy tubes, 255
Nausea, contrast agents-related, 8
Neck injury
 embolization treatment of, 145
 as internal jugular venous access contraindication, 161, 162
Necrosis
 coagulation, radiofrequency ablative therapy-related, 150
 pancreatic, 299
 tissue, radiofrequency ablative therapy-related, 152
Needles
 for aspiration biopsies, 319
 Chiba, 271, 273, 286
 gauge size of, 11
 for intraabdominal abscess drainage, 293
 micropuncture, 11
 for percutaneous transhepatic cholangiography, 268
 Potts, 11
 right femoral artery, 150–151
 trephine, 314
 trocar, 18
Nephrolithiasis, percutaneous nephrostomy in, 287, 288
Nephrostomy, percutaneous, 285–287
Nephrostomy tubes, 18
 changing of, 307
 size of, 287
Neuroembolic protection devices, 89, 90–91
Nitinol (nickel-titanium alloy), 16–17
Nitric oxide synthase, as cardiovascular disease treatment, 21
Nitroglycerin, in combination with vasopressin, 232
North American Symptomatic Carotid Endarterectomy Trial (NASCET), 84

NPO (*non per os*/nothing by mouth) status, 5
Nursing, interventional radiology, **4–6**

Obesity
 as atherosclerotic renal artery disease risk factor, 99
 as peripheral vascular disease risk factor, 53, 69
Obturator artery, in pelvic trauma, 140
Okuda, K., 268
Oligospermia, varicocele-related, 223
Olm's law, 225
Oral contraceptives
 as deep venous thrombosis cause, 192
 as uterine fibroid treatment, 125
Organ transplantation. *See also* specific types of organ transplantation
 nonvascular interventions in, **280–284**
Osler-Weber-Rendu syndrome, 202
Osmotoxicity, of contrast agents, 7
Osteoma, osteoid
 percutaneous bone biopsies of, 317
 radiofrequency ablation of, 314, 315, 317
Ostial renal artery lesions, 102, 103, 106
Outpatients, post-procedural care for, 6
Ovarian arteries, anastomosis with uterine arteries, 129, 130, 132
Ovaries, blood supply of, 129, 130
Oximetry, transcutaneous, 44
Oxygen therapy, for contrast reactions, 9

Paget-Schrotter syndrome, 195
Pain
 arterial occlusion-related, 79
 bone biopsy-related, 4
 interventional radiology procedures-related, 4
 liver biopsy-related, 324
 pelvic, 126, 128
 skeletal metastases-related, 316
 spinal, vertebroplasty treatment of, 311–313
 vertebrogenic, vertebroplasty treatment of, 312
Pallor, arterial occlusion-related, 79
Palmaz, Julio, 3
Palmaz stents, 106
 inventor of, 3
 as tracheobronchial lesion treatment, 257
Pampiniform plexus, in varicoceles, 220, 221
Pancreas
 abscess drainage in, 299–301, 305
 biopsy of, 324–325
Pancreatic cancer, as common bile duct obstruction cause, 275
Pancreatic duct, fistulas of, 301
Pancreatic islet cell transplants, 249–251
 Edmonton suspension infusion of, 251
Pancreaticoduodenal artery, aneurysm of, 114
Pancreatitis
 adrenal biopsy-related, 325
 nontarget embolization-related, 18
 pancreatic fluid drainage in, 305
Paralysis
 arterial occlusion-related, 79
 bronchial artery embolization-related, 98

Paresthesia, arterial occlusion-related, 79
Partial anomalous pulmonary venous return (PAPVR), 34
Partial thromboplastin time, 5
Patient education, for catheter and drain care, 310
Pelvic inflammatory disease, as uterine artery embolization contraindication, 127
Pelvic pain, 126, 128
Pelvic percutaneous interventions. *See also* Embolization, pelvic
  complications of, 142
Pelvis
  abscesses of, 297
    drainage of, 297–299, 305
    endocautery of, 299
    prevalence and causes of, 297
  arterial injuries to, arteriography of, 139–140, 141, 142
  arteriovenous malformations in, 40–41
Peptic ulcer disease, 231
Perclose system, of suture-mediated closure devices, 153, 154
Percutaneous entry technique, development of, 1
Perforator veins, 34, 215
Pericarditis
  as Budd-Chiari syndrome cause, 227
  as portal hypertension cause, 226
Peripheral vascular disease, **69–81**
  acute embolic *vs.* chronic occlusion in, 78
  atherosclerotic, 71–78
    interventional procedure treatment of, 72–78
    medical treatment of, 71–72
    as renal artery disease risk factor, 100
  definition of, 69
  diagnosis of, 69–71
  life expectancy in, 53
  lower-extremity arterial occlusive, 78
  risk factors for, 50, 52, 69
  treatment of, 53–56
Peritoneal cavity, as pancreatic islet cell deposition site, 250
Peritonitis
  secondary, 237
  spontaneous bacterial, as persistent ascites cause, 236
Peroneal vein, 34
PHACE syndrome, 37
Phlebography
  catheter-directed, 38
  direct percutaneous, 38–39
Phlegmasia alba dolens, 182
Phlegmasia cerulea dolens, 182
PIOPED (Prospective Investigation of Pulmonary Embolism Diagnosis) criteria, 198
Piperacillin, 271
Platelet count, assessment prior to arterial access, 71
Plethysmography
  arterial, 44–45
  impedance, for deep venous thrombosis diagnosis, 184
Pleural effusions
  malignant, 301–302

Pleural effusions *(cont.)*
  percutaneous management of, 301–302
Pleurodesis, as malignant pleural effusion treatment, 302, 303
Pneumoencephalography, 1
Pneumothorax
  adrenal biopsy-related, 325
  chest tube management of, 301, 305
  hemodialysis catheter-related, 166
  lung biopsy-related, 320–321
  venous access-related, 160
Polyarteritis nodosa, 106, 109, 119–120
  aneurysm associated with, 56, 109
  angiographic appearance of, 56
  gender differences in, 56
  treatment of, 56
Polycythemia rubra vera, as deep venous thrombosis risk factor, 182
Polymethylmethacrylate, use in vertebroplasty, 313
Polytetrafluoroethylene grafts
  for hemodialysis arteriovenous access, 171, 174, 175
  as pulmonary embolism cause, 16
  Trerotolo device placement in, 16
Polyvinyl alcohol
  as arteriovenous malformation treatment, 32
  as embolization agent, 148
    in bronchial artery embolization, 96
    in uterine artery embolization, 133, 134
  thrombogenicity of, 17
Popliteal artery
  adventitial disease of, 81
  gunshot wound to, 144
  occlusion of, femoropopliteal angioplasty treatment of, 76
  thrombus of, 80
Popliteal entrapment syndrome, 32, 80, 81
Popliteal vein, 34
Port-a-Cath, 164, 190–191
  malpositioning of, 169
Portal circulation, 225
Portal vein
  anatomy of, 225
  cavernous transformation of, 231
  intrahepatic bifurcations of, 234
  as pancreatic islet cell deposition site, 250
  as pancreatic islet cell suspension infusion site, 251
  stenosis of, in liver transplants, 249
  thrombosis of
    in children, 226
    in liver transplants, 248–249
    as portal hypertension cause, 226
    as transjugular intrahepatic portosystemic shunt contraindication, 235
Portography, 235
Portosystemic collaterals, in portal hypertension, 229–231
Portuguese School of Angiography, 1
Postembolization syndrome, 135–136, 148
Posterior tibial vein, 34
Postmediastinal mass, biopsy of, 321

Postoperative period, pseudoaneurysm occurrence during, 114
Postphlebitic syndrome, 185
Prednisone allergy, 214
Pregnancy
  after tubal recanalization, 292
  as aortic dissection risk factor, 62
  as deep venous thrombosis risk factor, 182
  renal arteriovenous malformations during, 111
  as uterine artery embolization contraindication, 127
  visceral aneurysms during, 114
Prostar XL system, of suture-mediated closure devices, 153
Prosthetic valves, as aortic dissection risk factor, 62
Protein C deficiency, as deep venous thrombosis risk factor, 182
Protein S deficiency, as deep venous thrombosis risk factor, 182
Proteus syndrome, 37
Prothrombin time, 5
Pseudoaneurysms, 111, 114, 115
  of arteriovenous fistulas, 174, 175
  of the extremities, embolization of, 144
  hepatic, in liver transplants, 116, 247
  renal, 144
    renal transplant biopsy-related, 280
    in renal transplants, 280
Pseudocysts, pancreatic, 299–300
Psychosurgery, "father" of, 1
PTD (percutaneous thrombectomy device), 16
Pulmonary arterial pressure, effect of low-osmolarity, nonionic contrast agents on, 198
Pulmonary arteries, 97
  foreign bodies in, 202
    removal of, 204
Pulmonary artery system, in massive hemoptysis, 92
Pulmonary disease, chronic, bronchial artery system in, 96
Pulse examination, 44
Pulseless disease (Takayasu arteritis), 56, 57
Pulselessness, arterial occlusion-related, 79
Pulse volume recordings, 44–45
PVA. *See* Polyvinyl alcohol

Radiation dose, during uterine fibroid embolization, 134
Radiation exposure, pelvic, as uterine artery embolization contraindication, 127
Radiation therapy
  for skeletal metastases, 316
  for superior vena cava syndrome, 186
RAS. *See* Renal artery, stenosis of
RBRVS (resource-based relative value scale), 24
Relative value unit (RVU), 24
Renal arteries
  acute occlusion of, 110
  anatomy of, 99
  arterial variants of, 99
  stenosis of, 99–107
    atherosclerosis-related, 104

Renal arteries *(cont.)*
    hemodynamically significant, 100
    ostial, 102, 103, 106
    pseudo-transplant, 241–244
    recurrent, 104
    stent treatment of, 101, 103, 104, 105, 106
    transplant, 109, 110, 241–244
Renal artery stents, 244
Renal cell carcinoma, vertebral bone biopsy contraindication in, 314
Renal dissection, renal transplantation-related, 244
Renal infarction, in renal transplants, 280
Renal injury, contrast agents-related, 7
Renal transplants
  arteriovenous fistula embolization in, 280
  percutaneous biopsy in, 280
  renal artery stenosis in, 109, 110, 241–244
  renal dissection associated with, 244
  vascular intervention in, **241–244**
Renal veins
  circumaortic, 209
    gonadal vein insertion into, 223
  left retroaortic, 209
Renovascular disease, **99–112**
  atherosclerotic, 99–100
Resource-based relative value scale (RBRVS), 24
Retinoblastoma gene product, 21
Retroviruses, as viral vectors, 22
Ribs
  anomalous first, 195
  cervical, abnormalities of, 195
  fractures of, 143
Right brachiocephalic vein, thrombosis of, 187
Right femoral artery, endoluminal treatment of, 217–218
Right femoral artery needles, 150–151
Right gastric artery, in chemoembolization, 148
Right hepatic artery, chemoembolization of, 148
Right proximal brachiocephalic vein, stenosis of, 187
Right renal vein, connection with inferior vena cava, 209
Right renal veins, multiple, 209
Riva-Rocci, Scipione, 44
Rosch, Josef, 2
RVU (relative value unit), 24

Salpingography, selective, 289, 290–292
Saphenous vein stripping, 217
Saphenous venous systems, 34
Sarcoidosis, as portal hypertension cause, 226
Scalenus anticus syndrome, 195
Scalenus minimus muscle, abnormalities of, 195
Schistosomiasis, as portal hypertension cause, 226
Sci-Med Sentinel, 90
Scimitar syndrome, 34
Scintigraphy, renal nuclear, with captopril, 100
Scion Filter, 91
Sclerosants
  as arteriovenous malformation treatment, 39, 42
  in varicose vein sclerotherapy, 216

INDEX 345

Sclerotherapy
  direct percutaneous ethanol, 39–40
  direct percutaneous venous, 39
  endoluminal, 224
  endoscopic
    complications of, 232
    as gastrointestinal hemorrhage treatment, 232
    as pelvic lymphocele treatment, 307
    in testicular vein embolization, 221, 224
    as varicose vein treatment, 216–217
Sedation, 4
Sedentary lifestyle
  as peripheral vascular disease risk factor, 53, 69
  as stroke risk factor, 84
Seizures, contrast agents-related, 10
Seldinger, Sven Ivar, 1, 268
Seldinger technique, 104, 293
Sepsis syndrome, as deep venous thrombosis risk factor, 182
Septicemia
  percutaneous abscess drainage-related, 295
  percutaneous transhepatic cholangiography-related, 269
Sharp recanalization technique, 189
Sheaths, 13, 14
Shunts
  direct intrahepatic portosystemic (DIPS), 239–240
  portosystemic, 233
  surgically-placed portosystemic, 235–236
  transjugular intrahepatic portosystemic, 229, 232, 233–236, 237–239
    complications of, 235
    contraindications to, 239
    as hepatic hydrothorax treatment, 302
    history of, 2
    as liver transplant portal vein thrombosis treatment, 248–249
    in liver transplant recipients, 240
    restenosis associated with, 238
    stents used in, 238
    technical and hemodynamic success rate of, 237
    variceal rebleeding after, 238
  vascular, use in hereditary hemorrhagic telangiectasia, 116
Sinograms
  of drainage catheters, 304
  of percutaneous abscess drains, 294, 304
S&I (supervision and interpretation) code, 24
Smoking
  as atherosclerotic renal artery disease risk factor, 100
  as Buerger's disease risk factor, 59
  as peripheral vascular disease risk factor, 50, 69, 71
  as stroke risk factor, 84
Smoking cessation, as atherosclerotic peripheral vascular disease treatment, 71
"Snowman" radiographic configuration, in total anomalous pulmonary venous return, 33
Society of Cardiovascular and Interventional Radiology, 3

Society of Cardiovascular Radiology, 3
Society of Interventional Medicine, 3
Society of Interventional Radiology
  manual on coding, 25
  Standards Committee of, 72–73
Solu-Medrol, 71
Spermatic veins, 220
Sphygmometer, invention of, 44
Spinal cord injury
  as deep venous thrombosis risk factor, 182
  as indication for vena cava filter placement, 209
Spinal cord paralysis, bronchial artery embolization-related, 98
Spinal pain, vertebroplasty treatment of, 311–313
Splanchnic vessels, microaneurysms in, 119
Spleen
  as pancreatic islet cell deposition site, 250
  traumatic injuries to, 143–144
Splenectomy, 143
Splenic arterial steal, 248
Splenic artery
  aneurysm of, 114
  collateralization of, 115
  embolization of, 143–144
    as liver transplant ischemia treatment, 248
  normal, 29
  pseudoaneurysm of, 115
Splenic vein, in hepatic portal circulation system, 225
Splenomegaly, as portal hypertension cause, 226
Stanford classification system, for aortic dissection, 62, 63–64
Steal phenomenon, in arteriovenous hemodialysis access, 172–174
Stem cells, 23
Stenosis. See also under specific arteries and veins
  blood velocity decrease in, 44
Stent grafts, 16
  differentiated from bare stents, 15
Stents
  as acute renal artery occlusion cause, 110
  as aortic rupture treatment, 65, 67
  balloon-expandable, 16, 78
  bare, differentiated from stent grafts, 15
  biliary
    in biliary strictures, 275
    migration of, 279
  carotid, 87, 88–89
    balloon angioplasty predilation prior to placement of, 86, 87
    complications of, 88, 89, 90
    as high-risk procedure, 82
    periprocedural complication rate for, 85
    thrombosis of, 89
  as chronic mesenteric ischemia treatment, 122
  colonic, 263–265
    comparison with surgical decompression, 264
    complications of, 264–265
    migration of, 265
  covered, as tracheobronchial lesion treatment, 258
  in direct intrahepatic portosystemic shunt procedure, 239

Stents *(cont.)*
  double-J, 18, 307, 308
  endotracheal, 257
  esophageal, 259–262
    cervical, 260
    comparison with laser therapy, 260–261
    as esophagorespiratory fistula treatment, 259–260
    "funnel phenomenon" of, 262
    as malignant esophageal lesion treatment, 261–262
    migration of, 261
  expandable, 2
  foreshortening of, 16
  gastroduodenal, 262–265
  in hepatic artery, 244, 248
  iliac, 53, 54, 55, 192
    patency rate for, 53
  as inferior vena cava stenosis treatment, 249, 250
  as inferior vena cava syndrome treatment, 193
  infrarenal aortic, 74–75
  major groups of, 78
  metallic
    biliary drain removal after placement of, 309
    as biliary stricture treatment, 275
    in biliary tract, 277–278
    as iliac occlusion treatment, 53, 55
    indications for placement of, 53
    occlusion of, 277–278
    placement in both right and left bile ducts, 276
    versus silicone, 257
  nephroureteral, 18, 19
  Palmaz, 106
    inventor of, 3
    as tracheobronchial lesion treatment, 257
  as peripheral vascular disease treatment, 72, 73
  as polyarteritis nodosa treatment, 56
  primary differentiated from secondary, 76
  as renal artery stenosis treatment, 101, 103, 104
    complications of, 105, 106
    contraindications to, 106
    indications for, 106
    stent restenosis in, 107
  in renal artery transplants, 244
  selection of, 76–77
  self-expandable, 78
    versus balloon-expandable stents, 189
    definition of, 16
  silicone, as tracheobronchial lesion treatment, 257
  as superior vena cava syndrome treatment, 188, 189
    restenosis of, 189
  tracheobronchial, 257–258
  in transjugular intrahepatic portosystemic shunt procedure, 238
  ureteral, 287–289
    internal, 287, 288–289
    internal-external, 288, 289
Stomach insufflation, in gastrostomy tube placement, 254
Stomach ulcers, nontarget embolization-related, 18

Strictures
  biliary, 271
    balloon dilation of, 271–272, 273
    coexistent with bile stones, 272
    liver transplantation-related, 280, 281–282
    malignant, 275
    postlaparoscopic cholecystectomy, 272
    stent placement in, 275
  colonic, 263
  esophageal, 261
  ureteral, 289
Stroke
  aortic arch atheromata-related, 83
  as deep venous thrombosis risk factor, 182
  etiology of, 84
  extracranial carotid artery disease-related, 82
  most common cause of, 83
Sturge-Weber syndrome, 37
Subclavian artery
  in giant-cell arteritis, 58
  in massive hemoptysis, 92
  occlusion of
    as subclavian steal syndrome cause, 61
    in Takayasu disease, 57
    in thoracic outlet syndrome, 32, 33, 194, 196
Subclavian steal syndrome, 60–61
Subclavian vein
  ipsilateral, occlusion or stenosis of, 188
  stenosis of, in hemodialysis arteriovenous access, 173
  in superior vena cava syndrome, 188–189
  thoracic outlet syndrome-related compression of, 194, 195
Subclavian vein access, inferior vena cava filters in, 160
Superficial femoral artery, stenosis of, 32
Superficial femoral vein, 34
Superior gluteal artery, in pelvic trauma, 140
Superior hypophyseal artery, 225
Superior mesenteric artery
  aneurysm of, 114
  arteriography of, in chemoembolization, 148
  in colonic ischemia, 120
  embolism of, 121–122
  endoleak at, 51
  mesenteric ischemia-associated occlusion of, 121
  normal branching pattern of, 30
  occlusion of, in Takayasu disease, 57
  stenosis of, 122
Superior mesenteric vein, in hepatic portal circulation system, 225
Superior vena cava syndrome, 186–189
  benign, 186, 188
  causes of, 186
  definition of, 186
  indwelling catheters in, 189, 190–191
  malignant, 186–188
  pseudo-, 186
  sharp recanalization technique use in, 189
  thoracic aneurysm-associated, 65
  treatment of, 186–189
Supervision and interpretation (S&I) code, 24

INDEX   347

Supracardinal veins, persistence of, 33
Supraduodenal artery, in chemoembolization, 148
Surgery. *See also* specific surgical procedures
  as deep venous thrombosis risk factor, 182, 184
Sutura system, of suture-mediated closure devices, 153, 154, 155
Syringes, hand injection pressure with, 19
Systemic lupus erythematosus, 119

Tachycardia, contrast agents-related, 8
  with bronchospasm, 9
Talc slurry, as malignant pleural effusion treatment, 301
Tandem trocar technique, of intraabdominal abscess drainage, 293
Tazobactam, 271
Telangiectasia, hereditary hemorrhagic, 116, 117
Tenecteplase (TNK), 79
Thoracic outlet, anatomy of, 32–33
Thoracic outlet syndrome, 61–62, 194–196
  causes of, 195
  definition of, 32–33, 194
  signs and symptoms of, 33
  treatment of, 195–196
Thoracic surgery, as superior vena cava syndrome treatment, 186
Thoracotomy, as pulmonary embolism treatment, 200
Thrombectomy
  as hepatic artery thrombosis treatment, 247
  as lower-extremity arterial embolic occlusion treatment, 79
Thrombectomy devices, percutaneous, 16
Thrombin, as embolization agent, 139
Thrombocytopenia, heparin-induced, 184–185
Thromboembolism
  inferior vena cava interruption-based prevention of, 206
  of lower-extremity arteries, 78, 79, 80
Thrombolysis
  catheter-directed, 189
  as meniscal embolism treatment, 80
  as peripheral vascular disease treatment, 72
  as pulmonary embolism treatment, 200
  renal artery, 110
Thrombolytic agents, commonly used, 79
Thrombolytic therapy
  for inferior vena cava syndrome, 193
  for thoracic outlet syndrome, 195–196
Thrombopoietin, 21
Thrombosis
  as acute renal artery occlusion cause, 110
  axillary-subclavian vein, 195
  of central lines, 164
  deep venous, **181–185**
    complications of, 185
    definition of, 181
    diagnostic tests for, 183–184, 200
    Homan's sign of, 181–182
    oral contraceptives-related, 192
    prevention of, 184
    risk factors for, 182, 197

Thrombosis *(cont.)*
    as thoracic outlet syndrome cause, 195
    treatment of, 184–185, 200, 205
    as varicose vein sclerotherapy contraindication, 216
    Wells Clinical Prediction Guide for, 183
    window of "clot" opportunity in, 181
  effort, 195
  exertional, 195
  generalized, protective mechanism against, 181
  of hemodialysis catheter-related, 165
  as mesenteric ischemia cause, 120
  primary, 195
  renal, 110–111
  superior vena cava syndrome-related, 189
  vascular gene therapy for, 21
  of venous catheters, 168
Thymidine kinase, 21
Thyroid metastases, vertebral bone biopsy contraindication in, 314
Tibial veins, 34
Ticlopidine, as stroke treatment, 84
TIPS. *See* Shunts, transjugular intrahepatic portosystemic
Tissue-plasminogen activator, 192
  recombinant, as malfunctioning catheter therapy, 169
Tissue plasminogen activator (TPA), 79
Torque devices, 12
Total anomalous pulmonary venous return (TAPVR), 33
Tracheobronchial lesions
  balloon dilation of, 258
  stent treatment of, 257–258
Tracheobronchial stenosis, 258
Tracheoesophageal interventions, 257–262
Tracheomalacia, 258
Transduction, differentiated from transfection, 23
Transfection, differentiated from transduction, 23
Transient ischemic attacks, 83
Transstenotic pressure gradient, 99
TRAS (transplant renal artery stenosis), 109, 110, 241–244
Trauma
  abdominal, 142
  as arterial injury cause, 139–142
  as deep venous thrombosis risk factor, 182
  endovascular management of, **139–145**
  as indication for vena cava filter placement, 209
  as pseudoaneurysm cause, 114
  as visceral aneurysm cause, 114
Trendelenburg position
  for air embolism management, 160
  during internal jugular venous access, 161
Trephine needles, 314
Trerotola device, 16
Trisomy 13, 37
Trisomy 18, 37
Trocar technique, in abscess drainage, 18, 293
Trousseau, Armand, 205
Troy, discovery of, 181
Tubal recanalization, 290

Tuberculosis, massive hemoptysis cause, 92
Tubes. *See also* Gastrostomy tubes; Jejunostomy tubes; Nephrostomy tubes
  general care and positioning of, 309–310
  indwelling, changing of, 307
  re-establishment of percutaneous tract of, 307
Turner's syndrome, 37

Ulnar artery, aneurysm of, 32

Ultrasound. *See also* Doppler ultrasound; Duplex ultrasound
  display modes of, 44
  in gene therapy, 21
  for percutaneous biopsy guidance, 322–323
  for percutaneous drainage guidance, 293
  for percutaneous pancreatic biopsy guidance, 325
  transducers in, 44
Ureteral obstruction
  causes of, 287
  ureteral stent treatment for, 287–289
Ureteral stones, percutaneous nephrostomy in, 287, 288
Ureteral strictures, 289
Urinary calculi, percutaneous nephrostomy of, 287, 288
Urinary frequency, uterine fibroids-related, 128
Urinary incontinence, uterine fibroids-related, 128
Urinary retention, uterine fibroids-related, 128
Urokinase, 79, 169
Urticaria, contrast agents-related, 9
Uterine artery
  absence of, 132
  anastomosis with ovarian arteries, 129, 130, 132
  anatomy of, 129, 131, 132
  diameter of, 129, 132
  embolization of, **124–138**
    arterial anatomic variants in, 31
    bilateral, 129, 130
    embolic agents for, 133, 134
    inadvertent leiomyosarcoma embolization during, 137
    medications used in, 134–135
    of pedunculated fibroids, 138
    pelvic anatomic variants of, 31
Uterus, arteriovenous malformations of, 42

Vagal reactions, to contrast agents, 10
Valsalva maneuver, during testicular vein embolization, 221, 224
Vanishing duct syndrome (ductopenia), 282–283
Varices
  anorectal, 230
  bleeding
    transhepatic embolization treatment of, 2
    transjugular intrahepatic portosystemic shunt treatment of, 236, 237–238
  gastroesophageal, 229, 231, 232
Varicoceles
  imaging of, 223
  testicular vein embolization of, **220–224**
Varicose veins, **216–219**

Vascular anatomy, **27–34**
Vascular anomalies, **35–43**
Vascular closure devices, **153–157**
  non-suture-mediated, 153, 154–157
  suture-mediated, 153–154, 155
Vascular diseases, types of, 69
Vascular endothelial growth factor, 21
Vascular lesions, congenital
  classification of, 35
  syndromes associated with, 36–37
Vascular malformations, 35–43
  definition of, 35
  differentiated from hemangiomas, 36
  growth of, 35
Vascular testing, noninvasive, **44–46**
  for renal artery stenosis, 100
Vascular tumors, as liver biopsy contraindication, 324
Vasculitis
  categories of, 56
  connective tissue disorders-associated, 56
  substance abuse, 119
  as visceral aneurysm cause, 114
Vasoconstrictive drugs, action mechanism of, 232
Vasopressin, in combination with nitroglycerin, 232
VasoSeal, 154, 155
Vasospasm, in uterine artery, 132
Venae comitantes, 34
Venography
  contrast, of deep venous thrombosis, 183
  endoluminal, of testicular varicoceles, 223
  left renal, during testicular vein embolization, 221
  lower-extremity, of deep venous thrombosis, 200
  in May-Thurner syndrome, 193
  prior to arteriovenous hemodialysis access, 171
Venous access, **158–170**
  as air embolism cause, 160
  arterial blood drawn during, 160
  catheter malfunction in, 168–170
  catheter tips for, 159
  devices used for, 158
  dysrhythmia during, 160
  for hemodialysis, **171–180**
  indications for, 158
  for peripherally-inserted central catheters, 33
  as pneumothorax cause, 160
  ultrasound use in, 159–160
  venous catheter materials for, 158
Venous malformations
  anatomic distribution of, 38
  sclerosant treatment of, 39
  venoarchitecture of, 38–39
Venous pressure, portal, 225
Venous syndromes, **186–196**
  inferior vena cava syndrome, 189, 191–193
  superior vena cava syndrome, 186–189
Venous systems
  deep, 34, 215
  lateral, 34
  superficial, 34
    insufficiency of, 215

Ventilation/perfusion scans, PIOPED (Prospective Investigation of Pulmonary Embolism Diagnosis) criteria for, 198
Vertebral compression, magnetic resonance imaging evaluation of, 311–312
Vertebral disease, implication for vertebroplasty performance, 312
Vertebral height, post-vertebroplasty, 313
Vertebrogenic pain, percutaneous vertebroplasty management of, 312
Vertebroplasty, percutaneous, 311–313
  cement extravasation in, 312–313
  combined with radiofrequency ablation therapy, 314, 316
Viral vectors, 22

Virchow, Rudolf Ludwig Karl, 181
Virchow's triad, 181
Visceral collateral arteries, 30, 31
Volvulus, sigmoid, 265
Vomiting, contrast agents-related, 8

Warfarin, as deep venous thrombosis treatment, 200
Westermark's sign, 198
Winslow pathway, 30
Wires. *See also* Guidewires
  hydrophilic, 11, 12
  safety, 15

Zeitler, Eberhart, 1
Zenith endoluminal graft, 48, 50